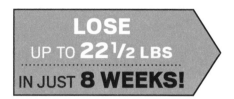
LOSE
UP TO **22 1/2 LBS**
IN JUST **8 WEEKS!**

WALK OFF
Weight™

Burn 3 *Times More Fat* with This Proven Program

MICHELE STANTEN, FITNESS DIRECTOR, **Prevention.**

RODALE

© 2010 by Rodale Inc.
Exercise and before/after photographs © 2010 by Mitch Mandel/Rodale Images

Rodale books may be purchased for business or promotional use or for special sales. For information, please write to: Special Markets Department, Rodale, Inc., 733 Third Avenue, New York, NY 10017

Prevention® is a registered trademark of Rodale Inc.
Walk Off Weight is a trademark of Rodale Inc.

Printed in the United States of America
Rodale Inc. makes every effort to use acid-free ♾, recycled paper ♲.

Book design by Donna Agajanian
Chapter opener photographs and author and individual test panelist portraits by Shannon Greer

Library of Congress Cataloging-in-Publication Data
Stanten, Michele.
    Walk off weight : Burn 3 Times More Fat with This Proven Program / Michele Stanten.
        p.   cm.
    Includes bibliographical references and index.
    ISBN-13 978–1–60529–564–0   direct hardcover
    ISBN-10 1–60529–564–7   direct hardcover
    ISBN-13 978–1–60529–563–3   trade paperback
    ISBN-10 1–60529–563–9   trade paperback
    1. Fitness walking.   2. Reducing diets.   3. Weight loss.   I. Title.
    RA781.65.S73 2010
    613.7'1—dc22   2010002496

Distributed to the trade by Macmillan
2   4   6   8   10   9   7   5   3   1   direct hardcover
2   4   6   8   10   9   7   5   3   1   trade paperback

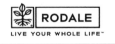

For more of our products visit prevention.com

FOR MY MOM, ROSALIE,

WHO HAS BEEN BY MY SIDE FOR THE MOST IMPORTANT WALKS OF MY LIFE—

MY FIRST STEPS, MY FIRST DAY OF SCHOOL,

DOWN THE AISLE, THE 3-DAY BREAST CANCER WALK,

AND ACROSS THE FINISH LINE OF OUR FIRST MARATHON—

AND EVERYTHING IN BETWEEN

Contents

Acknowledgments

I COULD FILL ALL OF THE PAGES of this book with thank-yous to the many people who helped to make it happen, directly or indirectly. I could not have done it without each and every one of their contributions and support.

To the Walk Off Weight test panel: Debbie Adie, Kathy Ashenfelter, Deb Baer, Theresa Bahnick, JulieAnne Bedard, Carmen Bell, Kathleen Caola, Laura Chiles, Lysa Delefeti, Kristina Donatelli, Stacey Geffken, Tammy Harding, Denise Jennings, Meg Kranzley, Geri Krempa, Joann Manuel, Susan Moyer, Mary Lou Phillips, Gail Rarick, Stacy Shillinger, Yvonne Shorb, Wendy Silfies, Lisa Stone, and Louise Wagner, who walked in the heat and rain to prove that this program works. Your efforts amazed me and will inspire millions of women like you!

To my colleagues: my editor, Andrea Au Levitt, for guiding me along the way; Donna Agajanian for designing a stunning book, and the rest of the art and photo team; Marianne McGinnis for her writing and research help; Heidi McIndoo, MS, RD, LDN, for developing a nutritious and delicious meal plan; Marielle Messing for coordinating the test panel and much more; Natalie Gingerich for reviewing the many versions of the program; Kelly Hartshorne and Tammy Strunk from the Rodale fitness center for testing our panelists; Diana Erney, Jen Keiser, and Krista Pegnetter from the Rodale library for their research help; Carol Angstadt, Susan Berg, Marilyn Hauptly, and the rest of the Rodale Books team for their meticulous attention to details; and to *Prevention's* former Editor-in-Chief Liz Vaccariello and Executive Editor Courtenay Smith for their never-ending support and belief in me—thank you!

To my mentors: Mark Bricklin and Maggie Spilner for turning me onto the powers of walking for exercise nearly 20 years ago; Lee Scott, Mark Fenton, Suki Munsell, and Casey Meyers for teaching me the techniques to turn a leisurely walk into a body-shaping workout; and Wayne Westcott, PhD, for his guidance and expertise in all things fitness.

To all of my fellow walkers, including Pat Schuppin, MaryPat Scorzetti, Rebecca Garson, Pam Jarrar, Beth Katcher, and all Team Prevention members— keep showing the world that walkers are athletes, too!

And most importantly, to my family and friends: my husband, Andrew, who has been my greatest supporter and fan for more than 20 years. Thank you for everything! I couldn't do it without you—and it means more to me to do it with you by my side. My son, Jacob, whose "big hugs with legs" kept me energized. My daughter, Mia, who learned to walk while I was writing this book; you always put a smile on my face, no matter how late I stayed up working. My dad, Gary, for always pitching in to help. Jessica Lievendag, Brenda McColgan, and their families for being there for my family on the many nights and weekends that I was busy with "the book." I love you all!

XOXO,

Michele

Introduction

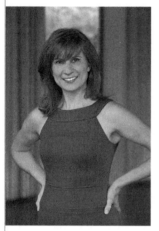

WELCOME TO *PREVENTION*'S WALK OFF WEIGHT (WOW) program. I've drawn on my nearly 20 years of experience as a fitness instructor and editor at America's leading healthy lifestyle magazine to create this unique 8-week exercise and diet plan that focuses on increasing the benefits of America's favorite type of exercise: walking! And to guarantee that it will work for you, I recruited about two dozen women just like you to road test it. Their results were amazing—and yours will be, too!

In just 8 weeks, these women lost as much as 22½ pounds and nearly 14 inches all over. So can you! Whether you've walked for exercise in the past or not, this program is designed to get you maximum results in minimal time by focusing on interval training. That means alternating high-intensity bursts of activity, such as fast walking, with lower-intensity recovery bouts of slower strolling. Scientific research shows that this type of training improves your body's ability to burn fat and can increase weight loss.[1] When our women put interval walking to the test under real-life conditions—while juggling work, family, volunteering, and more—they lost more than three times the weight that they would have through traditional, steady-paced walking.[2, 3, 4, 5] By comparing the weekly weight loss from walking studies, which ranged from ⅒ to ½ pound, to the results of our test panelists who lost up to 1¾ pounds a week on the exercise-only portion, I conservatively estimated that the WOW program could result in three times more weight loss.[6]

In addition to interval walks, the program includes moderate-intensity walks (to balance out the vigorous intervals) as well as strength training to build the muscle that fuels your metabolism and firms you up. Combining cardio and strength workouts has been shown to produce greater weight loss.[*] For even faster results, I enlisted Heidi McIndoo, a registered dietitian, to create an eating plan that will help you to consume fewer calories and still fuel your body for exercise—without feeling hungry. Testers who followed both the exercise and diet portions of the WOW program shed more than double the number of pounds on average and 65 percent more inches than the exercise-only group.

Now it's your turn. Picking up this book is your first step toward achieving a slimmer, firmer, stronger body and tons of energy. Let's get started!

*1.75 pounds per week of the biggest loser in the WOW exercise-only group divided by 0.5 pound per week based on the best results of studies equals 3.5 times more weight loss for the WOW program.

"My skin looks better. I have more energy.
And I'm almost never tired at my desk in the morning."
—*DENISE JENNINGS*

||||||||||

"I went dancing for the first time in years,
and I was fit enough to do it all night long."
—*SUSAN MOYER*

||||||||||

"I lost back fat! I never noticed
losing in that area on other programs."
—*KATHY ASHENFELTER*

||||||||||

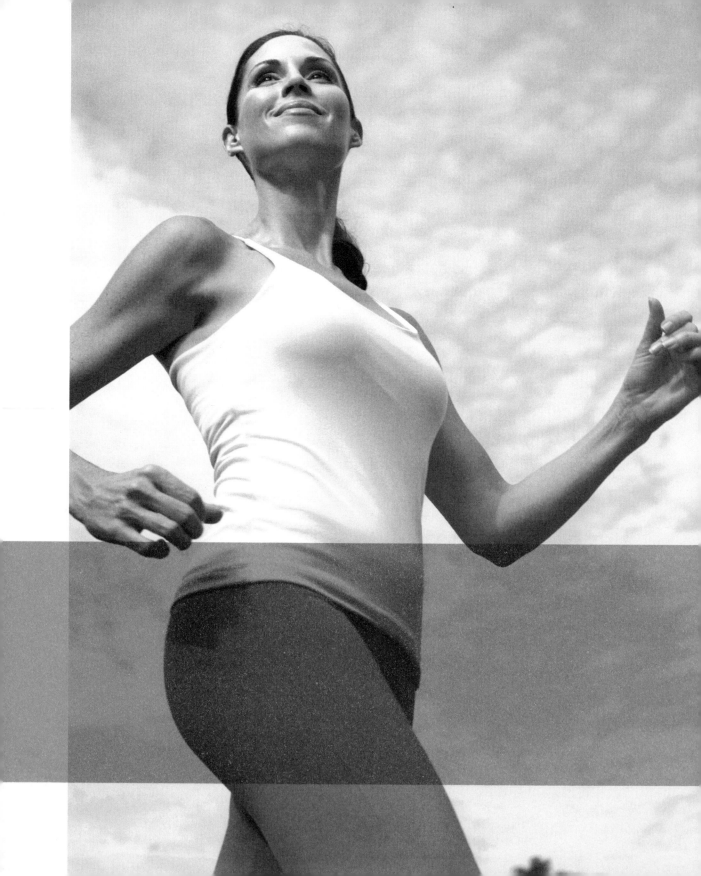

1

WHY
Walking?

I LOVE TO WALK! Whether it's strolling around my neighborhood with my husband and kids, speeding down a park path for a workout, or racking up the miles to complete a full or half marathon with *Prevention* readers, walking is my number one form of exercise. (And trust me, after nearly 20 years as a certified fitness instructor at *Prevention* magazine, I've tried just about every type of workout!)

I'm not alone in my love of walking. Over the years, I've gotten thousands of letters and e-mails from *Prevention* readers who are just as passionate about walking as I am. When I invited them to walk a marathon with me and other editors a few years ago, more than 500 signed up. In fact, *Prevention* readers are nearly 90 percent more likely to walk for exercise 2 or more days a week than other Americans.[1] And this love affair with walking isn't exclusive to *Prevention* readers; more than 100 million Americans walk for exercise.[2]

When you think about it, it's not surprising that walking is America's favorite way to work out.

- **IT'S EASY**—Most of us have been doing it since we were just about a year old.
- **IT'S CHEAP**—All you need is a good pair of sneakers (and socks!). And they don't have to be the most expensive kind. In one study, cheaper models scored just as well as, or sometimes even better than, pricier ones for support, cushioning, and comfort.[3]
- **IT'S BODY-FRIENDLY**—Unlike running, you always have one foot on the ground when you're walking. So the impact on your joints is low, which reduces your risk of injury. When you walk, you land with a force 1 to 1½ times your body weight, compared with about 3 times your body weight when you run. In a review of 28 high-quality scientific studies of exercise in women ages 50 to 65, researchers found that the rate of injury averaged just 3 percent for walking, compared with 23 percent for higher-impact activities like jogging—nearly 8 times more.[4]
- **IT'S FLEXIBLE**—You can walk around your neighborhood or nearby where you work. You can even do it when you're traveling. According to a Stanford University study, beginning exercisers who were able to work out at home were 45 percent more likely to still be exercising a year later compared with those who had to travel to a facility for their workouts.[5]
- **IT FEELS GOOD**—While all types of exercise can give you a mood boost, walkers report feeling better than runners while they're doing it, not just after they're done.[6]

That's not all! Walking is powerful medicine. The Harvard Nurses' Health Study, which has been tracking the health behaviors of more than 200,000 women for more than 3 decades, has shown that moderate walking for an average of 30 minutes a day can lower the risk of heart disease,[7] stroke,[8] and type 2 diabetes[9] by 30 to 40 percent, and the risk of breast cancer by 20 to 30 percent.[10] Walking also keeps your mind sharp, boosts your mood, fights off colds, revs up your energy level, improves sleep, reduces pain, helps you live longer, and even curbs food cravings.

But I know the *real* reason you picked up this book: You want to lose weight! And that's my goal, too—to help you walk off those pounds and leave them in the dust forever. After all, walking is the number one activity of successful losers.

The National Weight Control Registry is a study of more than 5,000 people who've managed to lose weight—66 pounds, on average—and keep it off for an average of 5½ years. When researchers asked these successful losers about their exercise habits, walking topped the list, with 54 percent of the women reporting that they walk a mile or more a day.[11]

WALKING POWERS WEIGHT LOSS

I WON'T LIE TO YOU. You don't have to walk—or do any other type of exercise—to slim down. In fact, most people will drop more pounds by dieting than by working out because of simple math. It's easier to cut calories from your diet than to burn them off with exercise. Skipping a single Caffè Mocha is a split-second decision that will save you 410 calories. To burn off that coffee drink, you'd have to walk for nearly 2 hours.

So why am I spending 300-plus pages telling you how to walk off weight? Because you'll look and feel better, be healthier, and improve your odds of maintaining your new slimmer figure over the long run if you combine diet and exercise to shed those extra pounds. Plus, I'm going to show you techniques that will power up your ordinary walks so you can blast those Caffè Mocha calories in about half the time!

Walk to Build Muscle—And Metabolism

One of the big problems with losing weight through diet alone is the loss of muscle that accompanies that approach. Generally, muscle uses up about three times as many calories as fat does to maintain your body. It also powers metabolism—the calorie-burning engine that generates the energy to fuel everything your body does throughout the day, from pumping blood and digesting food to walking and talking.

When you just eat less, the weight you lose tends to be a combination of fat and muscle. The more muscle you lose, the slower your metabolism becomes and the fewer calories you burn. This is probably one of the reasons that it's so hard to keep those pounds off over time. But including exercise in your weight loss program can minimize, maybe even halt, muscle loss.

In a University of Pittsburgh study, researchers compared the effects of weight loss with or without exercise in 64 overweight and obese seniors. The dieters cut 500 to 1,000 calories a day and followed a low-fat eating plan. The exercise group did the same, along with working out at a moderate intensity for 45 minutes, three to four times a week. After 4 months, both groups lost similar amounts of weight—45 pounds, on average—but the dieters lost about three times more lean body mass such as muscle, which can cause a dip in metabolism. In addition, the exercisers improved their fat-burning ability twice as much as the dieters. During a 1-hour exercise test, the exercise group burned nearly 40 percent more fat at the end of the study than at the beginning, while the dieters saw less than 20 percent improvement in their results.[12]

The other cool thing about maintaining muscle (or even gaining some): It's much more compact and firm than fat, so it looks a heck of a lot better. And even if you aren't losing as many pounds as you'd like, you'll be more likely to notice changes in how your clothes fit. Even before many of our testers saw any movement on the scale, they were reporting that their tight-fitting clothes weren't quite so snug anymore.

Walk Off Belly Fat

Canadian researchers found that women who walked briskly for about an hour a day reduced their belly fat by 20 percent over 14 weeks—without changing their eating habits.[13] On the WOW program, our walkers shrunk their waistlines by up to 8 percent, or 3 inches, in the first 4 weeks!

Walking may also help you slim down by curbing cravings, according to a new British study from the University of Exeter. When researchers had 25 regular chocolate-eaters take a test or handle a chocolate bar after either walking or sitting for 15 minutes, the walkers consistently reported less stress about the test or fewer cravings for the chocolate than the nonwalking chocoholics. Exercise may increase dopamine (a hormone that produces feelings of satisfaction and pleasure), which, in turn, may lower your desire for other normally crave-worthy foods, speculate researchers.[14]

WALKING IS POWERFUL MEDICINE

IF YOU HAVEN'T HEARD ENOUGH REASONS to get you off the couch, here are more amazing health rewards to inspire you. (And finding the right motivation to become more active can make you 70 percent more likely to stick with it, reports the American College of Sports Medicine.)

Keep Your Heart Healthy

Our WOW walkers showed amazing improvements in a number of heart disease risk factors. They cut their total cholesterol levels by up to 51 points, "bad" LDL cholesterol by up to 44 points, and triglycerides—a type of blood fat—by up to a whopping 75 points! They also lowered their blood pressure levels by as much as 30 points for systolic (top number) and 16 points for diastolic (bottom number).

Just like your biceps, your heart is a muscle, and exercise is key to keeping it strong and healthy. People used to believe that the heart had only so many beats in it, so if they raised their heart rates by exercising, they would die sooner. Of course, we now know better. In fact, the exact opposite is true. As you become fitter, your heart actually beats more slowly because it's able to pump more blood with each beat. So over time, it works less.

Numerous studies back this up, heartily. Researchers from Washington University who tracked overweight 50- to 60-year-olds for 1½ years found that those who burned 240 to 300 calories a day by walking (that's equivalent to 45 to 60 minutes at a moderate pace) lost an average of 22 pounds without dieting. Just as noteworthy, their hearts pumped blood and nutrients as efficiently as the hearts of people in their 30s and 40s.[15]

At Duke University, researchers found that moderate walkers outpaced joggers when it came to lowering artery-clogging triglycerides, a marker for increased risk of heart disease, heart attack, and stroke. These men and women—all over age 40—walked for 50 minutes, 4 days a week. Over 8 months of the study, they lowered their triglyceride levels by 25 percent, nearly twice as much as those who spent the same amount of time running. Lower-intensity workouts may do a better job of reducing bad fats like triglycerides and LDL cholesterol because they use fat for fuel, while high-intensity exercise primarily uses glucose (or sugar).[16]

Finally, researchers in Britain have found a link between heart-harming inflammation and walking—and it's all good. Just 30 minutes of walking at least 5 days a week lowered levels of TNF alpha, interleukin-6, and C-reactive protein, three markers of inflammation that are associated with heart disease.[17]

Stay Diabetes–Free

An estimated 23.6 million Americans (nearly 8 percent of the population) have some form of diabetes, and every year another 1.3 million people age 20 or older are diagnosed with the disease, according to the National Institute of Diabetes and Digestive and Kidney Diseases (NIDDK). But walking can go a long way toward preventing and even treating diabetes. For example, our WOW walkers reduced their fasting glucose levels by up to 22 points.

At the University of Michigan, researchers found that sedentary, prediabetic adults who walked for an hour daily improved their sensitivity to insulin by 59 percent and their ability to produce insulin by 31 percent in just 7 days.[18] Both measures indicate an improved ability to regulate blood sugar. Based on this study, if you keep on trucking, over the long haul, you could lower your risk of developing diabetes by 58 percent, especially if you drop a few pounds along the way.

Rev Up Immunity

When you exercise, powerful disease-fighting cells circulate throughout your body. On this program, you'll be walking most days of the week, and that kind of commitment gets you bonus benefits. The effects of regular exercise build up

Think beyond the scale. A University of Michigan study found that women who exercised with a goal of overall well-being were 34 percent more likely to stick with it than those interested only in weight loss.[19]

in a cumulative way that can lead to a lifetime of superior immune function. Keep going strong, and you'll experience fewer cold and flu bugs, and your body will be more effective at fending off conditions such as heart disease, cancer, stroke, and diabetes.

Appalachian State University researchers found that adults who walked regularly cut their number of sick days in half![20] Plus, your health-protecting arsenal remains elevated for a few hours after your workout.

Keep Joints and Bones Strong

An exercised body is a well-oiled machine. When you're active, your body does a better job of providing natural antioxidants, lubricants, and nutrients to your joints, muscles, and bones. If you sit still, it's like the body's maintenance man went on holiday; everything starts to rust. In a University of North Carolina at Chapel Hill study,[21] arthritis sufferers experienced 25 percent less pain and 16 percent less stiffness following 6 months of low-impact exercise like walking.

Almost all of the women on the WOW program reported fewer aches and pains. "My knees used to always hurt when I'd get up in the morning or after sitting for an extended period, but now I'm pain free," reports Geri Krempa, who lost nearly 12 pounds and 9½ inches all over.

"My doctor recommended knee surgery, but after WOW, I don't need it any more," says Susan Moyer, who had suffered from knee pain for more than a decade but now walks pain free.

In the bone department, women are more likely than men to run into trouble because they lose bone density at a greater rate as they age, putting them at higher risk for fractures. One Harvard Medical School study, however, found that women who walk a minimum of 4 hours a week are 41 percent less likely to suffer hip fractures than women who log 1 hour or less of walking per week.[22] Because walking is a weight-bearing activity (you do pound the pavement, even if it isn't as much as with running), researchers believe that it minimizes bone loss, keeping bones stronger.

Feel Energized

Whether you're looking to recapture that youthful, keep-going-and-going feeling or you need an instant pick-me-up, exercise is your best natural remedy. "I feel extremely alive and energized in my body—almost as if I were 20 years younger," Susan noted in week 5.

Another walker, Wendy Silfies, reported, "I had so much energy that I biked for 10 miles on top of my walking workouts."

That good feeling may last up to 12 hours after a mere 20-minute moderate-intensity workout, according to a University of Vermont study.[23] Plus, adults who walk for 30 minutes five times a week report that they have more energy to get through their daily tasks; they feel healthier; and they're more confident than those who walk infrequently, according to scientists at the Saint Louis University School of Public Health.[24]

Boost Your Mood

Every time you walk, your body releases hormones that make you feel good and reduce stress. That's a two-for-one emotional adjustment—and it's free! And I'm not just talking about everyday blues here. One of our WOW walkers, Stacy Shillinger, says that she was able to reduce the dosage of her antidepressant once she started our program. A study from the University of Texas at Austin seems to support this firsthand experience. Researchers there found that just 30 minutes of walking can give a temporary lift from even major depression. Walkers reported an 85 percent increase in energy and a 40 percent improvement in well-being, compared with study participants who rested quietly. Their improved mood lasted about an hour.[25]

Rest Easier

If you're looking for a better night's sleep, then WOW just might be your cup of chamomile. Most of our WOW participants reported that they were sleeping better. For one panelist, though, the program was a major breakthrough. "I'm sleeping at night! That's incredible because I've had insomnia for 2 years," wrote Lysa Delefeti, who lost about 5½ pounds and 5½ inches overall and nearly doubled her energy level.

It really isn't that hard to see the link between exercise and sleep: You expend energy, you get tired, and you doze off. But there's a lot more that walking does to help you sleep, such as improving your mood, lowering stress, reducing pain— all things that make for sound snoozing.

In one study published in the *Journal of Sleep Medicine*, women age 60 and older who walked a mere hour a week (about 9 minutes a day) woke up half as often and slept 48 minutes more a night, on average, than women who were sedentary.[26] In another study, when researchers asked more than 700 men and women about their exercise and sleep habits, they found that walkers were less likely to wake in the middle of the night, have nightmares, or experience an afternoon slump, among other sleep-related problems. Compared with those who didn't walk at all, people who walked at least six blocks a day at a moderate pace were one-third less likely to have trouble sleeping until their wake-up time. Those who walked the same distance at a brisk pace slashed their risk of any sleep disorder by 50 percent.[27]

Breeze through Menopause

The years before, during, and after menopause are a time of change, to put it mildly. Hot flashes, night sweats, cramps, mood swings, weight gain, headaches . . . oh, joy! But walking can help. "I'm not waking up as often with hot flashes," WOW walker Mary Lou Phillips reported.

Exercise appears to boost levels of feel-good brain chemicals called endorphins and ease the hormone fluctuations that are behind these symptoms. That's what one study found when researchers had sedentary women ages 42 to 58 do about 3 hours of moderate exercise (such as walking) per week.[28] Over a 2-year period, these women reported that they felt happier and more confident. And just like Mary Lou, they noticed a drop in hot flashes and night sweats. Even postmenopausal women will benefit from walking. In one study, the most active women in this age group, who walked about 25 minutes a day, reported less weight gain and 44 percent fewer headaches compared with their peers who exercised less than 10 minutes a day.[29] If you're not thinking about menopause yet, walking also helps ease PMS symptoms, according to researchers.

Boost Your Brainpower

Physical activity bathes your brain in oxygen-rich blood, increasing the production of chemicals that improve memory, attention, and problem solving. Italian researchers found that people age 65 and older who walked enough to burn 417 calories a week (about 5 miles at a moderate pace) were 27 percent less likely to develop dementia than more sedentary adults in the same age group.[30]

What if you aren't worried about dementia, but you'd just like to know where you left your car keys? Walking can help you, too. When University of Illinois at Urbana-Champaign researchers gave adults a mental task after 30 minutes of aerobic exercise like walking, 30 minutes of strength training, or no exercise, those who did the cardio session showed enhanced memory capacity and reaction time, while the other two groups didn't seem to increase their brainpower at all.[31] In a similar study, when sedentary adults exercised for a half hour three times a week for 12 weeks, their memories and ability to juggle tasks improved by a third, compared with their scores pre-exercise.[32]

Age Gracefully

Here are a few more surprising ways that walking can keep you feeling younger.

- You can have the ears of a 20-year-old if you stroll regularly. When Miami University scientists tested the hearing of 43 adults, they discovered that the people who were aerobically fit heard sounds at lower volumes than those who were unfit. Aerobic activities like walking enrich the blood with oxygen and may increase bloodflow to the ears, which can then improve their functioning, researchers speculate.[33] This is particularly important after age 40, since your ability to pick up whispers and high-pitched sounds declines with age.

- Working up a sweat and getting your heart rate pumping is also good for your eyes. Preliminary research from the U.S. Department of Energy's Lawrence Berkeley National Laboratory in California shows that vigorous exercise like running can reduce your chances of developing cataracts by more than one-third.[34] And in another study by the same research team, runners who logged nearly 2½ miles daily cut their risk of macular degeneration, a common cause of impaired vision as you get older, by as much as 54 percent.[35] Now you don't have to run to get these benefits. As long as you're pushing your intensity to that vigorous level like doing intervals, researchers believe that you'll benefit.

- For a brighter smile, get out there and aim for the government's guideline of 30 minutes of moderate activity five or more times a week. Adults who met this mark were 42 percent less likely to suffer from periodontitis, a gum disease that becomes more common with age.[36] Exercise may protect your teeth in the same way it does your heart—by lowering blood levels of inflammation-causing C-reactive protein.

Live Longer

If everything you've read here doesn't have you lacing up your sneakers, consider this: Thirty minutes of walking most days of the week can increase your life span by up to 3 years, according to a study published in the *Archives of Internal Medicine*.[37]

THAT GIVES YOU MORE than a dozen good reasons to make walking a habit. The next step is to learn how to take this everyday activity and turn it into a powerful weight loss tool.

WOW Winner
Susan Moyer

GROUP: Exercise and Diet

AGE: 51 HEIGHT: 5'6"
POUNDS LOST: 17 ¼
INCHES LOST: 11¾ overall, including 4 from her waist
MAJOR ACCOMPLISHMENT: Cured her knee pain; lowered systolic (top number) blood pressure by 10 points and diastolic (bottom number) by 8 points, bringing her almost out of the danger zone for high blood pressure

Back in the Game of Life

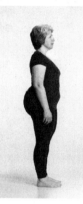

BEFORE

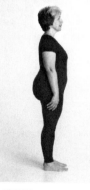

AFTER

SUSAN MOYER had been a high school athlete and continued to play softball much of her adult life, often being the only woman on the team. But all activity pretty much stalled when Susan and her husband, whom she played and coached with, got divorced in 2002. As she became more sedentary and gained weight, an old knee injury from her 30s started to act up.

The WOW program appealed to Susan because she has been a *Prevention* reader for years. "By committing to this program, I was making a promise to take care of myself for the first time in a long time," she said.

The first week was tough because her knee was sore and stiff. She had to wear her knee brace and modify many of the moves. But despite the pain, she pushed on (with her doctor's approval) and rediscovered the joys of being active. "I'd forgotten how much I like exercise," said Susan. After 2 weeks, "the stiffness and pain were gone, and I could tell that the muscles around my knee were getting stronger," reported Susan, who also noted feeling more energetic. "Not only was I able to do my walk, I weed-whacked and mowed my entire yard, and I swept out the garage—all in 1 day."

By the midpoint of the program, Susan started to see a thinner reflection in the mirror—the result of having lost 11¾ pounds and 5½ inches. She enthusiastically reported that she was able to bend her bum knee almost as much as her healthy one. In the final 3 weeks, she noticed that her elbows no longer bumped her hips when she walked, and she could see even more definition in her thighs and butt.

Despite thinking that she couldn't do this on her own, Susan loves her newfound independence. "The more physically fit I get, the more courageous and willing I am to take chances and do things that I haven't done before like hiking and mountain biking—all by myself!" said Susan. She's even led a church service—"I'd never done any public speaking before"—and found the confidence to go back to her one true love, writing. And she's already gotten published!

P.S. *Three months after the official end of the program, Susan recorded an additional 7½-pound weight loss and shaved another 5¼ inches off her figure, for a grand total of 24¾ pounds and 17 inches lost in 5 months.*

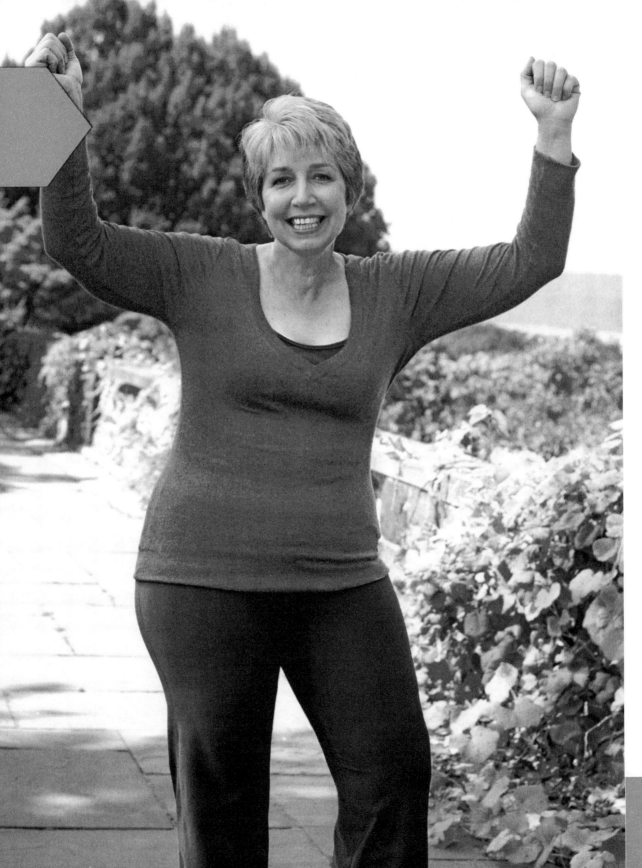

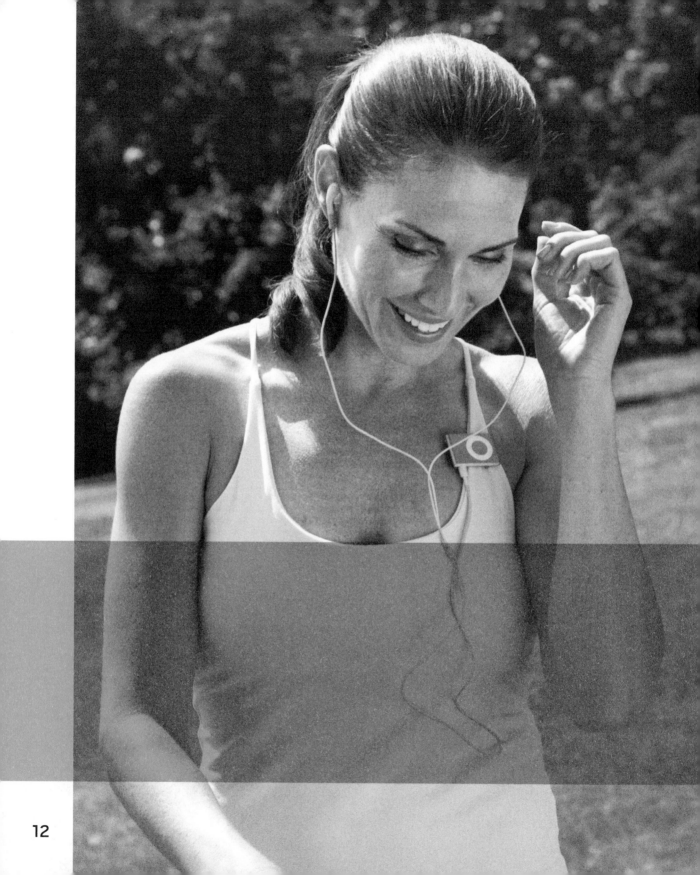

THE BEST WAY TO
WALK OFF
Weight

NOW THAT YOU'VE READ ABOUT all the amazing benefits of walking—and if you're already a walker, hopefully you've experienced some of them yourself—it's time to discover the best way to ensure that you achieve all these wonderful results as well as your personal goals. There's more than one way to walk, and not all types of walking will lead you down the path to weight loss. In fact, one complaint I frequently hear from women is that they walk regularly but aren't seeing results. That's why I wrote this book. I want to give you the tools to make walking work for you.

One of the reasons walking is an exercise favorite is that it's easy and comfortable to do—but that can also be one of its downfalls. We like to stay in our comfort zones, so most of us walk at an easy to moderate pace. That's not a problem when you first start exercising because any activity is an improvement from just sitting on the sofa.

This is what's known in exercise science as the overload principle. In other words, to achieve changes in your body as a result of exercise, the activity you do needs to provide a greater than normal stress. I'm talking about challenging your body beyond what it is accustomed to doing.

If you're like the average inactive person, just getting off the couch and moving more—taking a walk after dinner, squeezing in 10-minute strolls at work, increasing your number of steps throughout the day—is enough to challenge your body and get it out of its comfort zone. The result: You have more energy, your mood improves, you don't feel so stressed, your clothes may be looser, and you may even lose a few pounds.

After a few months of this (or less for some), though, the improvements slow and may even stop completely. You keep walking, but the scale won't budge. Exercise scientists refer to this as the adaptation principle; the rest of us call it a plateau. It means that the more you do a particular activity, the better your body gets at performing it. That's why you might feel sore when you try a new exercise or workout, but after a couple of sessions or weeks, your body becomes accustomed to the routine and you're no longer sore.

Thankfully, the body benefits of exercise don't stop that quickly. But eventually, they slow, too. Practice may make perfect, but when it comes to losing weight, you don't want perfection. As you get better at an activity, and your body becomes more efficient at doing it, you create a new comfort zone—and when that happens, you burn fewer calories while performing that activity. To become fitter and lose more weight, you need to change your routine (a training principle called periodization) and get out of your new comfort zone. By continuing to challenge your body—the overload principle—you'll continue to see results.

The WOW program is designed to keep you out of a walking rut and off those dreaded weight loss plateaus. The first step is to pick up the pace. Turn some of your one-speed walking workouts into fat-blasting interval walks in which you stride fast for a short period of time and then slow down to recover before cranking it back up. But that's not the only type of walking you'll be doing; remember, switching your routine will help to ensure that you lose more weight and get in the best shape possible. I've also included strength workouts using either your own body weight or an elastic exercise band to build muscle, maximize your metabolism, and burn more fat.

Here is an overview of the workouts you'll be doing:

- **INTERVAL WALKS**—By alternating fast and moderate/easy bouts of walking (if you graphed your speed, it would look like a series of peaks and valleys), you'll turn up your calorie burn by as much as 100 percent during your workout and afterward.[1] The length of these workouts as well as the intervals themselves will be altered throughout the 8-week WOW program to provide new challenges.

- **TONING WALKS**—Using an exercise band while walking will help firm your upper body and boost your calorie burn. Building muscle is the best way to stoke your metabolism long-term. When *Prevention* tested exercise bands in a head-to-head competition with dumbbells and other popular strengthening workouts, we found that the bands delivered faster firming.[2] Our band-users slimmed down and toned common trouble spots such as the belly, thighs, and butt by 30 percent more than women who did other types of strength training. (Check out the text starting on page 39 for more on the benefits of bands.)

- **LONG WALKS**—Endurance training (about an hour at a moderate intensity) has been shown to keep your calorie burn revved for up to 7½ hours postexercise.[3] There is also a dose response to exercise; that is, the more you do, the greater the benefits you'll receive. These will likely be the slowest walks you do in the program.

- **RECOVERY WALKS**—While they don't blast fat like intervals, these tried-and-true calorie-burners have an important place when you're trying to walk off pounds. They're the perfect workout in between vigorous interval days to keep up your calorie burn without risking an injury. You'll be walking as if you're in a bit of a hurry, so that you're slightly breathless.

- **SPEED WALKS**—During these shorter workouts, you'll maintain a high intensity for the entire session, striding as if you're late for an important appointment, so you're only able to speak in very brief phrases. This type of training has been shown to specifically attack belly fat better than longer, lower-intensity exercise.

- **STRENGTH TRAINING**—In addition to the toning walks that target your upper body, you'll do workouts for your lower body, core, and total body at various points in the program. Adding strength training to cardio workouts improves results: It boosts metabolism, increases weight loss, and can even help you eat less.

THE WOW FACTOR

Head uphill. If one of your walking goals is a toned rear, add hill climbs to your workouts. Research shows that walking uphill activates 25 percent more fibers in your backside than strolling on flat terrain. Search for a hilly route, or find one hill and repeat the climb a few times during your walk.[4]

AT-A-GLANCE WOW SCHEDULE

THE 8-WEEK WOW PROGRAM is divided into two 4-week phases. The first phase focuses on slightly longer workouts and intervals with more moderate intensities. During the second phase, the emphasis shifts to shorter workouts and intervals that you'll do at higher intensities. This is the training principle mentioned earlier, known as periodization—the systematic altering of your workouts every 4 to 8 weeks to continue to challenge your body and prevent plateaus. During each phase of the program, the workouts will progress gradually to help prevent burnout and injury.

Phase 1: AT A GLANCE

LOWER-INTENSITY, LONGER-DURATION TRAINING

WEEK	DAY 1	DAY 2	DAY 3	DAY 4	DAY 5	DAY 6	DAY 7
1	Basic Interval I 30 min Lower-Body Strength Workout 15 min **45 MIN TOTAL**	Toning Walk I (upper body) **20 MIN TOTAL**	Basic Interval I 30 min Core Strength Workout 15 min **45 MIN TOTAL**	Toning Walk I (upper body) **20 MIN TOTAL**	Basic Interval I 30 min Lower-Body Strength Workout 15 min **45 MIN TOTAL**	Long Walk I 45 min Core Strength Workout 15 min **60 MIN TOTAL**	Rest
2	Basic Interval I 30 min Lower-Body Strength Workout 15 min **45 MIN TOTAL**	Toning Walk I (upper body) **20 MIN TOTAL**	Basic Interval I 30 min Core Strength Workout 15 min **45 MIN TOTAL**	Toning Walk I (upper body) **20 MIN TOTAL**	Basic Interval I 30 min Lower-Body Strength Workout 15 min **45 MIN TOTAL**	Long Walk II 60 min Core Strength Workout 15 min **75 MIN TOTAL**	Rest
3	Basic Interval II 45 min Lower-Body Strength Workout 15 min **60 MIN TOTAL**	Toning Walk II (upper body) **25 MIN TOTAL**	Basic Interval II 45 min Core Strength Workout 15 min **60 MIN TOTAL**	Toning Walk II (upper body) **25 MIN TOTAL**	Basic Interval II 45 min Lower-Body Strength Workout 15 min **60 MIN TOTAL**	Long Walk III 75 min Core Strength Workout 15 min **90 MIN TOTAL**	Rest
4	Basic Interval II 45 min Lower-Body Strength Workout 15 min **60 MIN TOTAL**	Toning Walk II (upper body) **25 MIN TOTAL**	Basic Interval II 45 min Core Strength Workout 15 min **60 MIN TOTAL**	Toning Walk II (upper body) **25 MIN TOTAL**	Basic Interval II 45 min Lower-Body Strength Workout 15 min **60 MIN TOTAL**	Long Walk IV 90 min Core Strength Workout 15 min **105 MIN TOTAL**	Rest

ALL WALKS AREN'T CREATED EQUAL

THERE'S A COMMON MISPERCEPTION that you'll burn the same number of calories walking a mile no matter what speed you go. Not true! The faster you walk, the more muscles you use. For instance, as soon as you bend your arms and start pumping them forward and backward, you're activating more shoulder and back muscles. As you pick up the pace, your hips start to swivel, which engages more core muscles like your abs. And the more muscles that are working, the more calories you'll burn.

A 150-pound person who walks 1 mile at a 20-minute-per-mile pace (or

Phase 2: AT A GLANCE

HIGHER-INTENSITY, SHORTER-DURATION TRAINING

WEEK	DAY 1	DAY 2	DAY 3	DAY 4	DAY 5	DAY 6	DAY 7
5	Supercharged Interval Walk I	Recovery Walk 20 min **Total-Body Strength Workout** 20 min	Supercharged Interval Walk I	Recovery Walk 20 min **Total-Body Strength Workout** 20 min	Supercharged Interval Walk I	Speed Walk	Rest
	20 MIN TOTAL	40 MIN TOTAL	20 MIN TOTAL	40 MIN TOTAL	20 MIN TOTAL	30 MIN TOTAL	
6	Supercharged Interval Walk I	Recovery Walk 20 min **Total-Body Strength Workout** 20 min	Supercharged Interval Walk I	Recovery Walk 20 min **Total-Body Strength Workout** 20 min	Supercharged Interval Walk I	Speed Walk	Rest
	20 MIN TOTAL	40 MIN TOTAL	20 MIN TOTAL	40 MIN TOTAL	20 MIN TOTAL	<30 MIN TOTAL	
7	Supercharged Interval Walk II	Recovery Walk 20 min **Total-Body Strength Workout** 20 min	Supercharged Interval Walk II	Recovery Walk 20 min **Total-Body Strength Workout** 20 min	Supercharged Interval Walk II	Speed Walk	Rest
	30 MIN TOTAL	45 MIN TOTAL	30 MIN TOTAL	45 MIN TOTAL	30 MIN TOTAL	<30 MIN TOTAL	
8	Supercharged Interval Walk II	Recovery Walk 20 min **Total-Body Strength Workout** 20 min	Supercharged Interval Walk II	Recovery Walk 20 min **Total-Body Strength Workout** 20 min	Supercharged Interval Walk II	Speed Walk	Rest
	30 MIN TOTAL	45 MIN TOTAL	30 MIN TOTAL	45 MIN TOTAL	30 MIN TOTAL	<30 MIN TOTAL	

THE
WOW
FACTOR

Stand up straight!

Don't trudge through your workouts with slumped shoulders. Whether you're walking or lifting weights, research shows that exercising with proper posture can burn more calories and safeguard you from injury. It also allows you to take in more oxygen, so your workout feels easier.

3 MPH), a comfortable strolling speed, burns about 75 calories. Take it up to a moderate 15-minute-per-mile pace (or 4 MPH), and that same person burns an extra 10 calories—and finishes 5 minutes faster. In fact, walking at a speedy 12-minute-per-mile pace (or 5 MPH) burns a few *more* calories than breaking into a jog and running at the same pace. Push it to an 11-minute mile, and walking burns 16 percent more calories than jogging at the same pace.[5]

In just 8 weeks, our WOW testers were able to walk a mile an average of 2½ minutes faster than when they started the program. A third of the group was chugging along at 4½ MPH or more, with our speediest walker completing an entire mile in just 11 minutes, 40 seconds. That's 5.1 MPH!

As you can imagine, maintaining these high speeds for an entire workout can be difficult. That's where interval training comes in.

How Intervals Work

Interval training has been used by runners since the early 1900s,[6] and it's credited for many world-record performances.[7] One of the most popular is that of British runner Roger Bannister, who in 1954 used the technique to become the first man to run a mile in less than 4 minutes.[8] Some of the same physiological changes that interval training induces to help runners turn in record-setting times can help you achieve your weight loss goals—and your best body ever.

There are lots of fancy terms for intervals—sprint intervals, Wingate test, fartleks—but the basic principle is the same. High-intensity intervals push you into the anaerobic zone, where your body relies on the glycogen, or carbohydrate, stores in your muscles for quick energy. This produces greater improvements than steady-paced, aerobic-only training.[9]

Most exercisers, including walkers, work out in the aerobic zone, rarely or never utilizing the body's other energy-producing system—the anaerobic one. In the aerobic zone, your body uses oxygen to convert carbohydrate and fat throughout the body into energy. Because your body generally has an abundant supply of nutrients, you can sustain this type of activity for a long period of time.

The anaerobic system, on the other hand, doesn't use oxygen. It draws on only the carbohydrate (glycogen) stores in muscles to fuel short bursts of intense activity like sprinting or lifting heavy objects. Because there is a limited supply of glycogen, there is only enough energy for a brief period of this type of activity. The result is a buildup of lactate, which causes that achy, burning sensation in your muscles when you've pushed yourself really hard. Lactate can also inhibit fat burning.

So it's not surprising that most of us don't train anaerobically; it doesn't feel so good. It's out of our comfort zone. But getting out of that comfort zone for just a little bit is going to have dramatic results. When you first start pushing yourself, you may not even be getting to that anaerobic threshold, but every little push toward it works to your advantage.

The beauty of interval training is that foray outside of your comfort zone lasts only for a short time—in the WOW program, just 15 or 30 seconds. Then you have a recovery bout, which is a key component of interval training. During this time, you're back in the aerobic zone and your body is getting rid of the lactate. Then, when it's time for your next high-intensity interval, you're ready to go. Without these recovery bouts, you wouldn't be able to work out at such a high intensity long enough to see results.

The brief, repetitive challenges of interval training are enough to elicit changes in your body's ability to produce energy and burn fat. One of these adaptations is that your muscles increase the amount of energy (from food) they can store. That means less energy is available for storage as fat.

To understand one of the reasons intervals work so well, we have to go all the way down to the cellular level. Inside each cell are structures called mitochondria. They are often described as the powerhouses of cells because they're responsible for producing energy. Active cells, like those in muscles, have hundreds of mitochondria. As we age, however, mitochondria decrease in both number and activity, leading to a decline in the body's fat-burning ability.

Exercise can slow or even reverse this decline by increasing the number of mitochondria by 40 to 50 percent in just 6 weeks.[10] When you work out, your body needs more energy. To keep up with the demand, mitochondria simply divide in half to multiply. In addition, compared with straight-up aerobic exercise, interval training has been shown to produce greater improvement in the mitochondrial enzyme activity associated with fat burning and metabolism.[11] These enzymes may also increase adrenaline, a hormone that helps to burn belly fat.

The Fat-Burning Power of Intervals

A 2008 Australian study really highlighted the weight loss advantage of interval training[12] and is the basis of the interval workouts in the WOW walking program. University of New South Wales researchers divided a group of 45 women—all in their 20s and at a healthy weight—into two groups. One group pedaled on stationary bikes at a moderate intensity for 40 minutes, three times a week. The other group also did three workouts a week, but they cycled for only 20 minutes, doing 8-second speed intervals and 12 seconds of slow pedaling. Despite working out for only half the time, the interval exercisers burned just as many calories (about 200) per session as the women who cycled longer at one steady pace.

One of the top excuses I hear for not exercising, even out of my own mouth on occasion, is *"I don't have time."* So let me repeat: You can burn *the same number of calories* that you would exercising for 40 minutes in just 20 minutes by doing high-intensity intervals! I can think of at least a dozen things I could do with that extra 20 minutes; how about you?

Even better, the interval exercisers lost about six times more weight—a little over 3 pounds, versus not quite ½ pound for the noninterval exercisers—during the 15-week study. Now that may not seem like a lot, but keep in mind that these were young women who didn't need to lose any weight. The more pounds you're carrying around, the easier it will be to drop them (at least in the beginning). In our test panel, women who were 50 or more pounds overweight lost up to twice as much weight over 8 weeks as those carrying only an extra 10 to 15 pounds.

If you simply look at the number of calories the women burned from their workouts in the University of New South Wales study, you would expect them to have lost about 2½ pounds over 15 weeks. The math works like this: To lose 1 pound, you have to burn about 3,500 calories. Each woman did 45 workouts, burning about 200 calories per session, for a total of 9,000 calories. That equates to losing 2.6 pounds. In comparison, the interval exercisers shed 15 percent more weight, while the one-speed exercisers fell short by a whopping 80percent.

So how did the groups get such different results if they burned the same num-

INTENSITY MATTERS

A POPULAR FITNESS recommendation for more than a decade has been to take 10,000 steps a day. Whether it can actually get you the results you want is no longer quite so clear. When researchers reviewed nine high-quality studies of people who walked with pedometers, they discovered that, on average, people taking 10,000 steps a day lost only $\frac{1}{10}$ of a pound a week.[13] That can be really discouraging.

Don't get me wrong; it's a great place to start, and using a pedometer is a wonderful way to motivate yourself. In one study, pedometer-wearers increased the amount of walking they did by an extra 2,491 steps a day, or almost 1¼ miles.[14]

But unless you're moving at a moderate intensity, the 10,000-steps goal may not be enough to shed pounds, improve your fitness level, and reduce your risk of heart disease and other health problems. For instance, if you're logging most of your steps just strolling to and from the car, around the office and house, and running errands,

you're probably not working at a high-enough intensity.

A new study has quantified how many steps you need to take, and in what time frame, to ensure that you're walking at the minimum effort level required to improve your health. The goal is at least 1,000 steps in 10 minutes, or 3,000 steps in 30 minutes.[15] Now if you're following the WOW program, you'll far exceed that recommendation, I promise. Many of our testers were hitting 150 steps or more a minute—50 percent higher than the suggested pace.

ber of calories? While the study didn't track their eating habits, other research suggests that it's the most likely explanation for why the latter group didn't slim down more. Studies have shown that people often compensate for the calories they exercise off by eating more. (I'll tell you more about that in Chapter 5 because I don't want you to make the same mistake.)

One of the reasons the interval exercisers exceeded weight loss expectations is probably a revved-up postexercise calorie burn. Anytime you exercise, your body continues to burn calories at a higher rate after your workout until your energy expenditure returns to normal. This is called afterburn, and how long it lasts and how many bonus calories you get out of it depend on the type of exercise you do. Taking the dog for a half-hour stroll around your neighborhood might get you a 5-minute afterburn. But high-intensity exercise like intervals has been shown to keep your body's calorie-burning engines in high gear for at least an hour afterward, incinerating up to twice as many calories in the process.[16]

Walk Smarter, Not Longer

There are hundreds of studies of interval training, but one of the first to pique my interest came out of Laval University in Quebec and was published about 15 years ago.[17] Back then, the popular exercise prescription for weight loss was to do long, slow distances. This study showed that more isn't always better when it comes to fighting fat.

For the study, 27 men and women were assigned to one of two groups. The first group followed a 20-week endurance-training program consisting of 45 minutes of moderate-intensity activity, 5 days a week. The second group engaged in a 15-week high-intensity interval training plan with three interval workouts a week (each involving a total of 7½ minutes of vigorous activity and recovery bouts of various lengths) plus 30 minutes of easy to moderate, steady-paced exercise 4 days a week.

By the end of the training programs, the endurance group had burned twice as many calories on average as the interval group. However, the interval group lost three times more body fat. When researchers adjusted the outcomes based on the number of calories burned, they discovered that the interval group had lost nine times more fat for the amount of time they exercised—showing that you don't have to work out longer to lose more fat.

Intervals also train your body to be a fat-burning machine, so you blast more fat even when you're doing noninterval workouts. While all types of cardio exercise improve your body's fat-burning ability, interval training can get those results in less time with less exercise.[18]

In a study from the University of Guelph in Ontario, researchers tested the fat-burning capacity of eight young, moderately active women. Then the women did seven 60-minute interval workouts over the course of 2 weeks. Each workout consisted of cycling hard for ten 4-minute bouts, with 2 minutes of rest in between. After training, researchers retested the women by having them pedal at a moderate intensity for 60 minutes. The result: They burned 36 percent more fat than they had at the beginning of the study.[19] These types of changes usually take 6 to 12 weeks with typical 30- to 60-minute moderate-intensity workouts, but with interval training you can get them three to six times faster.[20]

With shorter workouts, it may also be easier to make exercise a habit. When researchers at Stanford University School of Medicine compared similar exercise prescriptions, they found that after 2 years, people who did short bouts of vigorous exercise were $2\frac{1}{2}$ times more likely to stick with their programs than those who engaged in more frequent, lower-intensity workout sessions.[21]

Interval training can also boost your endurance, so you can work and play longer. Everyday activities such as climbing stairs and chasing the kids or grandkids will feel easier. And you'll have more energy to give it your all during your workouts and blast even more calories. In a study at McMaster University in Ontario, researchers found that just six sessions of high-intensity interval training were enough to double endurance.[22] At the start of the study, the researchers tested 16 healthy young men and women to see how long they could bicycle hard before they tired out. They averaged 26 min-

"Just do it!"

Getting started was Mary Lou Phillips's biggest obstacle. "I had a major meltdown before I even began," said the 51-year-old nurse practitioner, who juggles two jobs, lots of volunteer work, and a teenage daughter. "Trying to do the program felt like one more thing on my very busy schedule. I didn't know if I could do it."

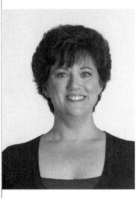

First, she couldn't get her sports watch to work properly for the intervals. Then she didn't think that she had a good place to walk. "I kept coming up with excuses," admitted Mary Lou, a self-described type A personality who needs to have everything planned out. But thanks to her husband's encouragement and practical advice, she got on her treadmill.

"I finally came to the realization that everything didn't have to be perfect," said Mary Lou. "What mattered most was that I made walking part of my daily schedule." And even when she didn't, she just got back on track the next day instead of throwing in the towel completely. Some of her incentive has been the results that she's seen: fewer hot flashes so she's sleeping better at night, dealing with stress more effectively, more energy, and tight calf and thigh muscles. "I have not had those since high school!" said Mary Lou.

utes—not bad when you're riding like someone is chasing you. Over the next 2 weeks, half of the group did six training sessions of sprint intervals, cycling all-out for 30 seconds and then either pedaling slowly or just sitting on the bike for 4 minutes to recover, repeating the intervals up to seven times. The rest of the men and women served as a comparison group and did not change their activity levels. After the 2 weeks of training, the researchers retested the exercisers to see how long they could cycle at a steady, hard pace. The interval exercisers improved more than 100%, lasting for an impressive 56 minutes.

MORE WOW WALKING WORKOUTS

INTERVAL WALKS ARE THE CORE of the WOW walking program, but they're not the only type of walking you'll be doing. Remember, mixing up your workouts is key to avoiding a plateau and reaching your goal.

Toning Walks

We all love to multitask, but every time I see someone carrying dumbbells while they're walking, I cringe! Any extra firming or calorie-burning benefits they think they're getting are tiny compared with the increased risk of a shoulder injury to which they're subjecting themselves. Your shoulder is already more susceptible to injury than other joints because of its wide range of motion. Start swinging even a light weight and the repetitive motion during a 30- to 40-minute walk can quickly fatigue these small muscles. And once you're out for a walk, there's no option for putting down those weights, further increasing your risk of injuring yourself.

There is a safer option: an elastic resistance band. According to a study reported in the *Journal of Strength and Conditioning Research*, bands have muscle-building effects that are very similar to what you'd get from working out on exercise machines.[23]

The concept of doing toning exercises with a band while walking was first introduced to me by Abbie Appel, a fitness trainer in Boca Raton, Florida. Knowing that *Prevention* readers are always looking for time-efficient workouts that provide maximum results, I asked Abbie to develop a routine for the magazine. The workout wasn't just a hit with our readers; I started taking my exercise band with me on my evening walks around my neighborhood. It revved up the intensity of my walks, and I got a super upper-body workout without exercising a minute longer—a big plus for a working mom. And since bands are lightweight, you'll be less likely to sustain a joint injury. So naturally I had to include toning walks in the WOW program. During the first 4 weeks of the program, you'll do these

THE WOW FACTOR
Reward yourself with a massage. According to research published in the *British Journal of Sports Medicine*, women who received a 10-minute leg massage following sprints were 49 percent less stiff afterward.[24]

double-duty workouts—heart-pumping, calorie-crunching cardio from the walking and body-sculpting, muscle-building strength training from the band moves—on days between interval walks.

Now I have to admit, when I first showed this routine to our test panel, some of the women told me flat out that I was nuts if I thought that they would walk in public doing band exercises. And I could tell that others were thinking the exact same thing. But in the end, about half of them proudly did their Toning Walks outdoors—and they may have inspired others to give it a try. "One woman stopped me and asked where I got the great idea," said Theresa Bahnick, one of our WOW panelists.

Some got over the embarrassment factor by walking at times when or in areas where there weren't a lot of people around. Others felt more comfortable where everyone else was exercising. Most of them just didn't care what others thought—love that! I think Wendy Silfies said it best: "At least I'm doing something to help with my fitness. I was more embarrassed before, when I wasn't doing any exercise." (The rest of the women did the Toning Walk indoors, either on a treadmill or around their houses, or they did the walk and the band exercises separately.)

This is all about you, not what anyone else thinks. So get out there and give it a try. You could be on the leading edge of a new exercise trend!

Long Walks

While interval workouts can produce more weight loss in less time, there are advantages to going longer occasionally. You'll be doing long walks once a week during the first 4 weeks of the WOW program. The results are worth it.

In a University of Wisconsin-Eau Claire study, 26 sedentary, postmenopausal women were prescribed either 30 or 45 minutes of moderate-intensity walking, 5 days a week, for 12 weeks. Guess who lost more weight? Not surprisingly, the women with the longer workout sessions did. But here's the kicker: They walked 50% longer, yet they lost five times more weight.[25] Not a bad return on their investment!

It gets better: The 45-minute walkers lost three times as many inches from their waistlines and twice as much body fat as the half-hour walkers. They also boosted their "good" HDL cholesterol twice as much. This change in HDL has been shown to equate to a 12 percent reduction in risk of heart attack. The 45-minute walkers also improved their fitness levels nearly twice as much—23.5 percent compared with 12.5 percent for the 30-minute walkers. According to other research, this change corresponds to a 20 percent decrease in the risk of dying from heart disease.[26]

Longer-duration exercise uses up more of your body's fuel stores. To replenish them and repair broken-down muscle fibers afterward, your body has to expend a lot of energy, sparking a bigger metabolic boost and greater than expected weight loss compared with shorter workouts. Researchers at the University of Victoria in British Columbia found that exercisers who chugged along for 60 minutes burned nearly five times as many calories postworkout as those whose workouts lasted only 30 minutes.[27]

These long walks are also an opportunity to see just what your body is capable of doing. Several of our WOW test panelists had never before walked for more than 45 to 60 minutes all at one time, and they were pleasantly surprised by the experience. "My legs were more powerful than I thought," wrote Mary Lou Phillips after her 90-minute walk during Week 4 of the program. "They seemed to 'kick in' and keep me moving when the rest of me was feeling tired." In fact, four of our test panelists were so inspired that after the 8-week program they trained for and walked a half marathon (13.1 miles). Bonus: When you do a shorter walk, it will feel so much easier.

Recovery Walks

During the second phase of the WOW program, you'll be doing a steady-paced, moderate-intensity walk to allow the necessary recovery time between your interval sessions while still keeping your calorie burn in high gear. You should be walking at a purposeful pace, you're in a bit of a hurry, about 3 to 4 cf^ . These are the perfect walks to ask family members, friends, or co-workers to accompany you. The camaraderie will help to keep you motivated.

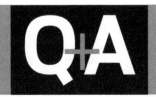

Q: Can men do this program?

A: Absolutely! Walking is a great workout for women or men. In fact, our test panelist Theresa Bahnick's husband, Dave, did just two or three interval walks a week—no dieting or strength training—and dropped almost 10 pounds in about 12 weeks. Guys can follow the walking workouts exactly as they appear, although they'll probably need heavier resistance bands for the strength training. They will also likely need to eat more, aiming for about 2,000 to 2,200 calories a day.

Speed Walks

During these sessions, you'll walk as fast as you can (probably 4 to 5 MPH) to complete 1 mile. Seeing the improvement in your time each week can give your confidence and motivation a huge boost. Straight-up speed workouts like this can also rev up your metabolism by targeting fast-twitch muscle fibers, the ones responsible for bursts of speed and power. Unfortunately, most traditional workouts don't activate these essential fibers. And if you don't use them, you lose them. Many women over 65 have virtually no fast-twitch muscle fibers left. Their disappearance is one of the reasons your metabolism takes a nosedive as you get older.

This type of workout is also supereffective at zeroing in on belly fat. In a University of Virginia study, researchers divided 27 obese women, average age 51, into three groups. One group did no exercise, while another walked or jogged at a moderate intensity 5 days a week. The third group did the same types of workouts 2 days a week, but on the other 3 days, they walked or jogged as fast as possible for a high-intensity workout. The exercise sessions lasted long enough for everyone in both groups to burn 400 calories.[28]

So, with all of the women burning 2,000 calories a week, both groups should have lost the same amount of weight, right? Wrong! The high-intensity group, who completed most of their workouts in less time, lost 67 percent more weight than the moderate-intensity-only group—8 pounds versus 5 pounds—over 16 weeks. The speediest walkers also lost five times more belly fat, three times more thigh fat, and four times more total body fat.

Vigorous exercise like this raises levels of fat-burning hormones more than moderate exercise does. And because you're working out harder, it takes longer for your metabolism to return to normal after a training session, which means your calorie burn stays cranked up about 47 percent longer than after less intense workouts. In one study, high-intensity exercisers burned 86 percent more calories during the 3 hours postexercise.[29]

STRENGTH TRAINING: A WALKING ALLY

ADDING STRENGTH-TRAINING WORKOUTS to your walking program will speed your results and ensure that you keep off those lost pounds long-term by building muscle. Muscle is key to maintaining a high metabolism and staying active as you get older.

Unfortunately, beginning in your 30s, you lose about 5 pounds of muscle every decade. By the time you're 65, you could be down by as much as 20 pounds of muscle, which can cause a steep decline in your metabolism and a decrease in strength that can make even getting out of a chair or climbing stairs more difficult. Both of these changes can undermine your weight loss efforts. The good news is, strength training can halt muscle loss and even build more muscle.

In a University of Rhode Island study, 23 women—all ages 19 to 44 and at a healthy weight—participated in twice-weekly strength workouts. During each session, they performed two or three 10-rep sets of six different exercises that targeted the major muscle groups of the body, such as the chest, back, legs, and glutes (the butt muscles). Although the women did not lose any weight (not surprising, since they were already at a healthy weight), they decreased their body fat by almost 10 percent in 12 weeks, replacing it with more than 4 pounds of firm, lean muscle to rev up their metabolism.[30]

Strong muscles also protect you against injury and help you to walk faster. In a recent study, strengthening your quadriceps muscles—key walking muscles in the front of your thighs—can increase your speed by as much as 15 percent.[31] That's equivalent to going from a 17-minute-per-mile pace (or 3½ MPH) to a 15-minute mile (or 4 MPH). And remember, the faster you walk, the more calories you burn, and the slimmer you get.

NOW THAT YOU KNOW WHAT you'll be doing for the Walk Off Weight program and why, it's time to get prepared for your workouts.

Positive Attitude, Powerful Results

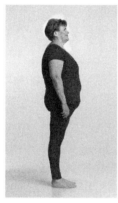

BEFORE

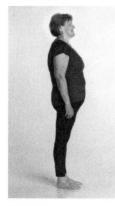

AFTER

KATHY ASHENFELTER will tell you two things about herself: She's a walker and an optimist. Unfortunately, neither weekend walks nor happy thoughts had helped her to keep the 60 pounds she'd lost a decade ago from creeping back on.

The WOW program gave Kathy the tools she needed to turn her walks into fat-fighting workouts. Combined with a doable diet that didn't leave her feeling deprived and toning workouts that made her feel powerful, Kathy now had a complete plan. And her fantastic attitude guaranteed her success—she lost nearly 23 pounds, the most weight of all our test panelists.

No matter how you lose weight, there will always be challenges; how you meet them can mean the difference between achieving your goals and not. Every step of the way, Kathy kept a positive attitude.

At first, she didn't like the toning exercises ("I felt clumsy and off-balance."), but as she got better at them, they made her feel more powerful. The walking techniques and posture tips took some getting used to as well, but Kathy noticed how following tips like "keep your eyes on the horizon" helped her walk faster and made her feel taller and thinner—even before the scale changed.

The diet was also a challenge at first, especially when it came to Kathy writing down everything she ate. But she stuck with it, and she quickly discovered that it helped her to avoid eating when she wasn't really hungry.

In addition to losing more than 10 percent of her body weight, Kathy shed nearly 8 percent body fat and reports that she no longer craves sweets. "Now it's no big deal to pass on dessert." Incredibly, she also has an even better outlook and more energy. "I know I believe in myself because I threw out my big clothes for the first time in my life," reported Kathy. "I didn't even wait to collect a bagful. As soon as something was too big, I donated it. This time, I know I can keep it off."

The difference? Kathy feels as if she's finally found a program that isn't restrictive or overwhelming. It's just a way of life—"*my* way of life," she said.

P.S. *Three months after the official end of the program, Kathy recorded an additional 5 1/2-pound weight loss and shaved another 6 3/4 inches off her figure, for a grand total of 28 pounds and 20 1/2 inches lost in 5 months.*

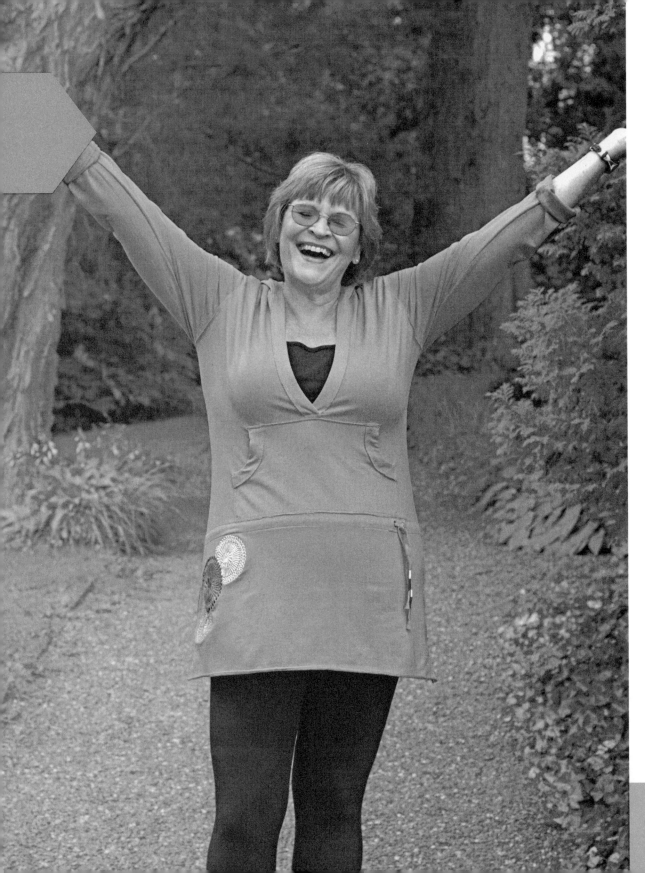

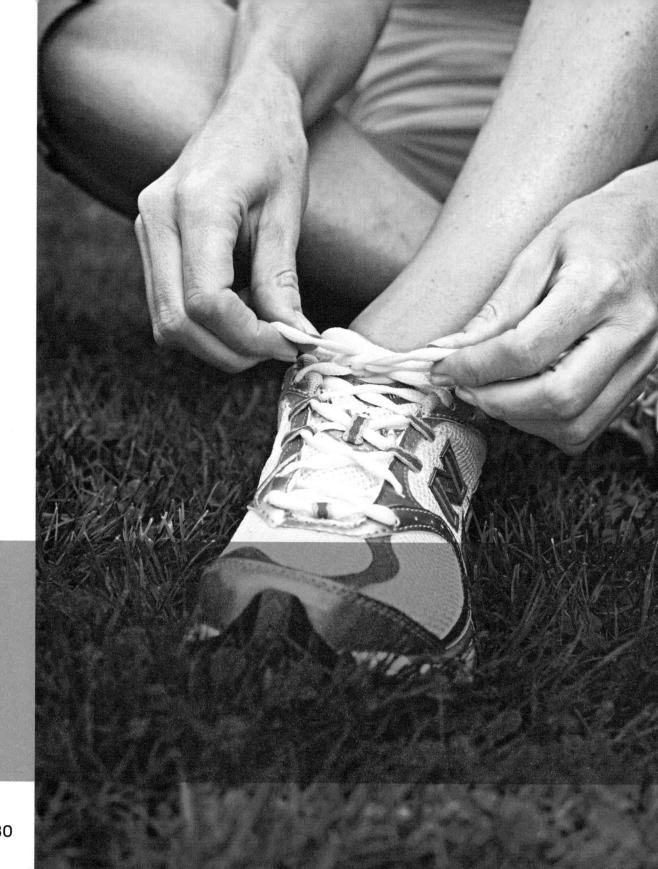

CHAPTER

3

PREP BEFORE YOU Walk

BEFORE YOU HEAD OUT for your first walk, I want to make sure that you're properly prepared so you get the most from your workouts—and you feel great doing them. Along with the gear that you'll need for the WOW program (don't worry, it's not a lot), I'm going to tell you about some other products—including clothes—that can make your workouts more enjoyable.

Also, you want to plan where you're going to do your walks. I'll give you the pros and cons of doing the WOW workouts indoors or out, plus tips to guarantee that you get a fabulous workout no matter where you walk.

One of the benefits of walking for exercise is that just about everyone can do it—and should do it. Our bodies are meant to move; it's a good thing. However, for some people, any form of exercise can be risky, especially when they're working at a

>> Good
supportive
walking shoes
($60–$120)

>> Comfortable
socks that fit with
your shoes ($3–
$12 per pair)

>> Timing device:
MP3 player ($30–
$300) loaded
with Walk Off
Weight podcasts
or a sports watch
with an interval
timer ($20–$65)

>> An elastic
resistance band or
tube ($4–$15)

*See Resources on
page 320 for more
information on
where to find these
products.*

higher intensity such as doing intervals. If you have any chronic medical condition (such as diabetes, high blood pressure, or arthritis) or risk factors (such as smoking or being more than 20 pounds overweight), and you have not discussed exercising with your doctor, it's important that you do so before beginning the WOW program. Pick up the phone and make an appointment right now. Then keep on reading and preparing so that as soon as you have the okay from your doctor, you can get started.

WALKING SHOES

IT REALLY ISN'T JUST A MARKETING PLOY. Back in the 1970s, when Nike made running and basketball shoes all the rage, you would have been laughed at if you had asked for a walking-specific shoe. "Every shoe is a walking shoe" is how a smug salesperson might have responded. But today, store shelves are stacked with shoes made for striding. The trick is finding the right pair both for your feet and for the type of walking you'll be doing.

First, walking shoes are specifically designed to support the heel-to-toe motion of walking and to help propel you forward. When you walk, you land on your heel—which is why walking shoes have a beveled or rounded heel, just like your foot. This allows you to roll smoothly through each step. And because your heel strikes the ground first, that's where you need the most cushioning. Runners, on the other hand, land more flat-footed in the middle of their feet, so the heels of running shoes aren't always as rounded, and they usually contain more cushioning in the midfoot area.

Next, walking shoes are designed to bend right where your foot naturally bends—in the forefoot, right behind the ball. This helps to facilitate the last part of the heel-to-toe motion, the push-off. Put it all together, and a good walking shoe will cushion and stabilize your feet for a smoother stride and a reduced risk of injury.

Everything from knee pain to a sore back can stem from poor foot mechanics or insufficient support and cushioning. One of our WOW testers, Gail Rarick, learned this firsthand. A few weeks into the program, Gail R finally purchased new walking shoes and almost immediately noticed an improvement in the knee and arch pain that she'd been having. "It used to hurt when I'd get up after sitting for a long time, but now my feet and knees never hurt," she said. That's why the right pair of walking shoes is the most important element of your walk.

When walking shoes hit the market in the late 1980s, they were primarily athletic sneakers designed for exercise walking. Today, companies are making sandals, dress shoes, and fashion sneakers with some of the same athletic technology, but often these don't have enough cushioning or support for the high-intensity walking that you'll be doing. Sometimes athletic shoes such as cross-trainers or even running shoes are being passed off as walking shoes. That's why it's important to educate yourself before you go shopping.

KNOW YOUR FEET No two pairs of feet are alike, so my favorite shoe might be a nightmare for you. And size is just one aspect; it's also important to know the shape of your foot and how your foot works in motion. The shoes that best support your foot type will feel better and last longer because you'll put less stress on both your feet and the shoes.

The shape of your foot is important for getting the right fit. The bottom of a shoe is called a last, and it's the mold on which a shoe is formed. It can be straight, semicurved, or curved. For a good fit, you want to make sure that the shape of the bottom of a shoe matches the shape of your foot. To do this, trace your feet on a piece of paper and take the cut-out tracings with you when you go shoe shopping.

DOES YOUR SHOE PASS THE TEST?

BEFORE YOU BUY, it's wise to take a closer look at the design of your shoe, especially if you have any question about whether it's a genuine walking shoe or if you're purchasing a running shoe (see page 37 for more on wearing running shoes to walk). Here are three simple tests that walking expert Mark Fenton recommends to ensure that the pair you choose will perform well when you're walking in them. *Note: These tests are meant only for athletic shoes. Some casual or fashion shoes may pass some or all of the tests, but lack the stability, cushioning, and support needed for walking workouts.*

1. Poke 'em. Place the shoe on a table and, using a pencil, push down firmly at the back of the shoe, inside the cup of the heel. If the heel is beveled sufficiently, the front of the shoe, where the ball of the foot resides, should rise off the table. Next, look at the toe of the shoe. The end of a smooth heel-to-toe roll is aided by a noticeable bend or curve upward at the toe of the shoe, called the toe spring. Poke down on the tip of the toe with the pencil; the heel should lift off the table.

2. Twist 'em. Grab the heel of the shoe with one hand and the toe with the other and twist it. The shoe should give only slightly. A stiff shoe impedes your foot's natural motion, while one that's super flexible lacks support, which could increase your risk of sprains and falls.

3. Bend 'em. Firmly grasp the heel of the shoe with one hand and push upward at the toes with the other to see where the shoe bends. You want it to bend at the ball, just like your foot. This flexibility will help to facilitate your push-off at the end of each stride. Be wary of a shoe that bends through the arch, which indicates a lack of support that can lead to discomfort in the bottom of your feet.

The shoes you buy should also accommodate your foot's natural movement. There are three basic levels of motion that your feet can have: rigid, or very little movement; flexible, or lots of movement; and moderate, which is in between. To determine which level best describes your feet and the type of shoes that are right for them, see "The Walking Wet Test" on the opposite page.

CHOOSE YOUR SOCKS All of this work to find the perfect shoe will be for naught if you don't wear a good pair of socks when you walk. There's a wide variety of styles and materials available today—everything from ultra-thin to extra-padded, which can affect the fit of your shoes. To find the right pair for you, see page 36 and, if possible, try out a few. Be sure to take them with you when you go shoe shopping.

HEAD TO A SPECIALTY STORE While you may get a better deal at a large chain store, you could pay the price by ending up with a poor-fitting, uncomfortable sneaker that leaves you more prone to injury. Technical running and/or walking stores usually employ more knowledgeable salespeople who will know how to evaluate your needs. They'll ask you questions about the type and amount of walking you do and watch you walk barefoot to help you find the best shoe for you. They'll also be more likely to allow you to road test the shoe before you buy it.

SHOP IN THE EVENING That's when your feet are biggest. Even if you walk in the morning, your feet swell during exercise because of increased circulation, temperature, and exertion. You want shoes that fit your feet at their largest.

GET MEASURED Getting older, having kids, and gaining weight can all cause your feet to expand, resulting in a half to a whole size increase. No wonder experts have found that women tend to buy shoes that are too small. No matter what your feet measure, don't get hung up on the number and try to squeeze into a smaller size. It's not like they're bowling shoes, with your size on display for everyone to see. If it makes you feel any better, I wear a size 10 or 10½.

FIND A MATCH Before you try on a shoe, compare the tracings of your feet with the bottoms of the shoe. Both should have the same basic shape—straight, curved, or semicurved—and none of the tracing should be off of the sole. If it is, move on to the next pair.

CHECK THE FIT Since athletic shoes can be sized quite differently from dress shoes, you may need to go up or down a size, depending on how they fit (I had to buy an 11 in one brand). You should have at least one finger's-width of space between your longest toe (usually your big toe) and the end of the shoe. Since you need to be standing up, someone else will have to test this. (A good salesperson will do it automatically.) Then wiggle your toes to make sure that you have enough room top to bottom. If you have chosen the correct last, the shoe shouldn't rub on the sides of your toes, either.

THE WALKING WET TEST

THIS SIMPLE TEST WILL HELP DETERMINE the amount of motion that your feet have when you are walking. If you've been a longtime *Prevention* reader, the test may look familiar to you, but don't skip over it. We've developed a new and improved version with the help of Mark Fenton, an internationally known walking expert who's done research on the biomechanics of walking and athletic shoes.

Instead of simply looking at your feet when you're standing, this test shows what your feet are doing when you're in motion. And that's how you should be spending the majority of your time in your walking shoes. (A podiatrist can do a similar assessment to determine your foot type.)

STEP 1: Locate a 5-foot-long area of cement, a piece of cardboard or brown packaging paper, or another surface on which you can make footprints. You'll also need a pan that's large enough for your feet. Fill the pan with water.

STEP 2: Dip your bare feet in the water, then walk naturally until you get a good print of your feet.

STEP 3: Match your walking print to the images below. (If your footprints look as if they are somewhere between moderate and flexible, use moderate as your guide. If you're between moderate and rigid, follow the advice for rigid. If your footprints are different patterns, aim to fit the more moderate one. Also go with moderate if you wear orthotics or insoles.)

Moderate: You'll see about a 1-inch strip of wetness in the arch area.

How you tread: Your feet are well balanced and roll, or pronate, almost perfectly (this is ideal for absorbing shock). They lengthen and spread out about a half shoe size when you walk, and they have good stability.

How to fit: Yours is the easiest foot to fit because many shoes are designed for your type. You can skip the models that boast a lot of motion control or cushioning. Make sure any shoe you buy feels good in the store—no rubbing or pinching.

Flexible: Your foot flattens out as you step. It will leave the fullest imprint, with the most arch area in contact with the walking surface.

How you tread: Your feet roll inward too much (overpronate) when you walk. They're unstable, but they absorb shock well because they spread out. They can change an entire size when you walk. People with flexible feet often report heel pain and may have trouble with alignment issues affecting their knees, hips, and overall balance.

How to fit: Because your feet tend to flatten when you put weight on them, you need a shoe that has less space between the laces and the sole. To judge height, move your feet up and down inside the front of the shoes while you're wearing them. You still want wiggle room, just not an excessive amount. You don't need a lot of cushioning, but you do need good arch support and stability or motion control.

Rigid: Your foot doesn't cave much as you put your weight on it. The arch stays so high that you'll see little, if any, imprint in the arch area.

How you tread: Your feet tend to roll inward only slightly, so you underpronate, meaning you walk more on the outsides of your feet. They're stable, but the shock isn't as evenly distributed as it should be. They tend not to lengthen and spread out much when you walk. Because people with rigid feet have poor shock absorption, they're more likely to experience heel, shin, and knee pain.

How to fit: You need shoes with lots of cushioning to absorb shock, and lots of flexibility to allow your feet to roll more. Go for a roomy upper to accommodate your high arches. If you have tight calves, choose the shoe with the highest heel.

TEST-DRIVE SEVERAL PAIRS Many specialty stores have a treadmill on-site for just this purpose. If your store doesn't, ask to go outside for a test-walk. At the very least, walk around the store. Taking a few steps in place isn't enough to thoroughly evaluate a shoe.

The best shoe for you will feel great right out of the box; you should never have to "break in" any type of shoe. If you feel any pinching or rubbing while you're walking, try on some others. Likewise, make sure that the heel of the shoe doesn't slip up and down when you walk.

When you have a shoe that's made a good first impression, try on another one or two for comparison. You may be surprised to find that another style or brand feels even better. And if you don't, it will confirm your first choice.

See Resources on page 320 for more information on where to find walking shoes.

SOCKS

NEXT TO YOUR SHOES, your socks are your most important piece of walking gear. A lousy pair of socks can ruin the feel of a great pair of shoes.

When you're buying socks, the most important thing to look for is a synthetic wicking material, such as CoolMax or Dri-Fit, or a lightweight wool designed for physical activity, such as SmartWool or Icebreaker. These types of fabric outperform cotton because they wick away sweat to keep your feet dry, comfortable, and blister free. Newer models of socks are boasting blends of different athletic materials such as SmartWool and CoolMax, and many walkers are finding these even better at wicking away moisture.

Don't forget to check the size. A sock that is too small is just as likely to cause a blister or a problem with your toenails as a shoe that is too small.

Many performance socks offer a variety of features. While they aren't necessary, depending on your foot issues, they may keep your feet a little bit happier. Here are some that might be of interest to you.

PADDING Some socks on the market that are specifically designed for walking, such as Thorlo, have extra padding in the heel and ball of the foot. Since the fatty foot pads on the bottoms of your feet diminish with age, you may find these types of socks more comfortable as you get older. They're also a good choice if you have diabetes or arthritis because they provide extra protection from bumps and bruises. If you do opt for padded socks, wear them while trying on shoes because the extra thickness may affect the shoes' fit.

Q+A

Q: How often should I buy new sneakers?

A: To protect your feet, replace your shoes every 300 to 500 miles, even if they don't look worn. (Aim for the lower end of the mileage range if you have foot, ankle, knee, or back problems or if you are obese.) Shoes lose their cushion and support on the inside long before they look old on the outside. If you walk about 3 miles, 5 days a week, you'll need a new pair after about 5 to 8 months. By the end of the 8-week WOW program, you'll have walked nearly 100 miles; if you continue at this or a similar activity level, then you'll be due for a new pair of shoes every 6 to 9 months or so. To help you remember, write the date when you start wearing your shoes on the underside of the tongue.

Q: Can I wear running shoes to walk?

A: Yes—and if you plan to do any running along with your walks, definitely purchase a running shoe. (Never run in a walking shoe, though, because they lack the cushioning you need for the greater impact.) Since there are more styles and brands of running shoes, some people may find a running shoe with a better fit. Others may prefer the extra cushioning of a running shoe, while speed demons may appreciate the lighter weight. No matter what type of shoe you buy do the Walking Wet Test (page 35) to make sure that you get a good fit, and subject your shoes to the three tests on page 33.

Q: Do toning shoes work?

A: Unfortunately, there haven't been any independent scientific studies to assess claims that sneakers with rounded bottoms will firm up your legs and butt without working out. The idea behind these shoes is that the unique soles cause you to be less stable, so more muscles have to work to keep you balanced. Studies by shoe manufacturers have shown increased muscle activation, but that doesn't guarantee a higher caloric burn or faster toning. In fact, it could backfire. If your legs become tired more quickly, you may end up walking less than if you weren't wearing the shoes—and some of the models are quite heavy, which can contribute to fatigue.

Even more worrisome is that this instablility could put some people at an increased risk for injury. That's why until there is more research, I can't recommend these types of shoes for walking workouts like the WOW program. For everyday walking, they may be fine as long as you gradually increase your wear time and don't have any foot, joint, or balance problems.

Q: Can I buy shoes online?

A: I don't recommend it unless you try them on at a store first—even if you already have a favorite brand and style and you want to order a replacement. While the brand may appear to be the same, companies often make changes from season to season that could affect the fit. Or your feet may change over time. Once you find a pair, feel free to look online for a better price. I won't argue with bargain hunting.

COOLING While some socks (like the padded ones I mentioned on page 36) are quite thick and provide extra cushioning or warmth, others are ultrathin to keep your feet cool and minimize bulk. Sample a few to see what you like best for your walks.

ODOR CONTROL Lightweight wool is a natural antibacterial, so socks made with this material can help reduce foot odor and fungal infections. Synthetic versions containing silver fibers, Cocona (a brand of fiber made from recycled coconut shells), or special coatings also have antimicrobial properties.

BLISTER PROTECTION Some of the newer trendy socks are infused with gels—such as the Adidas Aloe socks, which soothe dry patches and protect against blisters ($12 for two pairs; the aloe lasts about 20 washes). Just make sure to wear these socks on shorter walks, until you know how your feet react to the gel.

ANATOMICALLY CORRECT If you have trouble with socks that bunch, or if your feet are extra sensitive to bumps, seams, or ridges, give a brand such as the New Balance Marathon Trainer Left/Right a try. Because they're designed specifically for the left or right foot, they fit snugly without rumpling. See Resources on page 320 for more information on where to find socks.

TIMING DEVICE

MP3 PLAYERS If you don't already have an MP3 player, you'll need one to use the podcasts. While the iPod is by far the most famous MP3 player around, there

LACING TRICKS FOR A BETTER FIT

THE TRADITIONAL METHOD of crisscrossing laces works for most people. For others, the following lacing techniques, recommended by Tom Brunick, former director of The Athlete's Foot store's research and development center in Naperville, Illinois, may get you a better fit.

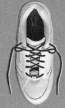

Narrow heel: Lace normally until the last set of holes. Instead of lacing across the shoe, pull the laces up toward your ankles and thread down through the last hole on each side, thus creating a loop by not pulling the lace all the way through. Cross the laces and thread through the loops, then tighten and tie.

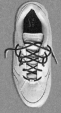

Low arch: Use crisscross lacing halfway up the shoe, then use the "loop lacing" technique (as described for the narrow heel, above) for the remaining holes.

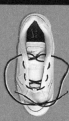

High arch: Make your first crisscross as usual, then thread straight up the next several holes on each side. Crisscross the last set of holes.

Wide foot: Thread straight up the first two or three sets of holes on each side. Start crisscrossing once you're past your forefoot.

are numerous ultralightweight models available (long gone are the days of bulky WalkMan players!). Some have built-in pedometers, watches, even GPS systems. For the WOW podcasts, you need only the most basic model. Take time to familiarize yourself with the options available. It helps to try on and test several varieties and sizes, including arm straps, waist clips, and earbuds to see what feels most comfortable to you. See Resources on page 320 for more information on where to find MP3 players.

WALK OFF WEIGHT PODCASTS As stated in the previous chapter, you'll be speeding up and slowing down for 15-second to 1-minute intervals during many of your workouts. To make this type of training easier, I created audio workouts for all of the Interval Walks and the Toning Walks. Just download them onto your MP3 player and head out the door. (If you don't already have an MP3 player, you can order one that's preloaded with the podcasts.) I'll tell you exactly when to speed up and slow down—no need to check your watch. Along the way, I'll offer technique advice, motivational tips, and words of encouragement to help you maximize your workouts—almost as if I were walking right next to you. And striding to fun, upbeat tunes will make your walks more enjoyable. Many women in our test panel reported that it was easier to kick up their intensity (that means burning more calories, too) when they used the podcasts. During the Toning Walks, I'll describe each move so you don't have to try to remember everything or carry notes. See Resources on page 320 for more information on how to get the WOW podcasts.

SPORTS WATCH If you're not using the podcasts for your interval walks, a sports watch is an invaluable tool, and the right one can make timing your speed and recovery bouts much simpler. I recommend a model that allows you to preprogram two different interval durations. Once you set your interval times, you simply hit start for your first interval; the watch will beep every time you need to slow down or speed up, so you don't have to keep checking the time.

Our test panel used the Timex Ironman 50-Lap Mid ($60–$65). "I liked it because I could walk with a friend and the interval beeps would let us know when to speed up or slow down without having to look at the watch," says Susan Moyer, who used the watch's interval function. See Resources on page 320 for more information on where to find sports watches.

RESISTANCE BANDS OR TUBES

CONFESSION TIME: UP UNTIL ABOUT 3 YEARS AGO, I wouldn't have been caught dead strength training with a resistance band. While I thought they had a place in strength training—for small muscles such as the rotator cuffs in your shoulders that don't require a lot of resistance or the adductors and abductors in your inner and outer thighs that aren't easily worked with dumbbells—I believed that it was dumbbells or nothing for serious firming. But then we tested my theory for a *Prevention* magazine article, and let's just say I'm glad I didn't put my money where my mouth is.

We recruited 18 sedentary women to evaluate five ways to get strong—weights, resistance bands, Pilates, yoga, and body-weight moves such as push-ups—to find out which could deliver a leaner, firmer figure the fastest. After 12 weeks, the women in our band group shaved 30 percent more inches off their bellies, hips, arms, and thighs than the other groups did, averaging a total loss of 15 inches. They also dropped 18 percent more weight—averaging 6 pounds each—while one of them built enough shapely muscle to rev up her metabolism by about 120 calories a day.

I was shocked until we looked at our results a little more closely. In our experiment, the band-users exercised more. Some felt that the bands were less intimidating than weights, while others enjoyed the novelty of them. Because the bands are lightweight and portable, they're easy to use at home or on the road—so no more excuses. And they deliver what experts call functional training; in other words, they mimic real-life actions, such as taking out the garbage—and target more muscles for faster results in the process.

Unlike dumbbells, where your muscles are working hardest during only part of the range of motion, resistance bands keep the tension on the entire time if you use them properly. That means resisting against the pull of the band as you release it. If you let the band snap back into position, you're not getting the full toning benefit, and you're risking an injury. Bands also provide resistance as you move in all kinds of directions, whereas dumbbells work best only when you're moving them against gravity.

According to research, resistance bands can increase strength—10 to 30 percent in 6 to 12 weeks of training—as much as other modes of resistance training.[2] A study from the University of Valencia in Spain and Appalachian State University shows that they're just as effective at firming you up and slimming you down. When researchers had 35 women, average age 53, strength-train twice a week using either bands or weight machines, both groups showed similar gains in fat-free mass (such as muscle) and similar losses of body fat.[3]

Compared to weight machines, bands offer more flexibility, as one of our testers found. "When I stopped using the weight machines at my gym, the sore spot on my elbow stopped hurting," said Denise Jennings. "The band allowed me to make adjustments. If I felt pain, I'd move my wrist or elbow half an inch, and I was good. You can't do that with a steel bar."

For the WOW program, you'll be using resistance bands or tubes for your strength training workouts. They provide the versatility to combine strength training with walking and target some muscles more effectively than if you were using dumbbells.

You can choose from flat bands or tubes with handles. It's really a matter of personal preference. Just like dumbbells, bands and tubes come in a variety of resistances that are harder or easier to lift (or stretch). I recommend that you start with two 5-foot or longer bands or tubes—a light to medium resistance one, and a medium to heavy resistance one—because you'll need more resistance for some moves. Plus, as you get stronger, you'll want to continue to challenge yourself. For more information on using resistance bands, see page 81. See Resources on page 320 for more information on where to buy resistance bands.

OPTIONAL GEAR

SPORTS BRA About 60 percent of women experience breast pain during exercise—but many times the right bra can help. When British researchers tested 70 women with cup sizes ranging from A to F, they found that encapsulation-style bras, which have separate molded cups, reduced pain the most. The key is that they stop motion in all directions—not just up and down—for better support and more comfort.[4] Other sought-after comfort factors are wicking and compression fabrics, as well as front-adjustable straps for easy reach. For D+ sizes, look for extra back support from wide straps—not from something that will squeeze, pinch, or bind you like a corset. (Remember, you don't want an exercise bra that restricts your breathing!)

HOW TO BUY Try on several styles, jogging or marching in place to see how they perform when you're moving. Look for one that is formfitting and supportive, but doesn't squeeze or pinch. See Resources on page 320 for more information on where to find sports bras.

HYDRATION PACK It's important to stay hydrated, but carrying a water bottle in one hand can create muscle and motion imbalances that slow you down and possibly contribute to aches and pains. That's why a waistpack or backpack is essential if you're carrying water. You can find a variety of models and sizes at sporting goods stores—everything from a simple waistpack for a single water bottle to carriers that hold multiple bottles to backpacks with water bladders for hands-free sipping. Many styles have room for keys, a cell phone, your ID, and even snacks for longer walks.

HOW TO BUY Before you choose, try on a few different brands and styles—with full water bottles, if possible—and walk around the store to see which one feels the most comfortable. See Resources on page 320 for more information on where to find hydration packs.

OPTIONAL
GEAR

>> Sports bra ($15–$60)

>> Hydration pack ($15–$150)

>> Heart rate monitor ($25–$300)

>> GPS (global positioning system) ($80–$500)

>> Pedometer ($20–$100)

HEART RATE MONITOR While purely optional, these watches with chest straps keep tabs on your heart rate throughout your workout without your having to stop and check your pulse. Heart rate monitors are wonderfully useful devices because they teach you to exercise at the right level to maximize your fitness and fat-burning benefits. They can also help you get comfortable with pushing yourself a little harder for the high-intensity intervals and keep you from slacking off too much during the recovery ones.

HOW TO BUY Choose a model that has a chest strap; they tend to be more accurate than the ones without straps and the ones on exercise equipment. The watch-only monitors can also be difficult to use when you're trying to maintain your speed. See Resources on page 320 for more information on where to find heart rate monitors.

GLOBAL POSITIONING SYSTEM (GPS) You can find many watch or cell-phone styles of these little satellite-powered gadgets, which tell you where you are and how far and how fast you are going—no more driving your walking route to clock your mileage. Depending on the device, you can get many other facts, too, including the time, the temperature, even the number of calories you've burned.

HOW TO BUY Once you find a style you like, take it for a test-walk to see how it feels while you're in motion. Something too clunky or uncomfortable may end up getting left at home in the junk drawer. See Resources on page 320 for more information on where to find a GPS.

PEDOMETER This little gadget can be a powerful motivator. In one study, pedometer-wearers racked up nearly 2,500 more steps a day compared

A WORD ABOUT WATER

MORE THAN 50 PERCENT of your entire body is made up of water. Some parts have even more: Your brain, for example, is 70 percent water, and your muscles, 75 percent. So as you can see, water is absolutely essential for a properly functioning body. But when you work out, you sweat, which causes you to lose fluids. That's why it's particularly important to make sure that you're drinking enough before, during, and after your workouts.

As you'll see, the WOW diet guidelines in Chapter 7 recommend drinking at least five 8-ounce glasses of water a day, in addition to other fluids. If you drink less than that, it can make exercise feel harder, and it may even slow your metabolism.

To make sure that you're properly hydrated for your walks, drink one or two of those glasses 1 to 2 hours before your workout. Then either carry water with you (in a waistpack or backpack, not in your hand) or make sure that you can get water along your route, and sip every 15 to 20 minutes. Replenish with another 8 ounces at the end of your walk. (You may need more in hot weather.)

with when they weren't tracking their steps.[5] That's equivalent to walking almost 1¼ extra miles a day.

While you can monitor all of your steps, the best use of a pedometer for the WOW program is to wear it when you're not doing the workouts. I know it sounds counterintuitive, but one of the biggest mistakes beginning exercisers make is to decrease the amount of activity they do throughout the rest of the day, such as getting up from their desks or couches more often, taking the stairs, or parking far away from their destination. This reduction in activity can be enough to slow or even stall your weight loss.

To prevent this from happening, record your daily step counts on 3 or 4 days before you begin the program. Then calculate your average daily step count by adding up your daily totals and dividing by the number of days tracked. Once you start the program, wear your pedometer whenever you're not doing a WOW workout to make sure that you're maintaining your preprogram activity level. If you aren't, your fat-burning ability will decline. For instance, if you normally log 5,000 steps a day but skip half of them on the days when you walk, it could slow your weight loss by up to 50 percent—even though you're exercising.

HOW TO BUY For the WOW program, a simple step-counting pedometer is all you need. However, there are now a variety of styles of pedometers to choose from—everything from the traditional clip-on-your-waistband style to superslim ones that slide in your pocket to ones you can toss in your purse or wear around your neck. Consider your lifestyle and the types of clothes you wear to decide which one will work best for you. If you're into über-gadgets, you can find pedometers with a watch, a timer, a calorie counter, and/or the ability to download and graph your steps. Just be sure to try them out to make sure you can easily operate your device while walking. See Resources on page 320 for more information on where to find pedometers or calorie-burn devices that also track your activity level.

WHAT TO WEAR

WHILE THE ONLY ESSENTIAL PIECES of equipment for walking are a good pair of sneakers and socks, outfitting yourself with a few key pieces, along with season-specific clothing, will make walking more enjoyable, so you'll be more likely to stick with your workouts year-round.

Rain Gear

With today's high-tech, breathable, waterproof fabrics, you can keep walking even when it's wet outside. A good waterproof (such as Gore-Tex) jacket and pants will help you stay dry. Also:

- **GET A BRIM** Look for a jacket with a brim on the hood, or wear a hat with a brim to keep the rain out of your eyes.
- **RAMP UP YOUR SHOES** If you live in a climate that gets a fair amount of rain, you may want to invest in a pair of waterproof shoes. They often have a heavier, more rugged tread that can help you navigate slippery terrain gracefully.
- **RAINPROOF YOUR SHOES** For occasional showers, you can enhance the water resistance of your shoes by treating them with a waterproofing shoe spray, available in most shoe stores.

Hot Weather Gear

When the temperature rises, it's best to wear light-colored, loose-fitting breathable fabrics, such as Dri-Fit or CoolMax. Avoid cotton, which tends to get soggy. (Trust me: Once you try wicking fabrics, you'll never go back.)

- **CHOOSE CLOTHES WITH COVERAGE** While you'll want to wear the bare minimum when it's sweaty weather, you still should protect yourself from the sun's skin-damaging rays. Look for athletic apparel that comes with an SPF (or UPF, ultraviolet protection factor) rating of 30 or higher. They are available at many sporting goods stores, or search "sun-protective clothing" online. (And don't forget the sunscreen on exposed body parts.)
- **SWITCH SHOES** For warm-weather workouts, you need lightweight, ventilated walking shoes and socks that wick away sweat. Mesh is cooler than leather and dries faster when your feet sweat. You might also get an extra pair of shoes and alternate between them every other day so that each pair has a chance to dry out completely. This helps to prevent fungal infections, blisters, and smelly feet.
- **WEAR A HAT AND SUNGLASSES** Besides the obvious protection from UV rays, these two sun-blocking items can ensure that you maintain good walking posture. A common response to sun shining in your eyes is to look down at the ground in front of you, which is one of the most common walking mistakes. It puts pressure on your neck and upper back—and slows you down.

Night Gear

It takes more than just a white shirt or a few reflective strips to be noticed at night. A driver going 50 MPH needs nearly 300 feet to see you, react, and get his vehicle to come to a complete stop on dry pavement. If you're wearing a white T-shirt, he won't spot you until he's 224 feet away. Reflective wear makes you four times more visible.[7] (The key is to illuminate yourself from head to toe. The more of your body shape that drivers can see, the more quickly they will recognize you.

- **WEAR A BRIGHT HAT OR HEADBAND** This ensures that your highest point is visible.
- **FIND A REFLECTIVE JACKET OR TOP** Look for ones with reflective material on at least two of these key areas: waist, shoulders, and arms.
- **SLIP ON A VEST** It will turn any top or jacket into a visible shield. The more reflective strips, the better—especially around the waist and shoulders.
- **MAKE SURE THAT YOUR SHOES AND GLOVES ARE VISIBLE, TOO** Drivers will see you sooner when the body parts that you move the most—your hands and feet—are illuminated. See Resources on page 320 for more information on where to find reflective gear.

Cold Weather Gear

For wintertime walking, you want to dress in layers. That way you can easily take some clothes off as you warm up and then put them back on as you cool down. And thanks to high-tech synthetic fabrics like CoolMax, you won't look or feel bulky. Synthetic materials also do a better job of keeping you warm and dry than either wool or cotton. You'll be amazed at how comfortable you can be, even at extremely cold temperatures.

- **START WITH A LIGHT INNER LAYER** The one closest to your skin should be made of a light synthetic fabric such as CoolMax or polypropylene to wick sweat away from your body so you stay dry.
- **ADD A MIDDLE, OR INSULATING, LAYER (OR TWO)** A sweater, a sweatshirt, or a pullover made of a lightweight fleece fabric such as Polartec will keep you warm.
- **CHOOSE A PROTECTIVE OUTER LAYER** A top layer of waterproof, breathable fabric such as Gore-Tex will buffer you from the elements and let sweat escape. You want a garment that protects you from wind and cold, but it should also be breathable, meaning that it allows water vapor to escape without actually letting water in.
- **WEAR A PAIR OF WATERPROOF SHOES OR BOOTS** For icy conditions, the athletic strap-on cleats available at many sporting goods stores—such as STABIL-icers and Yaktrax—can give you more traction. See Resources on page 320 for more information on where to find strap-on cleats.

- **DON'T FORGET A HAT, GLOVES, AND SUNSCREEN!** You can still get sunburned in the winter, especially when sunlight is reflecting off snow.

WHERE TO WALK

YOU CAN DO THE WOW WALKING WORKOUTS INDOORS OR OUT, depending on the weather or simply your mood or preference. Here are some things to consider when choosing the locations of your walks.

Outdoors

Research has actually shown that you may push yourself harder without even noticing it when you exercise outside. And in addition to the scenery being more appealing, you'll boost your mood and your brainpower more than if you work out indoors. The great outdoors also offers lots of options for walking—parks, city sidewalks, country roads, and athletic tracks, to name just a few. Some locations will be better than others for certain types of walking. Here are some things to keep in mind when planning your routes.

- **FOR SHORT WORKOUTS** If you have a half hour or less, stay close to home or work. Increasing your total workout time by driving to and from your walking location may make it harder to stick with your workouts. Save farther-away parks and trails for longer walks so you're walking more than you're driving.
- **FOR INTERVAL TRAINING** Try to choose routes with fewer interruptions. Routes with lots of hills, traffic, and stoplights can make interval training difficult. Because hills increase your intensity, you might not get adequate rest if you're climbing one during a recovery interval. And stopping for traffic or a light during a vigorous interval can be frustrating and counterproductive.
- **FOR SPEED WALKS** Athletic tracks are ideal when you need to walk a specific distance. And the flat, smooth surface without any traffic makes them a great choice for interval workouts. However, going around in circles can get boring, so it's best to use these facilities for shorter workouts.

Wherever you choose to walk, use a little common sense to avoid dangerous situations. Here are some reminders and additional steps (pun intended) that you can take to stay out of harm's way.

- **AVOID RUSH HOUR** You'll reduce your risk of injury and exposure to carbon monoxide.
- **FACE TRAFFIC** If you walk in an area without sidewalks, stay on the left side of the road, so you can see oncoming traffic. The exception: as you come to the top of a hill or a curve. In these spots, approaching cars aren't able to see you from a distance. You'll be more visible if you temporarily switch sides of the street. If you're on a two-lane road and cars are coming both ways, step onto the shoulder or off the road until they pass.
- **LOWER THE VOLUME** If you listen to music or a podcast, keep it low or use only one earbud, so you can hear if a car or another person is approaching. Skip the tunes altogether if you're in an unfamiliar area.
- **BE BRIGHT** Any time of the day, wear white or bright-colored clothes to stand out against whatever environment you're walking in. If you're out at night, dusk, or dawn, wear reflective gear (see page 45).
- **INFORM, AND BE INFORMED** Let someone know where you're going and when you'll be back; know where you are and where you are going; and carry ID and a cell phone.

WOW WINNER Debbie Adie 47, Lost 15 pounds and 11 inches overall

"I have more energy."

In an inconvenient twist, Debbie Adie went from being a stay-at-home mom to a full-time working mom the same day she started the WOW program. But thanks to a little planning, Debbie was able to overcome her biggest obstacles, such as fitting everything in, and succeed at both. "After work, I'd walk in the house, change my clothes, and walk out again for my workout," she said. "I knew if I sat down, I'd never get up to exercise." To avoid temptations like chicken fingers and French fries, she packed her own lunches.

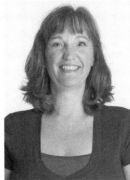

Within 2 weeks, Debbie noticed that she had more energy, felt stronger, and was happier. "I was sure I'd be completely overwhelmed. But instead I felt great—and then my clothes started getting looser. One day, my husband said, 'That's the best that suit's ever looked on you!' That felt so good," she said. And to Debbie's surprise, her success was influencing some of her co-workers to adopt similar healthy habits.

"Even though I wasn't looking forward to going back to work and changing my diet and exercise habits, and it was scary, everything turned out fine," Debbie said. "Now I work full-time, exercise 6 days a week, and manage my family—and I have more energy than when I was unemployed and sedentary." She even trained for and walked a half marathon (13.1 miles)!

- **GET A BUDDY** If you're walking after dark or you feel less than safe, it's an especially good idea to have someone else with you.
- **WARD OFF DOGS** If there are a lot of unfamiliar canines along your route or you're walking in an unfamiliar area, carry pepper spray or a noisemaker. We like the Dazer II; it lets out high-frequency bursts of noise that can't be heard by humans but are extremely annoying (but harmless) to dogs. See Resources on page 320 for more information on where to find the Dazer II.

Indoors

Your best bet for doing the WOW program inside is on a treadmill because of the versatility it offers. If you have one at home, you can work out anytime and in any kind of weather without worrying about your safety. Position it in front of a TV if you need an extra incentive to get moving. On the downside, treadmills are costly and you need to have the space for one.

Doing the WOW Interval Walks on a treadmill will take a little modifying. Since there's a lag when the treadmill speeds up and slows down, consider adding an extra 5 to 10 seconds to the speed bursts to ensure that you're hitting your maximum pace for the recommended time. For instance, if it takes 5 seconds for your treadmill to hit the 4.8 MPH pace you use for a 15-second high-intensity bout, that means you're really only getting a 10-second speed burst unless you lengthen the interval.

Here are some tips to help you feel more comfortable on a treadmill and maximize your workout.

- **START SMOOTHLY** Plant your feet alongside the belt and hold on to the handrails. Wait until the speed is at least 1 MPH before you step on the belt (unless your directions tell you otherwise). As soon as you're comfortable, let go of the handrails to ensure good walking form. Gradually increase your speed.
- **DO INTERVALS** Because treadmills can't switch speeds as quickly as your body, increase your fast intervals by 3 to 5 seconds to be sure that you're at top speed for the recommended amount of time. This isn't as critical for the recovery bouts, since they're longer and decreasing your pace a bit more slowly won't affect your workout. Another option on the treadmill is to use the incline for your intervals. It adds some variety and is a great way to firm up your legs and butt.

- **FINISH STRONG** After you've cooled down at a slower pace, continue to reduce the speed until the belt stops. When you get off, you may feel a bit unstable, so don't move too quickly.

If you don't have access to a treadmill, other options are to walk at a mall, a convention center, an office building, or even in your own home. (Yes, some of our testers did this to get in their workouts when the weather wasn't cooperating.) These are probably best reserved for when you really need an indoor alternative. Unless it's quite large, strolling around the same space can quickly get boring. And if there are a lot of people around, it can make it difficult to maintain your pace. But if it's the only way to get a workout in, go for it! (I've already stepped up and down off of a low step stool while watching TV.) It's better than nothing.

ON THE TREADMILL

IF YOU LIVE IN AN AREA that gets lots of rain, ice, or snow or has more than a few days a year with high humidity and a heat warning, a treadmill can be a good investment in your health. In a University of Pittsburgh study, women who had a treadmill at home lost twice as much weight as those without one.[9]

You can expect to spend at least $1,000 for a decent treadmill, so make sure that you're comfortable on the model you choose. That means putting on your walking shoes and spending no less than 5 minutes on several brands, testing out the speed controls, inclines, and any other features. Here are some key things to look for:

- **Motor** Look for at least 1.5 continuous horsepower for a smoother performance; you don't need to worry about peak horsepower. The motor casing should be far enough forward that you're not hitting it when you walk. Also, pay attention to how loud the motor is, especially if you want to watch TV while you walk or if you have young children who might be disturbed if you use the treadmill after their bedtimes.
- **Belt** It should be at least 18 inches wide and long enough that you can stride comfortably without feeling like you're going to fall off.
- **Deck** Cushioned ones reduce the impact on joints. Look for ample space on either side of the belt for sure-footing when getting on and off the treadmill.
- **Control panel** Check for large, easy-to-read displays and controls that change smoothly without sticking or jumping ahead.
- **Handrails** They should be easy to grab, if needed, but you don't want them to hinder your arm swing.
- **Size** Make sure that you have enough space at home for the model you're considering. Put the treadmill in a room that you'll enjoy working out in; otherwise, you'll be less likely to use it.
- **Additional features** One I recommend is a cup holder, so it's easy for you to stay hydrated while you work out. A fan is also a nice option, but don't choose a treadmill for that reason alone.

From Bookworm to Bicyclist

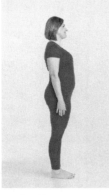

BEFORE

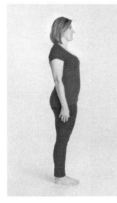

AFTER

THANKS TO DINING OUT more after she got married, 38-year-old Stacy Shillinger went from a slim size 6 to a size 16 over the past 5 years. But after just 8 weeks on the WOW program, she shrunk 2 sizes and is still losing, thanks to finding an exercise plan that she could live with.

"I've never stuck to an exercise program in my life," said Stacy, who recently left her marketing job to pursue a career in health care. "I knew I needed to walk the walk. How do I tell someone else to get moving and lose weight if I'm not doing either?"

The only athletic activity she'd ever done with any consistency was some golfing with her husband. "I'd rather be reading a book on the porch," she proclaimed. "I hate to sweat, and my asthma acts up when I work out. But I knew I needed to do something."

By the 4th week of the program, she was fitting back into some of her skinny clothes, and this self-proclaimed nonsporty type was zipping around on a 45-minute hilly bike ride with her husband—in addition to her regular workouts. "I never would have had the confidence to go before," she said.

Stacy credits her success to the simplicity of the program. While she's still not leaping out of bed in the morning to work out, she does feel as if she's established a habit that will last her a lifetime. "Now I understand that I *will* feel better afterward—and often during—my walks," explained Stacy. And the sweat? Well, she still doesn't love it, but she realizes that the results are worth it.

And she herself will be proof to her future patients that exercise pays off: Her cholesterol has dropped 20 percent from a dangerous 216 to a healthier 184; her lung capacity has increased and her asthma symptoms have decreased; her energy level is higher; and her moods have improved to the point that she's been able to cut back on her antidepressant medication.

"For the first time in my life, I'm a real exerciser, and I'm the role model I want to be," exclaimed the new, athletic Stacy, who's proud of wearing through her first pair of sneakers ever. Next up: She's training to walk/run her first 5-K.

P.S. *Three months after the official end of the program, Stacy recorded an additional 2 1/2-pound weight loss and shaved another 2 inches off her figure, for a grand total of 10 3/4 pounds and 11 1/2 inches lost in 5 months.*

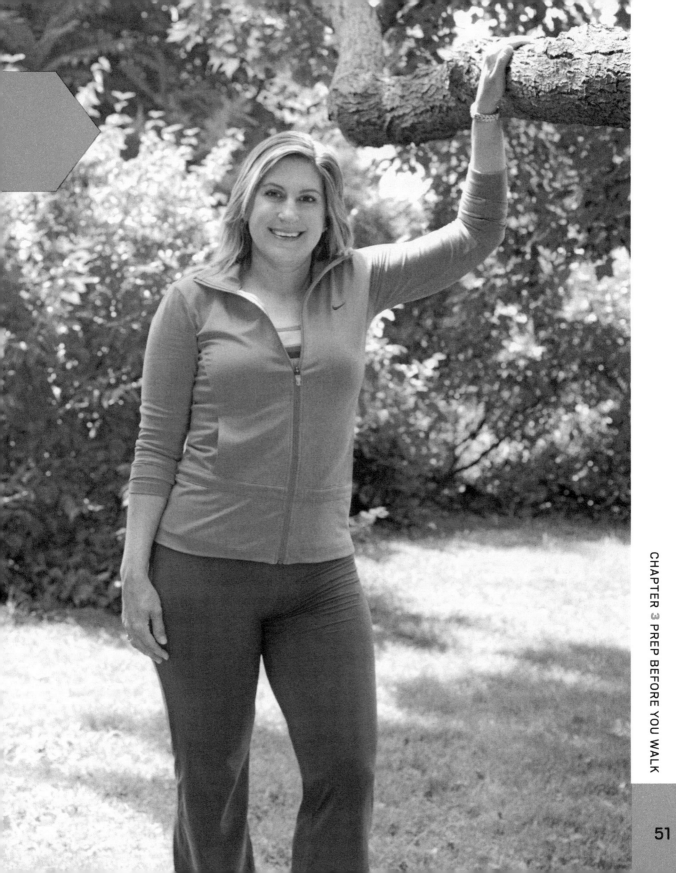

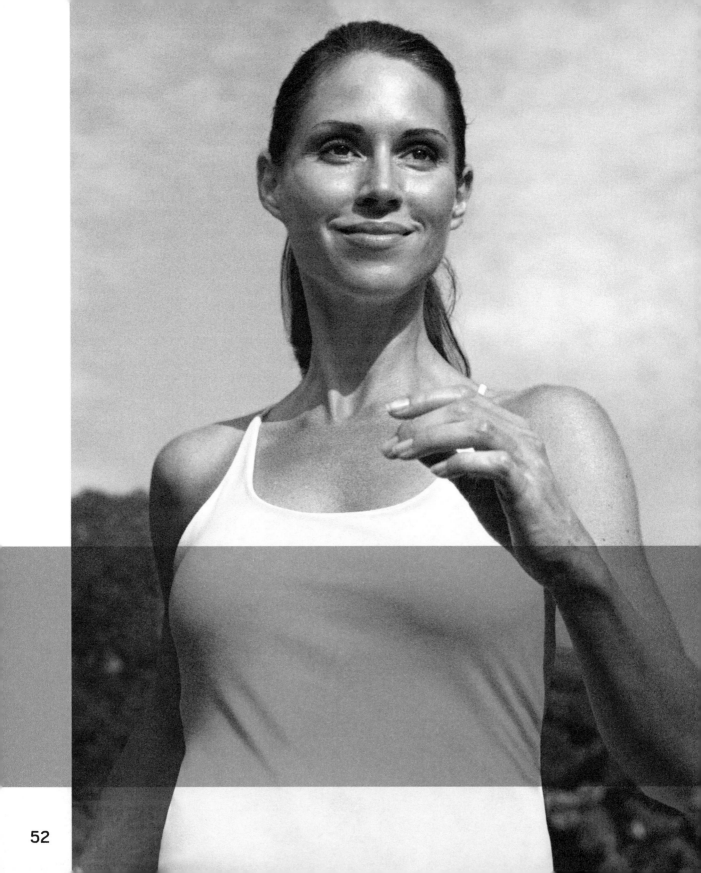

4

GET UP TO
Speed

A KEY TO GREAT RESULTS on the WOW program is fast walking. That doesn't mean you have to clock a 12-minute mile (or 5 cf^), though some people may walk that fast or even faster. Some will move a little slower; others, slower still. It's all relative—to your cardiovascular fitness level, flexibility, strength, even your nervous system (that is, how fast your neurons fire to contract your muscles).

Your walking speed can even change from day to day or week to week, depending on how fueled you are, how well you slept the night before, the weather, and especially your menstrual cycle. You know what I'm talking about—those days when you feel so bloated and blah that even if George Clooney (or write in your favorite hunk) was waiting for you around the corner, you couldn't get yourself to walk any faster.

Don't get hung up on a number. Listen to your body and do what's right for you—not what someone else may be doing. The important thing is that you're seeing improvements in your pace over time.

The first step to walking faster is good posture. Once you've established that, you want to add some technique to help you hit your maximum speed. Even when you're just moving at a brisk pace or doing a Toning Walk, this advice is useful because good form and proper technique will protect you against injury, give you a better workout, and make your walks feel easier.

Here are some of the elements that will apply to all your workouts throughout the program.

WORKOUT BASICS

THERE ARE THREE ESSENTIAL STEPS to optimize any type of exercise.

1. Warm-up
2. Cool-down
3. Stretch

Warm-Up

Starting slowly is key to improving your performance and results and reducing your risk of injury. All of the walking routines in the WOW program lead off with a 3- to 5-minute warm-up in which you'll be strolling at an easy pace. This gradual start will raise your heart rate, send blood to your working muscles, ramp up your respiration, increase your body temperature, and boost your calorie burn.

For each degree your body temp goes up, your metabolic rate (your body's calorie-burning engine) rises by about 13 percent. Warming up also increases circulation, bloodflow, and muscle temperature, which improves your range of motion and protects you from injury. It supplies your muscles with extra oxygen, too, so you'll feel more energized.

By giving your body a chance to acclimate to exercise, you'll feel more confident in your ability to complete the workout. You might even push yourself to exercise at a higher intensity.

Note: If you do the strength workouts separately or before a walk, make sure you include a warm-up. See the individual routines for warm-up suggestions.

Cool-Down

Finish all of your walks by gradually slowing your pace to an easy intensity for 2 to 5 minutes. During exercise, blood accumulates in your working muscles. Easing out of your workout, instead of stopping abruptly, prevents the blood from pooling in your legs, which can cause dizziness or nausea. It also helps remove lactate that can build up in muscles, so you'll feel less fatigued. By taking some time to cool down, you'll feel better, and you'll be more likely to look forward to your next workout, since you're finishing your current one on a good note.

Stretch

The best time to stretch to increase flexibility is after your cool-down, when your muscles and joints are their warmest. This will help to counter the decrease in range of motion that occurs as you get older and makes everyday tasks, such as reaching for things on high shelves and bending over to put on your socks, more difficult. The following exercises stretch all of your walking muscles without the hassle of getting down on the ground, so you can easily make them a habit by automatically adding them to the end of your walks, after your cool-down, when your muscles and joints

Q+A

Q: Can I stretch at the beginning of my workout, too?

A: Sure, as long as you do it after your warm-up. When it comes to stretching, the rule is to make sure your muscles are limber and pliable before you stretch. If they aren't, you may be more likely to injure yourself. Stretching before or during your workout can also provide on-the-spot relief for areas that feel tight such as your hips, shins, or thighs. Several of our WOW test panelists found this particularly helpful for shin pain, a common complaint for new walkers (see page 228 for an example of a shin stretch).

Q: I'm more likely to stick with my walks when I do them with someone else. But my neighbor, whom I always walk with, isn't able to go as fast as I am on the intervals. What do you suggest?

A: Try walking at a track, on a looped path, or even around a particular block. Stick together for the warm-up, then go at your own pace for the intervals and join back up for the cool-down. It may take a little practice to get the timing right, or one of you may have to cut across the track or turn around and head in the opposite direction to catch up with the other. Either way, this will allow you to benefit from the camaraderie and still push yourself at your own level.

are still warm and pliable. Think of stretching as the finishing touch to a perfect workout. Hold each stretch for 10 seconds, pause for a second, then repeat two more times for a total of 30 seconds. According to research from San Diego State University, this method stretches muscles as effectively as holding the moves up to four times as long.[2]

Lunge & Reach
(stretches calves, hips, and sides of torso)

Stand with your right foot 2 to 3 feet in front of your left, toes pointing straight ahead. Bend your right knee, keeping your left leg straight and your heel on the ground, stretching your calf and hip. Reach your left arm overhead and toward the right to feel a stretch along your left side. Hold, then switch sides.

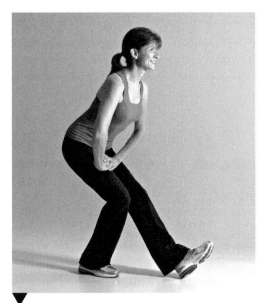

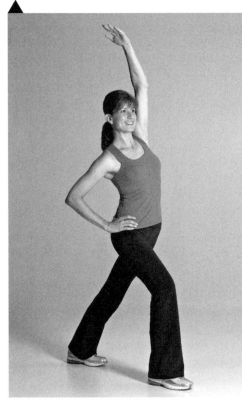

Sit Back
(stretches back and hamstrings)

You can segue from the preceding stretch directly into this one. Stay in the same position, with your left leg in front, but move your right foot forward a few inches. Straighten your left leg, raising your toes off the ground. Place your hands on your right thigh and bend your right knee and hips. Press your left heel into the ground, stick out your butt, and sit back until you feel a stretch in the back of your left leg. Hold, then switch sides.

Bent-Leg Balance
(stretches quads and hips)

Balance on your left leg (hold onto something sturdy for support, such as a tree or the back of a bench, if you need to). Bend your right knee, grasp the top of your foot, and pull your heel upward toward your butt. Keep your right knee pointing toward the ground, and press your right foot against your right hand to feel a stretch in the front of your thigh. Hold, then switch sides.

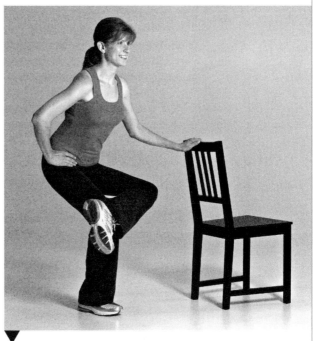

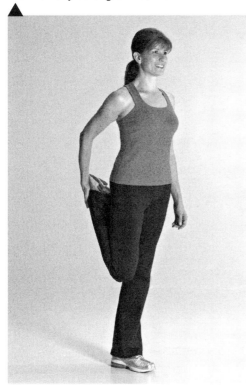

Figure 4
(stretches hips and glutes)

Hold onto something sturdy for balance and rest your left ankle on your right thigh. Place your right hand on your hip and slowly sit back until you feel a stretch in your left hip and glute area. Hold, then switch sides.

FAST-WALKING TECHNIQUES

PERFECTING YOUR WALKING POSTURE and adding some simple technique will help you increase your speed, burn more calories, and firm up more than just your legs.

There are many aspects to walking posture and technique. It might seem a bit overwhelming at first, but don't panic! You don't have to do everything at once. For now, just review the information and try some of the exercises. Then when you begin the 8-week program, you'll focus on just one or two things each week, building as you go along.

Stand Tall

Proper posture doesn't just increase your speed, it also ensures that you'll feel good while you walk. Standing tall helps to prevent aches and pains and makes breathing easier, so you can take in more oxygen to fuel your muscles and boost your energy.

When you have good posture, your skeletal system is doing most of the work to hold you upright, so your muscles can put all of their power into moving you forward. In order for this to happen, your bones need to be stacked properly one on top of the other.

Let's start with your pelvis and hips, since this is the area where all walking actions originate. You want your pelvis in a neutral position, not tucked under

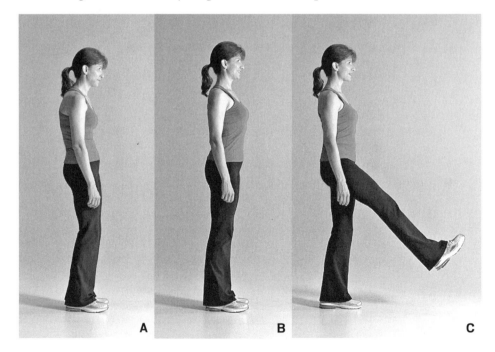

A   B   C

so that your lower back is rounded or tilted forward so that your back is over-arched. To find the right position, tilt your pelvis forward and back a few times in exaggerated motions. Look in a mirror as you do this and notice how your lower body shifts forward when your pelvis is tucked. As you tilt your pelvis forward, your upper body goes forward. The changes are slight, but even these minor misalignments make your muscles work harder to hold you up and can lead to aches and pains when you're walking. Tilt your pelvis a few more times, reducing the range of motion until your pelvis is in about a midpoint, or neutral, position. In this position, your spine forms an S shape, with a slight arch in your lower back.

Working your way down your body, your knees should be directly under your hips and your ankles directly under your knees. As you move up from your pelvis, your shoulders should be directly above your hips and your ears above your shoulders. Stacking your body in this way aligns your skeleton properly so your bones can do their job of supporting you.

To help you get into alignment, imagine a wire attached to the top of your head, gently pulling you upward. Holding your chin level, think of creating a little extra space between the vertebrae in your spine. Lift out of your hips, raising your rib cage. Actually slide your hands from your hips up to your rib cage, lifting and lengthening your torso. This helps to give your legs more room to swing. To get the feel of this, try the exercise below.

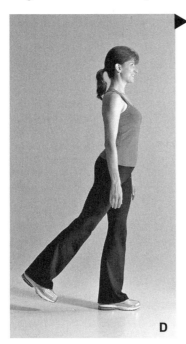

D

▶ Relax into a slouchy posture, letting your upper body sink into your hips (A). Balance on one leg and swing the other leg forward and back. Switch legs. Now stand up tall, lift out of your hips (B), and swing each leg forward (C) and then back (D). You should notice that your leg swings more freely. This simple change can make walking more enjoyable and going faster easier.

Ears in line with shoulders
don't jut head forward

Chin level
don't look down at your feet

Chest lifted
don't collapse forward and round
shoulders

**Shoulders relaxed,
down, and back**
don't pull them up
toward ears

**Hands cupped
loosely** don't
clench fists

Arms bent 90 degrees
don't let them swing down
at your sides

Abs tight
pull them in and up like you're
zipping a snug pair of jeans

Hips under shoulders

Pelvis neutral
don't tuck or overarch back

Knees pointing forward
not in or out to sides

**Lean forward slightly
from ankles**

**Feet parallel
to each other**
not pointing
in or out

60

Shirt Pull

To help you maintain good posture during your walks, practice this Shirt Pull exercise that I learned from Suki Munsell, PhD, a movement therapist and creator of Dynamic Walking, a program designed to restore your body's natural, balanced posture. Aim to do it about every 10 minutes during a walk (after a speed interval is always a good time), or whenever you feel as if you're slouching or you notice any achiness.

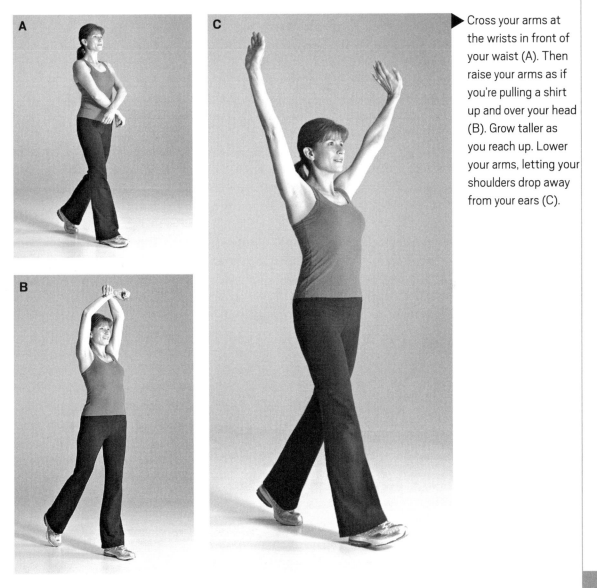

Cross your arms at the wrists in front of your waist (A). Then raise your arms as if you're pulling a shirt up and over your head (B). Grow taller as you reach up. Lower your arms, letting your shoulders drop away from your ears (C).

Bend Your Arms

You wouldn't run with your arms down at your sides, so why walk with them in that position? The easiest way to speed up is to simply bend your arms. These limbs act as pendulums, and the shorter the pendulum, the faster it swings. As your arms swing more rapidly, your feet automatically want to keep up.

Get in front of a mirror and practice. Start by bending your elbows 90 degrees. Imagine that your arms are in casts and you have to maintain this bent-arm position throughout your walk. Now swing your arms forward and back. The action should be coming from your shoulders, not your elbows. Keep your shoulders relaxed and down; don't pull them up toward your ears.

Turn sideways and look in the mirror. Your hands should be making an arc from your chest to your hips. Keep your elbows in and your hands close to your body so they almost skim your sides. On the backswing, bring your hand all the way back to just past your hip. As your hand comes forward, let it swing to about chest height. Imagine a shelf extending out from your chest and keep your hands from hitting it.

Face forward and make sure that your hands aren't passing the midline of your body. Swinging your arms across your body and letting your elbows flail out to the sides slows you down (not to mention that it makes you look like a chicken flapping its wings). Imagine you have a headlight on the front of each hand. You want to keep that light shining straight ahead to light your way. If you swing too high, it will be shining up into the sky. If you're letting your wrists drop or you're straightening your arms on the backswing, the light will be shining toward the ground. The more streamlined and forward focused your body and energy are, the faster you'll go.

To make sure that you're keeping your arms bent, try this exercise. Put your

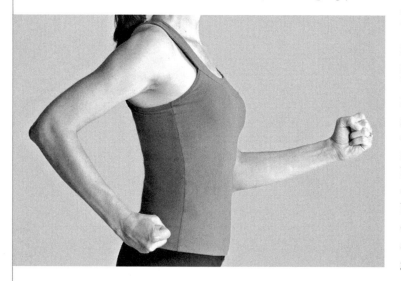

exercise band around your neck, bend your arms into position, grab an end with each hand, and go. If you're keeping your elbows bent, the band should not be sliding side to side on your neck (and getting tangled in your hair—ouch!). If it is, focus on swinging from your shoulders and not bending and extending your elbows with each swing. Remember, you have a light in the front of each hand; you want to keep it shining forward, not down at the ground.

Roll Heel to Toe

When you walk, your feet act kind of like the rockers on a rocking chair, rolling from heel to toe with every step. To some extent, you do this without even thinking about it. But now that you're focusing on increasing speed, you need to pay a little more attention to the heel-to-toe movement.

When your foot comes forward, you want to land on your heel and lift your toes toward your shin. This allows a greater range of motion in your ankle joint for more power. I'll warn you now: You're going to feel this in your shins. But that's not a bad thing; it's actually a sign that you're doing it right. Sit in a chair and try it. Pull your toes toward your shins, lifting your entire foot off the floor except for your heel, like you're tapping your toes. Keep tapping, and you'll feel your shins working, I promise.

Most of the women in our test panel experienced shin pain during the first 2 weeks of the WOW program, so be prepared. But know, too, that the pain will go away as your shins get stronger.

To ease some of the soreness in the meantime, Toronto-based walking coach Lee Scott taught me this trick: Concentrate on squeezing your glutes as you plant your heel. Activating these powerful muscles may take some of the

WOW WINNER Kristina Donatelli 37, Lost 7¼ pounds and 6½ inches overall

"Challenging myself kept me motivated"

Kristina Donatelli set a goal at the beginning of the WOW program, just as she had during previous weight loss attempts. But this time it had nothing to do with the scale. After completing our 1-mile walk test in 16 minutes, 24 seconds, she said, "I want to do this in 15 minutes by the end of the program." Along the way, Kristina discovered the amazing power of setting the right goal.

Instead of turning to the bathroom scale for motivation, this full-time working mother of two focused on her speed. She celebrated the small improvements—every tenth of a mile increase for intervals—and the big ones—walking a 3½-mile route 10 minutes faster than when she started. "It felt good pushing myself, and I

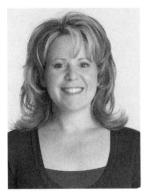

have more energy and confidence than I've had in a long time," she reported, adding that for the first time she was actually looking for more opportunities to be active, like cutting the grass for her husband, taking her kids for more walks, and doing extra housework. At Week 5, she beat her goal and walked a mile in less than 15 minutes. She then set a new goal: doing it in less than 14 minutes.

While she wasn't focusing on the scale, she did have to weigh herself for the program and was often feeling frustrated by the slow improvements despite how wonderful she felt. Finally, at Week 6, Kristina was rewarded for her efforts: She was able to slip back into her size 10 pants, and a snug-fitting shirt now had some extra room. At the end of the 8-week WOW program, Kristina had lost 14% of her body fat—and she smashed her goal, finishing the 1-mile walk test in just 13 minutes and 37 seconds!

pressure off your shins—or, at the very least, it helps direct your attention away from your achy shins. (For more tips to help your shins, see page 228.)

Now don't overthink this next part. It happens naturally, but I want you to be aware of it. As your foot lands, your weight shifts from the outside of your heel, up along your foot, across your toes, and finally onto your big toe as you roll forward and then push off. It happens so quickly that it's almost imperceptible, but if you pay attention, you'll notice it.

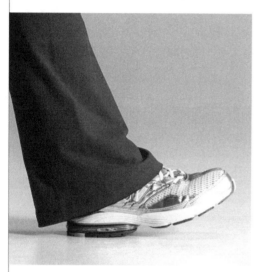

Throughout the landing (remember toes up) and rolling, keep your leg straight but not locked. Bending your knee will cause you to bounce up and down and slow your forward motion. And avoid taking big steps, which make the heel-to-toe motion more difficult. If you notice your upper body swaying, make sure your feet are positioned under your pelvis. They should be as parallel as possible and close together, no more than 4 inches apart. Walking with your feet spread wide will cause your upper body to sway from side to side, which slows you down. In fact, the faster you walk, the closer your feet will come to landing one directly in front of the other, along an imaginary line directly beneath your body. So, a slower walk has wider footfalls, while a faster walk has a narrower stride. (This is due to the natural increase in rotation of the pelvis at higher speeds.)

10 TIPS FOR TACKLING HILLS

OF COURSE, GOOD WALKING posture applies—head up, arms bent—but here are some specific tips that will have you powering up hills in no time!

GOING UP

- Don't bend at your waist and lean into the hill; stay as upright as possible. A slight lean from your ankles is fine.
- Take shorter steps.
- Land on your heel with your toes lifted, not flat-footed.
- Maintain your posture.
- Make sure your back leg is extended as you push off with your toes.

GOING DOWN

- Don't lean back.
- Keep your feet under you.
- Take short, quick steps, landing on your heel and rolling through to your toes.
- Don't let your feet pound into the ground; stay light on your feet.
- Soften your knees just a bit to absorb impact, but not so much that you're bouncing.

Push Off Strong

This is the ending of the heel-to-toe action that powers you forward. As you roll onto your toes, your upper body is passing over top of your front foot, so that leg moves behind you. As you push off of the ground with your toes, you propel yourself forward. You can really feel this action when you're walking up a hill.

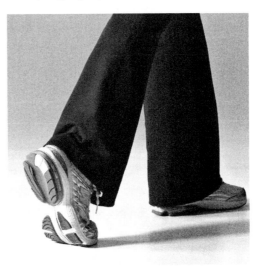

The key to getting maximum acceleration from your push-off is to wait until your foot is behind you. You should have a longer stride behind you than in front of you. If your foot is too close or under your pelvis, you're more likely to push your body up instead of forward, which results in a bouncy walk.

I learned a great tip from Mark Fenton, former coach of the U.S. Racewalking Team and coauthor of *Pedometer Walking*, to ensure a strong push-off: Think of lifting your heel so that someone who is walking behind you can see the sole of your shoe.

Shorter, Quicker Steps

One of the most common mistakes people make when they try to walk faster is that they take steps that are too long. While your stride does lengthen as you pick up the pace, most of the increase should come from keeping your back foot on the ground longer, not taking bigger steps with your front foot. The real secret to speed is taking more, quicker steps, not excessively long ones.

This is why it's possible for someone with shorter legs to walk faster than someone with longer ones. At the 2008 Olympics in Beijing, 5'3" Russian Olga Kaniskina left 5'8" American Joanne Dow in the dust to take the gold and set a new Olympic record in the racewalking 20-K. Dow finished 31st. In fact, long legs can be a disadvantage because the longer they are, the more time and energy it takes to swing them forward, which slows turnover or step count.

No matter how tall you are, taking strides that are too long also causes your foot to act as a brake, which—in addition to slowing you down—may increase your risk of injury. And the farther apart your feet are, the harder your legs have to work, and the more quickly they'll fatigue.

Think of it this way: There are two parts of the walking stride, single support and double support. Single support is when one leg is supporting your body weight as the other leg swings forward and your body passes above the basically upright supporting leg. Double support is when your two legs form a triangle supporting your body, one leg extended in front, contacting the ground with your heel, the other behind you on your toes.

For the most efficient stride, don't think of the double support phase as a balanced triangle, with the front leg reaching forward just as far as the back leg is extended behind you. Instead, think short as you step forward, keeping that side of the triangle shorter and your stride more underneath and behind your body. Overreaching as you step forward means that you have to expend more energy to rise up onto that leg for the single support phase, slowing you down like a brake would. It can also increase injury risk by requiring the hamstrings and glutes of your forward leg to absorb more impact and do more work.

Likewise, if your stride length is too short, you'll notice that you're bouncing up and down as you walk. Focus on keeping your forward steps short and keeping your back foot on the ground as long as possible to extend that portion of your stride. Try overstriding and understriding for a few minutes, and adjust your stride to find the length that feels natural for you.

A great way to push yourself to take quicker, shorter steps is to count your number of steps for a particular interval and then work on beating it over the course of the WOW program. Or use a pedometer to track your steps for an entire workout. You can also estimate your walking speed by counting steps; for instructions, see page 68.

Here's another exercise to find your perfect stride length:

Stand with your feet parallel and walking distance (about 4 inches) apart. Balance on one foot and lift the opposite knee in front of you to hip level so your lower leg is perpendicular to the ground. Now plant the heel of your raised leg straight down in front of you (your body weight will shift forward as you do this). That's your natural stride length at a moderate speed.

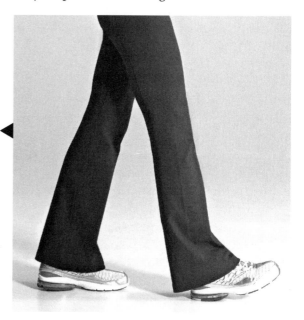

INTENSITY LEVELS

Here are the effort levels that you'll be aiming for throughout the various WOW walking routines. They are based on a 1 to 10 scale, with 1 being equivalent to sitting and 10 being as if you're sprinting for your life.

Intensity levels are very subjective and are affected by your current fitness level. Beginners may not have to go as fast to hit the appropriate intensity but will still get similar benefits. As you become more fit, you may find that you need to speed up to be working out at that same level. That's a good sign because it means that your heart and body are becoming better conditioned. Most important, listen to your body and walk at a pace that's appropriate for you.

ACTIVITY	INTENSITY LEVEL	PACE	HOW IT FEELS	SPEED ESTIMATES**
INACTIVE	1–2	Barely moving	Easy; you could do it for a very long period of time	<2.0 be]
EASY*	3–5	Leisurely stroll	Light effort, rhythmic breathing; you can sing	2.0–3.5 be]
MODERATE	5–6	Purposeful	Some effort, breathing somewhat hard; you can talk in full sentences	3.0–4.0 be]
BRISK	6–7	In a bit of a hurry	Hard effort, slightly breathless; you can only talk in brief phrases	3.5–4.5 be]
FAST	7–8	Late for an appointment	Very hard effort, breathless; yes/no responses are all you can manage	4.0–5.0 be]
VERY FAST	8–9	Trying to catch a bus as it's pulling away	Maximum effort; no breath for any talking	4.5–5.5 be]
SPRINT	10	Racing for your life	All-out effort; you can't maintain it for more than a minute	5.5+ be]

*Use this for warm-up and cool-down.
**These are only rough estimates, with the midpoint based on someone who is moderately fit. If you're just starting out, you'll probably hit each intensity level at a slower pace, closer to the lower end of the speed range or even below. If you've been walking regularly and you're very fit, you may have to walk faster, aiming toward the higher end of the range, to achieve the recommended effort levels. Pay attention to your body and do what feels right to you.

HOW EXERCISE SHOULD FEEL

Any time you're doing something that's out of your comfort zone—which is the intention of exercise in order for your body to change—it's going to be uncomfortable. That's normal, but some symptoms aren't normal and shouldn't be ignored. Here are guidelines for how exercise should feel, what's abnormal, and what to do if you experience any abnormal symptoms.

NORMAL	ABNORMAL	WHAT TO DO
Heart pumping rhythmically harder and faster	Chest pain, pressure, or tightness; skipped heartbeats or palpitations	Stop immediately and call 911.
Breathing faster and harder	Difficult or uncomfortable breathing that doesn't improve when you decrease your intensity or stop exercising	Stop immediately and call your doctor.
Muscle soreness or burning	Sharp, shooting pain or pain in a joint	Stop and rest and ice the area. If pain persists, call your doctor.
General fatigue	Light-headedness or dizziness	Stop immediately.

HOW FAST ARE YOU WALKING?

Count the number of steps you take in 1 minute. (If it's easier, you can count for a 30-second interval and multiply by 2 or count for 15 seconds and multiply by 4. Either calculation will determine your total number of steps per minute.) Next, find your height in the left-most column of the chart below. Move across the chart to the right until you find the number closest to your 1-minute step count. Follow that column to the top, and you'll see how fast you're walking. If you are between the heights in the chart, take the average of the speeds for the heights above and below yours.

MINUTES PER MILE	24 MIN	20 MIN	17 MIN	15 MIN	13 MIN
SPEED	2.5 MPH	3 MPH	3.5 MPH	4 MPH	4.6 MPH
HEIGHT					
5'0"	109	119	128	137	148
5'2"	108	117	127	135	146
5'4"	107	116	125	133	144
5'6"	106	114	123	131	142
5'8"	105	113	122	129	140

Source: W. W. K. Hoeger, "One-mile step count at walking and running speeds," American College of Sports Medicine's Health & Fitness Journal 12 (January/February 2008): 14–19.

Recruit Your Backside Muscles

Surprisingly, a secret to moving forward faster is to focus backward or on what's behind you. I'm talking about your back and butt muscles. Your glutes are the most powerful muscles in your body, so the more you use them, the faster you can go—and the firmer you'll look from behind. Your back muscles are also large and can power up your arm swing, which, as I mentioned earlier, can get your feet moving quicker.

Here's an even more enticing reason to get those arms in on the act: Several of our test panelists noted that during the WOW program, they lost back fat—you know, those rolls around your bra straps. Now we all know that it isn't possible to spot reduce—and they didn't; they slimmed down all over—but I think powering up their arm swing helped by firming up that problem area.

Start with your glutes, or butt muscles. Put one hand on your butt and pull that leg back. Feel the muscle contract. That's a lot of butt power! Take advantage of it. Every time your heel strikes the ground in front of you, squeeze your glutes. (Remember, this may help ease any shin pain, too.) Now think of using those butt muscles to pull your body forward over your front leg. Walking isn't just about propelling your body forward by pushing off with your back foot. By using both legs, the back one to push you forward and the front one to pull you forward, you'll have a faster, more powerful stride.

If you have a hard time feeling your butt contract as you walk, stand still and practice. Squeeze both cheeks together, pulling them forward and up. Then try them separately.

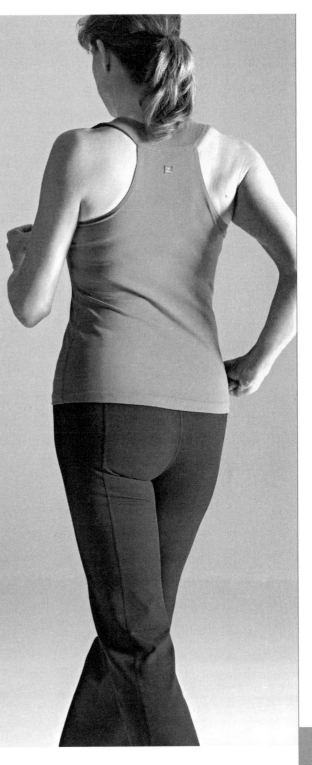

For your back, stand or sit tall and squeeze your shoulder blades together. These are the muscles you want to activate to power up your arm swing. When you're walking, imagine that you're pulling on a rope as you swing your bent arm behind you, contracting your back muscles. Then let your arm naturally swing forward. Keep your shoulders relaxed and down; don't pull them up toward your ears.

Move Your Hips

Your arms and legs will get you only so far (or should I say fast?). Now it's time to get your hips in on the action. Don't worry—I won't have you waddling around your neighborhood like a racewalker. But I am going to teach you how to adapt some of those techniques to your walking workouts.

You'll know that it's time to focus on your hips when you become "peg-legged" or stiff as you try to speed up, or you feel as though running would be easier. The hip action you want to strive for is forward and back—not side to side, like you're shaking your booty on the dance floor. Remember, you want to keep your body

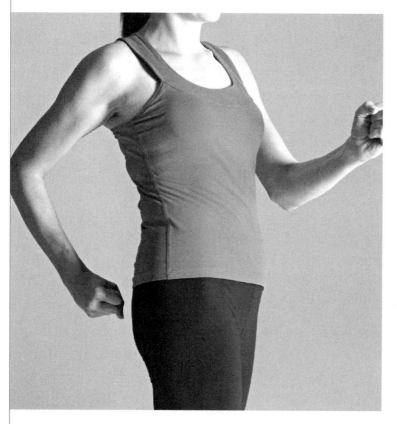

as streamlined as possible, with all motion going forward and back, not side to side or up and down. Once our WOW tester Denise Jennings learned to focus on moving her hips, she increased her pace for her fast intervals by an extra 10 steps per minute.

To help with this hip action, imagine that your leg starts up around your navel and that your hip is an extension of your leg. Here are two exercises from walking coach Lee Scott, creator of the DVD *Simple Secrets for a Great Walking Workout.*

1. Stand with your feet a few inches apart and place your hands on your hips. Now pull your right hip back, allowing the left one to go forward. Your right leg will straighten and your left one will bend. Just make sure your hips, not your legs, are driving the action. Your hips will be moving only an inch or so back and forth.

2. As you walk, allow your feet to cross over the midline of your body (like a runway model). Place your hands between the bottom of your rib cage and the top of your hip bones to feel how your abs are working and your hips are rotating. Then walk normally to compare. Once you get the hang of the hip action, transition back to a normal walk where your feet aren't crossing the midline but you maintain the hip movement. This is a good exercise to practice during your warm-up and cool-down.

Getting your hips in on the action may actually extend your stride length slightly, and that's okay. This type of extension is smoother and will actually speed you up, not slow you down.

I KNOW THIS IS A LOT to try to remember. That's why I want you to take the tips one at a time, as I've outlined in the 8-week WOW program (see Chapters 5 and 6). If you have the opportunity for someone to watch you—or better yet, to videotape you—as you walk, it can be very helpful for improving your walking technique.

Most important, remember that a key to good technique—and an enjoyable walk—is to stay relaxed. Don't overthink it or try too hard. Just keep practicing a little at a time, and it will all come together.

WOW Winner
Gail Rarick
GROUP: Exercise and Diet

AGE: 48 HEIGHT: 5'1½"
POUNDS LOST: 15½
INCHES LOST: 10¼ overall, including 3 from her waist
MAJOR ACCOMPLISHMENT: Significantly reduced her risk of heart disease by lowering her total cholesterol 44 points, "bad" LDL cholesterol 21 points, and triglycerides 49 points

Rediscovering Her Athletic Spirit

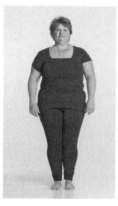

BEFORE

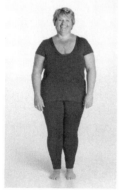

AFTER

GROWING UP, GAIL RARICK played sports—lots of sports: volleyball, basketball, softball, and golf. But that was more than 2 decades ago.

For the last 20 years, Gail and her husband have been dedicated to raising, carting, and coaching their three kids (now ages 20, 17, and 13) in all of their various life, school, and sport activities. Along the way, Gail's exercise dwindled to just occasional walks. "I rollercoastered," Gail explained. "Even though I love walking, one thing or another would always come up, either with the kids or work. So I'd blow off [my walks]." As a result, she had added nearly 60 extra pounds to her 5'1½" frame. But the WOW program reignited her inner athlete.

Right from Week 1, Gail loved the walking. "I was so happy to be moving again; it reminded me of training for sports," she said.

The WOW podcasts were particularly helpful; they reminded Gail to maintain good posture and practice the walking techniques. "Now, even if I'm walking without my iPod, I straighten up if I notice that I'm slumping."

She also loved the variety of workouts. "This wasn't any kind of walking I'd known before—you know, just head out for a walk, chat with your friends, and head home. This is real exercise."

In addition to her workouts, Gail would have her husband drop her off several blocks ahead of the field where her son was playing baseball, and she started walking when invited to the parties and barbecues she loves so much. She even joined her girlfriends for extra walks several times a week.

"The other day, I was trucking up a hill and a neighbor gave me the thumbs-up," reported Gail. "It made me smile, and at the same time, I noticed that I wasn't even out of breath." And she's increased her walking pace by about 33 percent. "Now it only takes me 40 minutes to finish a loop that used to take me an hour!" she said.

"At first, I'm sure my family thought, 'Here goes Mom again.' But now I think they know I'm hooked," said Gail. "Anytime there's an opportunity, I'm like, 'See ya, I'm going walking!' It just feels so good!"

P.S. *Three months after the official end of the program, Gail recorded an additional 4¼-pound weight loss and shaved another 5¼ inches off her figure, for a grand total of 19¾ pounds and 15½ inches lost in 5 months. Six weeks later, she walked Philadelphia's half marathon (13.1 miles) in 3 hours 28 minutes.*

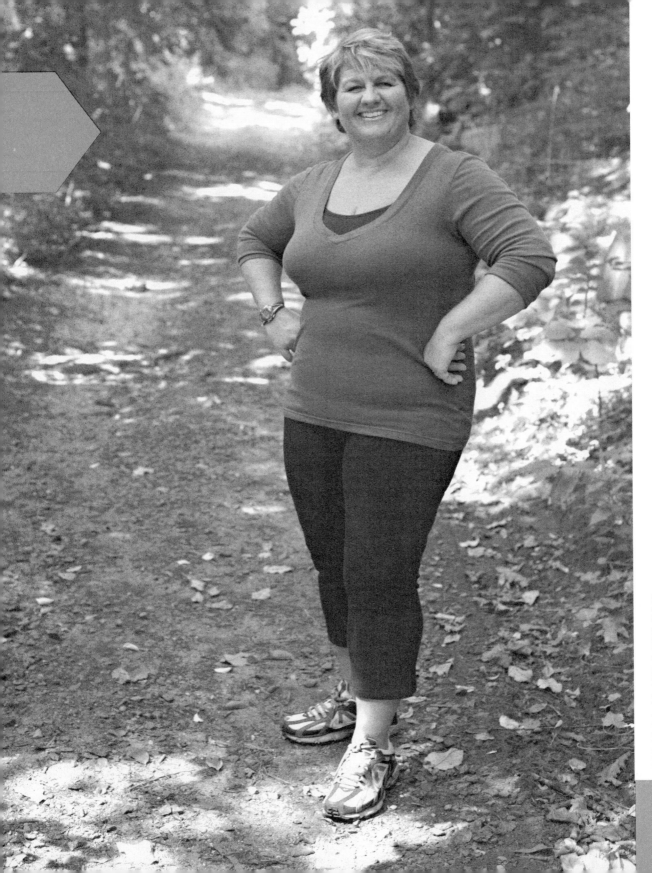

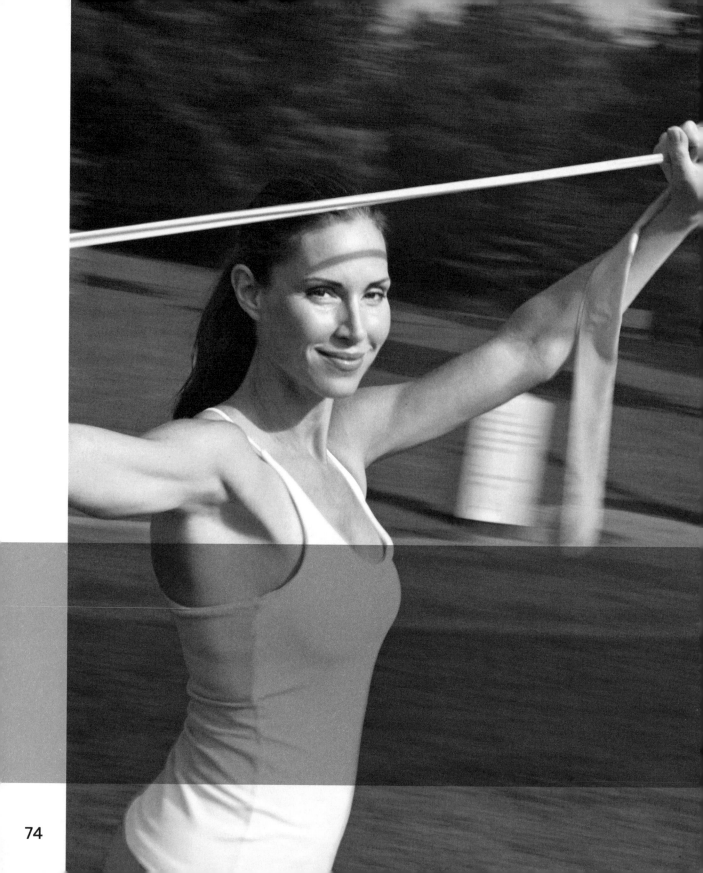

5

WOW PHASE 1: WEEKS 1–4

NOW LET'S GET STARTED on the first phase of *Prevention*'s Walk Off Weight program. The primary focus here is to build your endurance with increasingly longer walks and to introduce you to interval training. During the first 4 weeks, you'll work up to doing 45-minute Basic Interval Walks that alternate 60 seconds of moderate walking with 30 seconds of fast walking. Each week, you'll also challenge yourself to see just how far you can walk. The strength-training portion includes body-part specific routines, one each to target your upper body, core, and lower body; to firm you from head to toe; and to power up your walking stride.

Before you get started, I want you to make your commitment to yourself and the WOW program official and capture your enthusiasm at this very moment. Taking these little steps now will help you to stay on track or make it easier for you to get back on track if you ever stray. Fill out the form below, then share your plans with at least three people and ask them to support you in reaching your goal (heck, you can even have them witness your contract). Be as specific as possible. As the program progresses, review your contract anytime you need a motivation boost.

I also suggest completing the pretests that appear on page 299. Then watch as these numbers improve—a sure sign that you're getting fitter with every step.

Now lace up your walking shoes and get ready for a journey that's going to take you to a healthier, happier way of life.

My Get Healthy Contract

I, _____,
do solemnly swear to make myself a priority and to follow the Walk Off Weight program.

My goal is _____
_____
_____

Being overweight or out of shape makes me feel _____
_____
_____

I want to achieve this goal because _____
_____
_____

Achieving this goal means _____
_____
_____

With my stronger, slimmer, fitter body, I plan to _____
_____
_____

X_____
(Sign your name here.)

Phase 1: AT A GLANCE

LOWER-INTENSITY, LONGER-DURATION TRAINING

WEEK	DAY 1	DAY 2	DAY 3	DAY 4	DAY 5	DAY 6	DAY 7
1	**Basic Interval Walk I** 30 min **Lower-Body Strength Workout** 15 min **45 MIN TOTAL**	**Toning Walk I** (upper body) **20 MIN TOTAL**	**Basic Interval Walk I** 30 min **Core Strength Workout** 15 min **45 MIN TOTAL**	**Toning Walk I** (upper body) **20 MIN TOTAL**	**Basic Interval Walk I** 30 min **Lower-Body Strength Workout** 15 min **45 MIN TOTAL**	**Long Walk I** 45 min **Core Strength Workout** 15 min **60 MIN TOTAL**	Rest
2	**Basic Interval Walk I** 30 min **Lower-Body Strength Workout** 15 min **45 MIN TOTAL**	**Toning Walk I** (upper body) **20 MIN TOTAL**	**Basic Interval Walk I** 30 min **Core Strength Workout** 15 min **45 MIN TOTAL**	**Toning Walk I** (upper body) **20 MIN TOTAL**	**Basic Interval Walk I** 30 min **Lower-Body Strength Workout** 15 min **45 MIN TOTAL**	**Long Walk II** 60 min **Core Strength Workout** 15 min **75 MIN TOTAL**	Rest
3	**Basic Interval Walk II** 45 min **Lower-Body Strength Workout** 15 min **60 MIN TOTAL**	**Toning Walk II** (upper body) **25 MIN TOTAL**	**Basic Interval Walk II** 45 min **Core Strength Workout** 15 min **60 MIN TOTAL**	**Toning Walk II** (upper body) **25 MIN TOTAL**	**Basic Interval Walk II** 45 min **Lower-Body Strength Workout** 15 min **60 MIN TOTAL**	**Long Walk III** 75 min **Core Strength Workout** 15 min **90 MIN TOTAL**	Rest
4	**Basic Interval Walk II** 45 min **Lower-Body Strength Workout** 15 min **60 MIN TOTAL**	**Toning Walk II** (upper body) **25 MIN TOTAL**	**Basic Interval Walk II** 45 min **Core Strength Workout** 15 min **60 MIN TOTAL**	**Toning Walk II** (upper body) **25 MIN TOTAL**	**Basic Interval Walk II** 45 min **Lower-Body Strength Workout** 15 min **60 MIN TOTAL**	**Long Walk IV** 90 min **Core Strength Workout** 15 min **105 MIN TOTAL**	Rest

WORKOUT SCHEDULES

CRAZY BUSY SEEMS TO BE THE NORM THESE DAYS, so it's not surprising that fitting in exercise can be tough, especially when you're just starting out. I'll be giving you a sample schedule for each week's workouts, but I would encourage you to adjust it to fit into your life instead of the other way around. Then you'll be more successful at sticking with it.

Here are some guidelines to follow when creating your own workout schedule.

- Choose any day of the week as your rest day. You might decide to schedule it for when your calendar is so jam-packed that trying to exercise would feel like just one more thing you need to do. Or use it as a reward at the end of the week for doing all the recommended workouts. Sometimes it may happen by default—say, when it's 9:00 or 10:00 p.m. and you're finally winding down, only to realize that you didn't squeeze in your workout. That's okay, but you'll need to be extravigilant for the remainder of the week because you have only that one rest day.

- You can move the Long Walk to a day that's more convenient, probably on a weekend. Ditto for the Speed Walks in Phase 2 of the program.

- During Phase 1, you can rearrange the strength workouts—for instance, doing the core and lower-body routines on the same day. You could even do them on the same day as the upper-body Toning Walk. However, don't do any one workout on back-to-back days—for example, don't do the lower-body routine on Monday and Tuesday. Muscles get stronger by having time to rest and repair. You could do the core routine on Monday and the lower body on Tuesday because you're working different muscles each day.

- In Phase 2 of the program, you have only one toning routine, which you'll do two or three times a week. Again, just make sure not to do it on consecutive days. A good way to schedule these is every other day, such as Monday, Wednesday, and Friday—but no more frequently than three times a week.

- Just like strength workouts, don't do your interval workouts on consecutive days. Alternating high-intensity workouts with more moderate ones will help prevent injury and burnout.

Q+A

Q: What if I don't have time to do an entire workout?

A: "Some is better than none" is my mantra, and I hope you'll make it one of yours. If you're supposed to do a 30-minute Interval Walk, for example, but you have only 20 minutes, lace up your sneakers and go. You'll get more benefits from a partial walk than from none at all. You may be thinking *"no-duh,"* but so many of us get stuck in an all-or-nothing mind-set—if we can't do every last second of a workout, we think it's not worth it, and so we skip it entirely. Do as much as you can; even as little as 10 minutes will rev up your calorie burn, boost your mood, and help you to make exercise a habit. And if you find some extra time later in the day, sneak in another short workout for even more benefits.

Q: Can I split up my workouts?

A: Absolutely! Numerous studies have found that doing multiple short exercise bouts, such as three 10-minute sessions, provides fat-burning, fitness-boosting, and disease-fighting benefits comparable to one longer 30-minute workout.[1] While this hasn't been tested with interval workouts, it's reasonable to believe that they'd deliver similar results.

One difference, however, may be how hard you're able to push on the high-intensity intervals. Some of our WOW test panelists noted that they pushed harder about midway through their walks, once they were really warmed up. In that case, doing the interval workouts in their entirety would likely produce better results. Other panelists reported that they couldn't push as hard toward the end of their walks. If you notice this, too, then breaking up your workouts might leave you feeling fresher, with more energy to push really hard on all the intervals.

Either way, the difference in calorie burn is probably small, so it comes down to what's going to fit into your life better. What's most important is that you're doing *all* the workouts, because that's what's going to get you the best results. You can break up your toning workouts, too, if you want.

Q: I'm struggling with the core (or lower-body) routine. Help!

A: That's not uncommon, since you're working similar muscles during each exercise instead of alternating muscle groups and giving them a break, like you do during a workout targeting your total body. By the third or fourth move, your muscles are becoming fatigued, so the exercises feel more challenging and you may be having trouble maintaining good form. Here's how to stay fresh so you can get the most out of all the moves without getting hurt.

- **Modify the moves** Try the easier versions for some or all of the exercises.
- **Split them up** Do two or three of the moves in the morning and the remaining ones later in the day.
- **Rearrange the sequence** If you're struggling with a particular exercise, start with that one so you're fresher. Or each time you do the routine, change the order.

Q+A

Q: Can I use handweights instead of a resistance band for the Toning Walks?

A: Please don't. Since you can't put them down in between the toning exercises, you're not giving your upper-body muscles a chance to rest. And while walking with dumbbells does increase your calorie burn a little, the risk of injury from swinging your arms while holding weights is greater. Besides, most of the exercises in the Toning Walk won't be effective with handweights because the weights don't offer the same type of resistance.

Q: When is the best time to exercise?

A: Whatever time you're most likely to stick with it. Some surveys have shown that morning exercisers are more consistent, probably because there are fewer opportunities to get sidetracked than if they were working out later in the day. But if you're not a morning person—and I'm not one myself—the snooze button may be all it takes to distract you. Instead, find the time that you're most willing and able to exercise. Fit your workouts into your life when you have your best shot of keeping other activities from getting in the way. The time of day has no significant impact on the calories you burn or how quickly you see results. What matters most is that you exercise consistently.

Q: Is it better to exercise before or after a meal?

A: In terms of weight loss, it really doesn't matter. The most important thing is to make sure that you're properly fueled so you have the energy to give it your all during your workout. That means if it's been more than 2 hours since your last meal, you should eat something. The best choices are foods that provide both carbohydrates and protein, such as a banana and yogurt. Also, limit yourself to 150 to 200 calories so you feel energized, not weighted down. The closer you eat to the time you're working out, the lighter your snack should be.

On the flip side, if you just had a meal—especially if it was a heavy one—you should wait about 2 hours for your body to finish digesting it. Exercise diverts bloodflow away from your stomach and intestines, impairing digestion, which can leave you feeling not so good and result in a so-so workout. But an easy stroll after dinner is a good way to help digestion and ease that too-full feeling.

Q: Should I use a sports drink?

A: If your goal is to lose weight, skip the sports drinks. Unless you're walking really hard for more than an hour, or if the weather is very hot and humid, your body doesn't need all the extra nutrients, and your waistline doesn't need the extra calories. For the workouts in the WOW program, water should be your beverage of choice. And make sure that you're drinking enough—at least 8 ounces before and after you exercise, plus sips of water every 15 to 20 minutes during activity.

LOWER-BODY STRENGTH WORKOUT

THESE MOVES TARGET ALL OF YOUR MAJOR WALKING MUSCLES from your butt down. A recent study found that simply doing one move to strengthen your quads (the fronts of your thighs) could increase your walking speed by 15 percent.[2] That's equivalent to increasing your pace from 3.5 MPH to 4 MPH! Imagine what you could do if you shape up all of your lower-body muscles. These exercises also challenge your balance, giving your core muscles an extra workout, and improve your posture for a stronger, pain-free stride.

During Phase 1 of the WOW program, you'll be doing this routine twice a week, taking a 30- to 60-second break between moves. Each week, you'll be increasing the number of repetitions of each exercise. Here's what you should try to aim for, repeating on each side when appropriate:

WEEK 1: 6–8 reps
WEEK 2: 8–10 reps
WEEK 3: 10–12 reps
WEEK 4: 12–15 reps

If you're doing this workout separate from your walks, start out by taking about 5 minutes to warm up by walking at an easy pace.

Lightly hold onto something sturdy such as a chair back or the wall to help you maintain your balance if you find that you're wobbly when doing any of these moves. You'll get more muscle building and firming out of the exercises and reduce your risk of injury if you're steady. Over time, even within just a few weeks, your balance will improve, and you can eventually try the moves without holding on.

How to Use the Resistance Band

You'll need a resistance band for at least two of the following moves. Position the band as described, and check that it's secure before you begin the exercise. If you're instructed to make a loop from the band, be aware that the larger the loop, the easier the resistance will be; the smaller the loop, the harder it will be. You can also increase the resistance by moving farther away from the anchor point.

If you need to tie the band in a loop around your lower legs for an exercise, you can wrap it around your legs twice for maximum resistance. Just remember, don't sacrifice good form for increased challenge. Stretching and releasing the band's resistance with control is key to maximizing toning and avoiding injury. Don't let the band snap back once you've reached the top of the move; pause, then slowly release, resisting against the band's pull as you do.

Cross Leg Swing
(targets inner thighs)

MAIN MOVE

Attach the resistance band near the floor around a sturdy furniture leg, a railing, or under a heavy piece of furniture so that it forms a loop. Stand so that the band is on your left. Put the band around your left foot near your ankle. Step away from the anchor point until the band is taut when your left leg is extended out to the side, toes pointed. Flex your left foot, contract your inner thigh, and swing your leg across the front of your body toward your right leg. Hold, then slowly return to the start without letting your left foot touch the floor between reps.

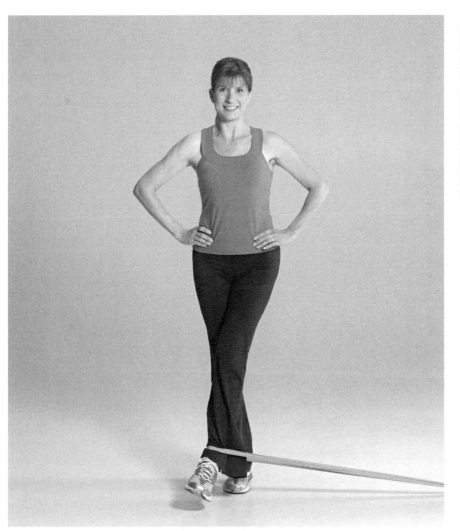

TRAINING
TIP

Lead with your heel as you raise your leg. And really concentrate on your inner thigh, even putting your hand on it to feel it working.

Make it harder:
Hold your leg in the up position and pulse it twice, lifting and lowering an inch or so, before returning to start for your next rep.

Make it easier:
Lower your foot to the floor between reps.

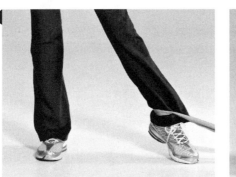

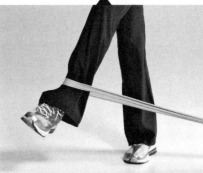

One-Leg Squat

(targets quads, glutes, and hamstrings)

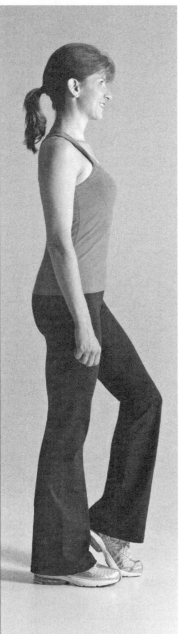

MAIN MOVE

Balance on your right leg with the toes of your left foot lightly touching the floor and your arms at your sides. Bend your hips and right knee and sit back as if you were lowering halfway into a chair. Let your arms swing forward to about chest height. Keep your right knee behind your toes. Press into your right foot and stand back up.

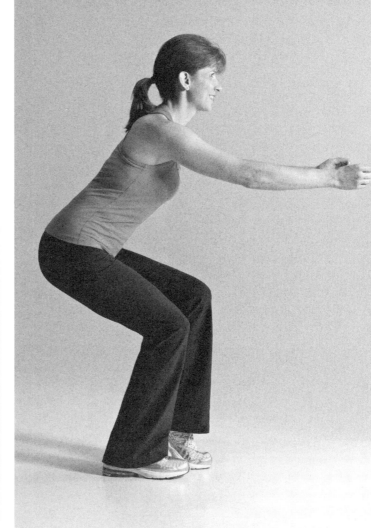

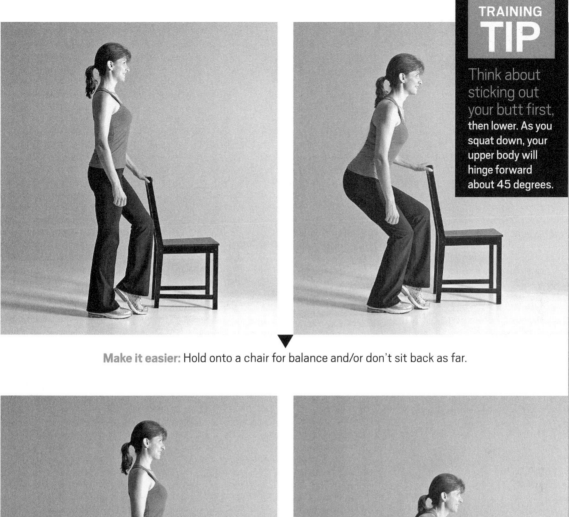

TRAINING TIP

Think about sticking out your butt first, then lower. As you squat down, your upper body will hinge forward about 45 degrees.

Make it easier: Hold onto a chair for balance and/or don't sit back as far.

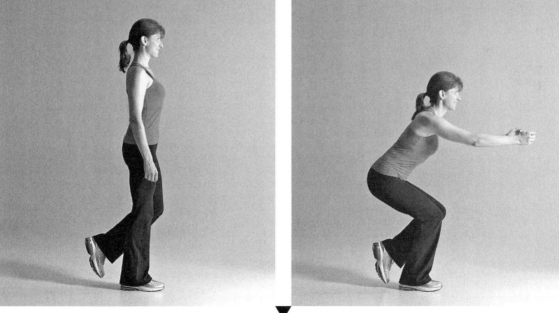

Make it harder: Balance on your right leg with your left foot completely off the floor.

Rear Kick
(targets glutes and hamstrings)

MAIN MOVE

Attach the resistance band near the floor around a sturdy furniture leg, a railing, or under a heavy piece of furniture so that it forms a loop. Stand facing the anchor point and put the band around your right foot near your ankle. Step backward if needed so the band is taut. Balancing on your left leg, with your left knee slightly bent, press your right leg back, with your foot flexed, and squeeze your butt. Hold and slowly lower without touching your foot to the floor between reps.

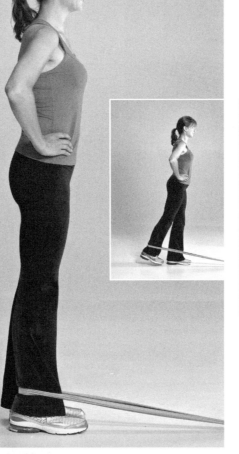

TRAINING TIP

Don't lean forward as you raise your leg. You don't have to lift your leg high to target your glutes, and they work harder if you stand tall.

Make it harder:
Hold your leg in the up position and pulse it twice, lifting and lowering it an inch or so before lowering it completely.

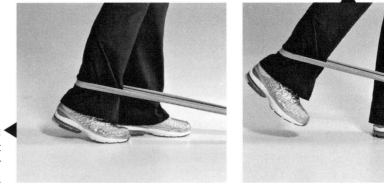

Make it easier:
Lower your foot to the floor between reps.

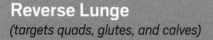

Reverse Lunge
(targets quads, glutes, and calves)

MAIN MOVE

Stand with your feet together and your arms at your sides. Step 2 to 3 feet behind you with your right foot, toes pointing forward, and bend your knees so that the right one is almost to the floor (your right heel will come off the floor). Simultaneously, swing your arms forward to about chest height. Keep your left knee directly over your left ankle; if it's coming forward, shift your hips back or take a bigger step back. Press into your front foot and stand back up, bringing your feet together. Repeat, stepping back with the left leg. Continue alternating legs until you complete the recommended number of reps with each leg.

TRAINING
TIP

Don't bend at your waist or lean forward as you lower. Your torso and head should be straight up and down.

Make it harder:
Add a heel lift. As you stand back up and bring your feet together, rise up onto your toes. Hold for a second, then lower and step back into the next lunge.

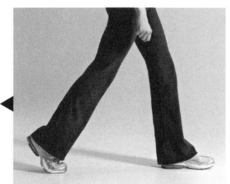

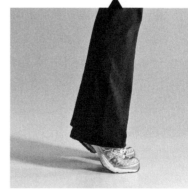

Make it easier:
Do stationary lunges, with your left foot 2 to 3 feet in front of your right foot (heel will be up the entire time).

Moving Squat
(targets quads, glutes, and outer thighs)

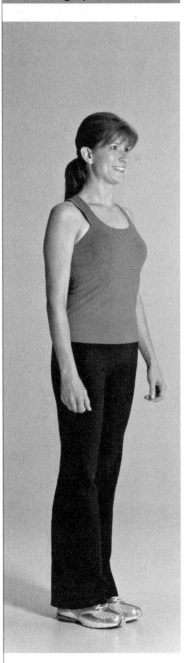

MAIN MOVE

Stand with your feet together and your arms at your sides. Step your right foot out to the side 2 to 3 feet, bend your hips and knees, and sit back as if you're lowering into a chair. Simultaneously, swing your arms forward to about chest height. Keep your knees over your feet, not out past your toes or rolling in toward each other. Your upper body will lean forward about 45 degrees. Stand back up, bringing your left foot toward your right. Step to the right again. Continue moving to the right until you run out of space or you've completed all of the reps. Then repeat to the left. You may need to alternate going side to side, depending on how much space you have.

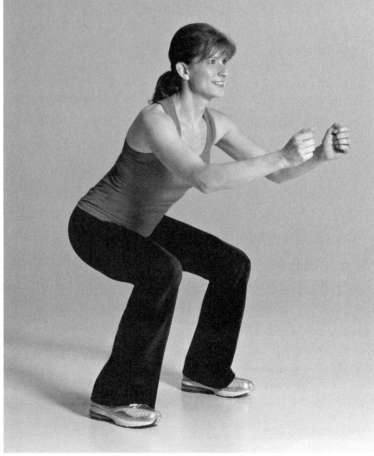

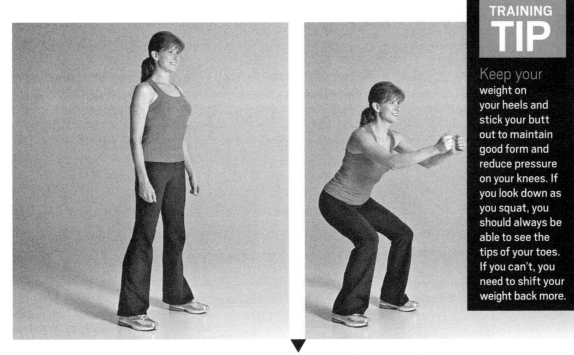

Make it easier: Do stationary squats with your feet about shoulder-width apart the entire time.

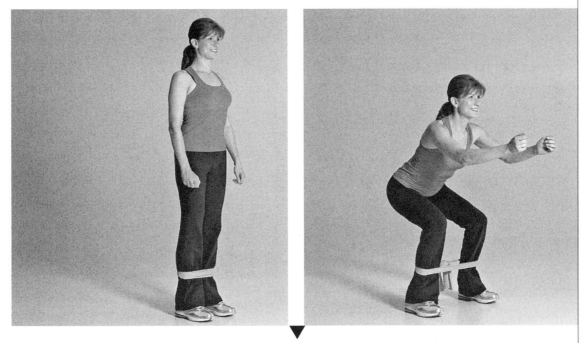

Make it harder: Tie a resistance band around your lower legs so that it's taut, then step and squat.

TONING WALK MOVES

FOR ON-THE-GO FIRMING, you'll do these upper-body moves with a resistance band while you walk. Don't worry—with a little practice you can do it—all of our test panelists did. It's also a great way to improve your coordination.

Do this routine twice a week. Instead of counting reps like you do for the Lower-Body and Core Strength routines, you'll be doing each exercise for a specific time interval (45 seconds during Weeks 1 and 2, and 60 seconds during Weeks 3 and 4). Using controlled movements, you'll complete as many reps as possible in that time (usually 20 to 30), then you'll drape the resistance band around your neck and walk briskly for 1 minute before doing the next exercise.

How to Use the Resistance Band

To increase the resistance, shorten the band by folding it lengthwise, adjusting your hand position by moving them closer together, or wrapping the band around your hands. Or you can give yourself more slack and less resistance by moving your hands farther apart. Controlled stretching and releasing of the band is key to maximizing toning and avoiding injury. Don't let the band snap back once you've reached the top of the move; pause, then slowly release, resisting against the band's pull.

Pull-Down
(firms lattisimus dorsi muscle in upper and mid back and biceps)

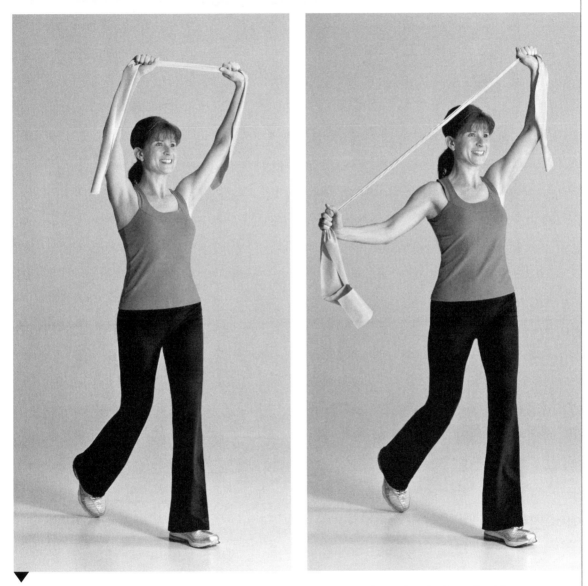

▼

With arms extended overhead, hold the center of a resistance band with your hands about shoulder width apart, palms forward, and elbows bent slightly. Keeping your left hand stationary, pull your right arm down and out to the side, without bending your elbow, until your hand is at about shoulder level. Hold for a second, then slowly return to the start position.

Front Press
(firms pectoral muscle in chest and triceps)

Loop a resistance band around your upper back and under your arms. Grasp an end of the band in each hand. Position hands near your chest, palms forward, and elbows bent out. Extend your arms straight in front of you at chest level. Hold for a second, then slowly return to the start position.

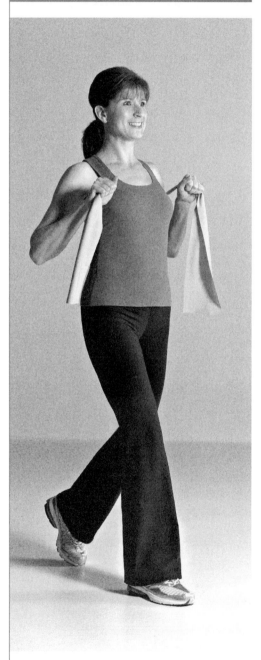

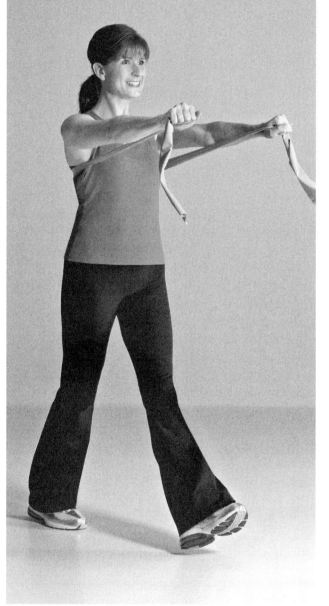

Row
(firms lats and rhomboid muscles in mid back and biceps)

With your arms extended in front of you at chest level, hold the center of a resistance band with both hands. Keeping your left arm stationary as an anchor, bend your right elbow and pull your arm back, keeping it close to your body, until your hand is near your hip and your elbow is pointing behind you. Hold for a second, then slowly return to the start position.

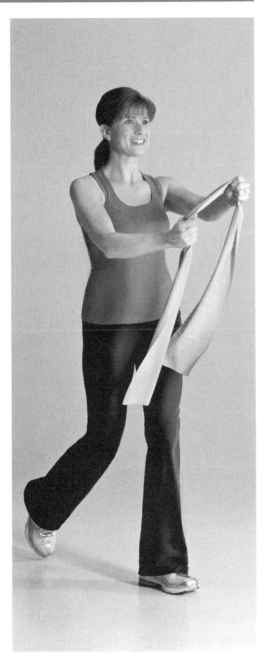

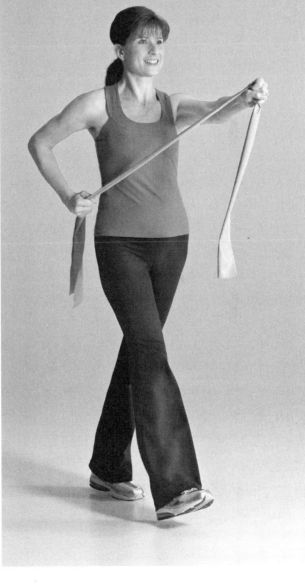

Overhead Press
(firms deltoid muscles in shoulders and triceps muscles in backs of upper arms)

Loop a resistance band around your upper back and under your arms. Grasp an end of the band in each hand, with your elbows bent and pointing down and out to the sides. Your hands should be near your shoulders, palms forward. Press your hands straight up overhead. Hold for a second, then slowly return to the start position.

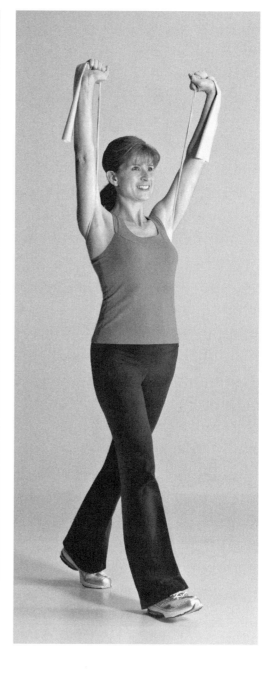

Front Pull
(firms rear deltoids in backs of shoulders and rhomboids)

With your arms extended out in front of you, hold a resistance band at chest height with your hands about shoulder width apart. Keeping your arms straight, pull your hands apart, squeezing your shoulder blades together and bringing your hands almost directly out to the sides. Hold for a second, then slowly return to the start position.

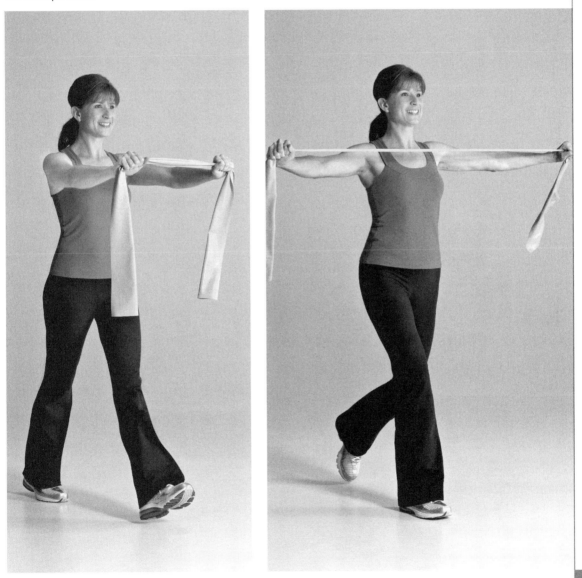

Arm Pull

(firms triceps muscles in backs of upper arms)

Drape a resistance band around your neck and grasp each side with your arms bent and your hands by your shoulders. Press your hands down and straighten your arms. Hold for a second, then slowly return to the start position, keeping your upper arms stationary throughout.

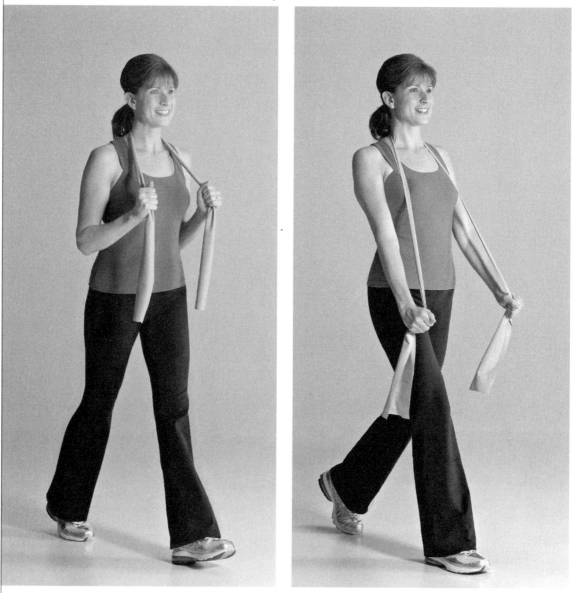

CORE STRENGTH WORKOUT

WALKING MAY SEEM LIKE A LOWER-BODY-ONLY EXERCISE, but the action of walking really starts within your core with the psoas muscles, which lie deep in your pelvis and attach your spine to your thighs, and the abdominals. In fact, research shows that strengthening your abs and back muscles—exactly what these exercises target—helps you to walk faster.[3] Strong core muscles also keep your pelvis in neutral position, which is important for good walking posture.

Do this routine twice a week, taking a 30- to 60-second break between moves. Each week, you'll be increasing the number of repetitions of each exercise. Here's what you should aim for (unless otherwise noted), repeating on each side when appropriate:

WEEK 1: 6–8 reps
WEEK 2: 8–10 reps
WEEK 3: 10–12 reps
WEEK 4: 12–15 reps

If you're doing this workout separate from your walks, make sure that you warm up first by walking at an easy pace for about 5 minutes. Then do these upper-body moves to prepare your torso muscles for their workout: Roll your shoulders forward and back; twist your torso to the left and right, reaching the opposite arm across your chest; and reach each arm overhead, stretching to the opposite side.

Plank

(targets abs, back, glutes, shoulders, chest, and triceps)

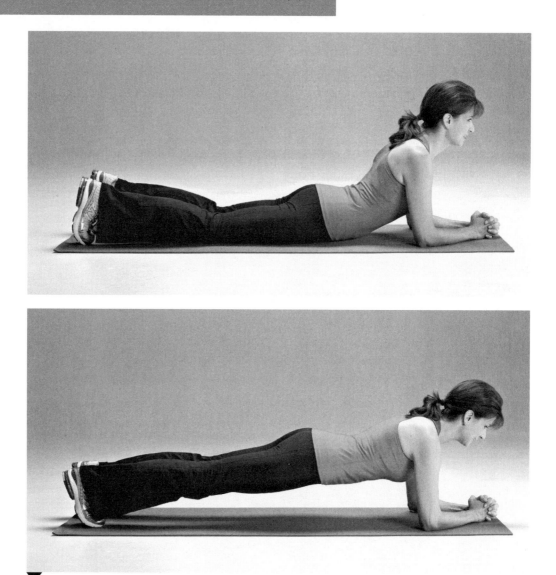

▼
MAIN MOVE

Lie facedown with your forearms on the floor, hands clasped, elbows under your shoulders, and toes tucked. Contract your abs and raise your belly, hips, and legs off the floor, keeping your body in line from head to heels. Don't bend at the waist. Hold for 15 seconds the first week, then increase by 15 seconds each week. Do just one time.

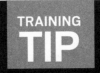

not rounding your upper back and pulling your shoulders toward your ears. This often happens when you try to hold the plank position longer. To prevent this, think of lengthening your body, pulling your head and heels in opposite directions, and pulling your shoulder blades down your back.

Make it easier:
Instead of tucking your toes under, bend your knees so your feet are completely off the floor. Keep your knees on the floor as you raise up, keeping your body in line from head to knees.

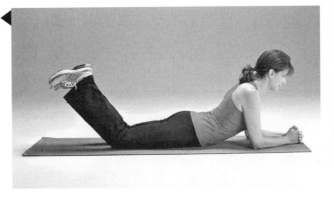

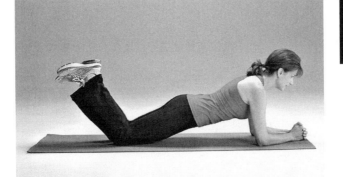

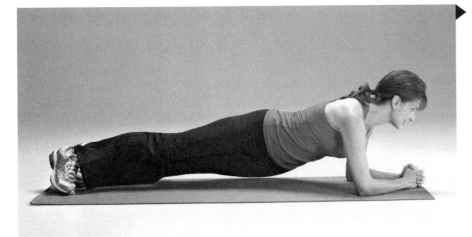

Make it harder:
Add a dip. Slowly twist your torso, lowering your left hip toward the floor, and then come back up. Repeat the dip with your right hip.

Tabletop Balance
(targets back, abs, glutes, hamstrings, and shoulders)

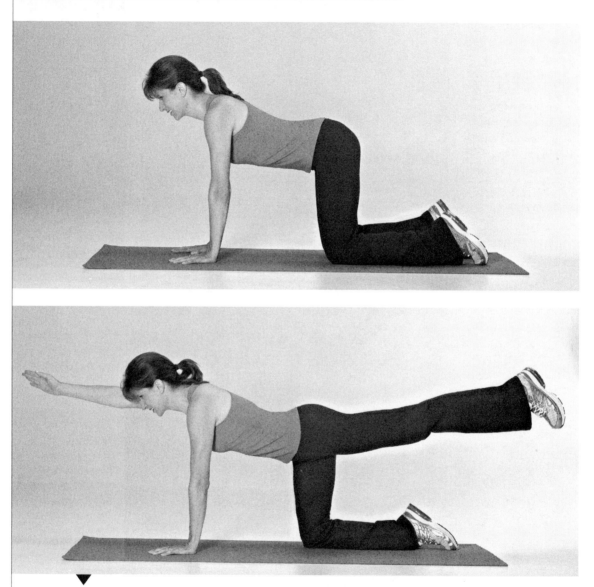

▼ MAIN MOVE

Get down on all fours, hands under your shoulders and knees under your hips. Keeping your abs tight, raise your right arm and left leg simultaneously until they are in line with your spine, squeezing your glutes as you do. Hold for a second, then lower. Repeat with the opposite arm and leg.

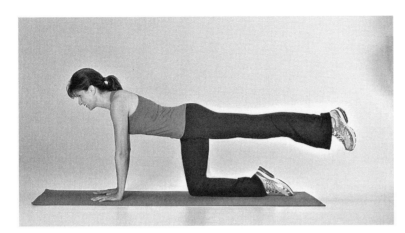

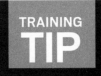

TRAINING TIP

Look at the floor a few feet in front of you to keep your head in line with your spine.

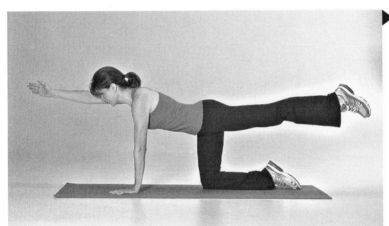

Make it easier: Raise your leg first. When you are balanced, raise your arm. Hold and lower together.

Make it harder: Once you've raised your arm and leg, pulse them three times, lifting and lowering about an inch.

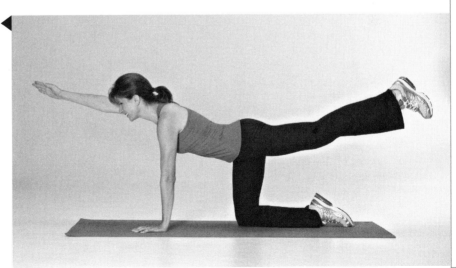

Side Plank
(targets back and side abs)

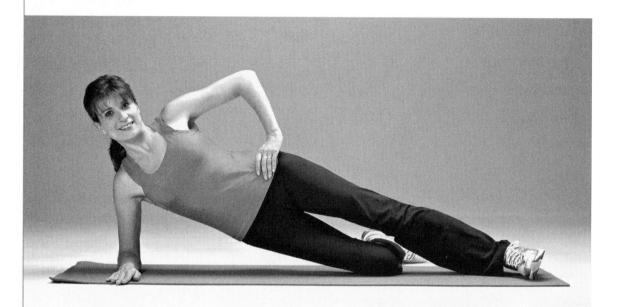

▼

MAIN MOVE

Lie on your right side with your legs stacked and the bottom one bent behind you. Prop yourself up on your right elbow with your right palm flat on the floor and your left hand on your left hip. Contract your abs and raise your right hip and leg off the floor. Slowly lower your right hip toward the floor without touching, then lift back up.

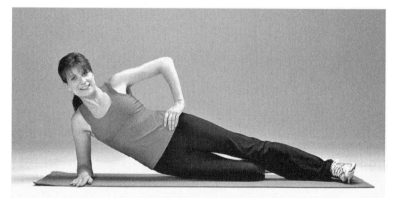

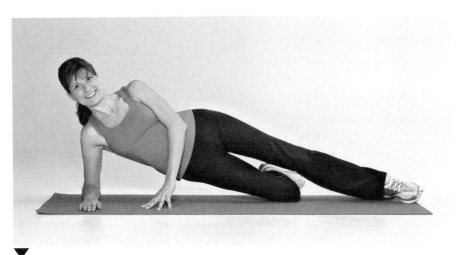

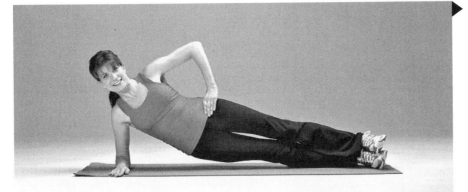

▼

Make it easier: Place your free hand on the floor to help you raise your hip. Return that hand to your opposite hip and hold for as long as possible, working up to a total of 60 seconds.

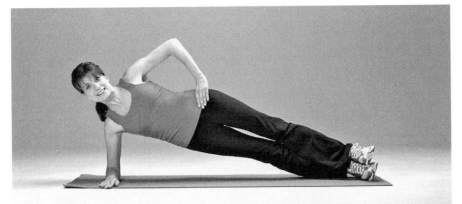

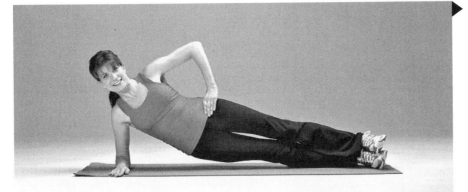

▶

Make it harder: Straighten both legs and stack them, feet flexed. Raise your bottom hip off the floor so that you're balancing on the bottom foot, elbow, forearm, and hand.

TRAINING TIP

Make sure your elbow is directly under your shoulder. If your arm is too far away from your body, it will be harder to lift into the plank and you'll be less stable. You may need to bring your elbow a little closer to your body before you lift to ensure the proper position.

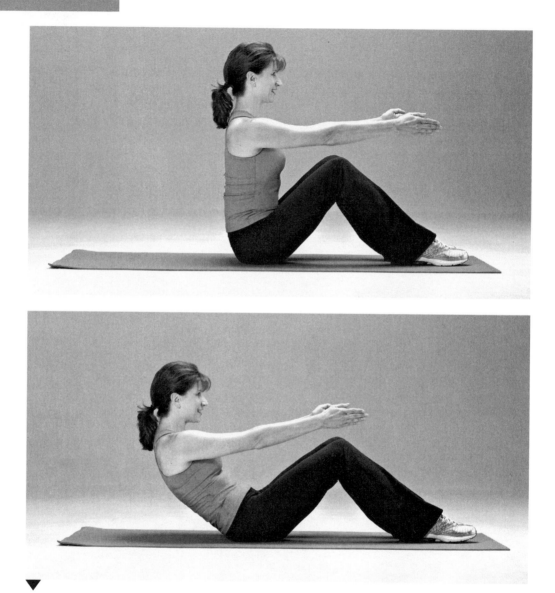

▼

MAIN MOVE

Sit on the floor with your knees bent, feet flat on the floor, and arms extended in front of you. Pull your abs in, round your back, and inhale as you roll down about halfway toward the floor. Exhale and slowly roll back up, sitting tall.

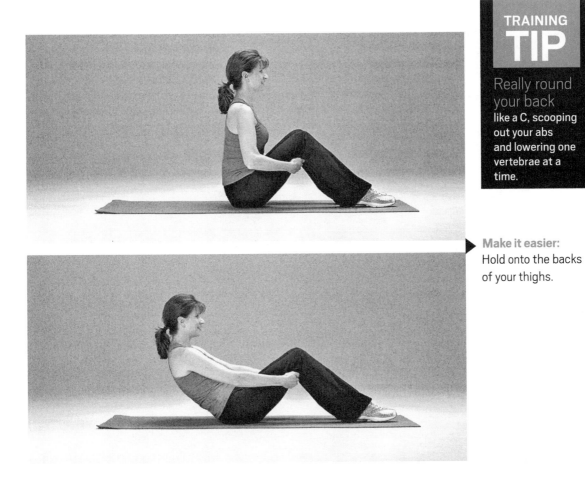

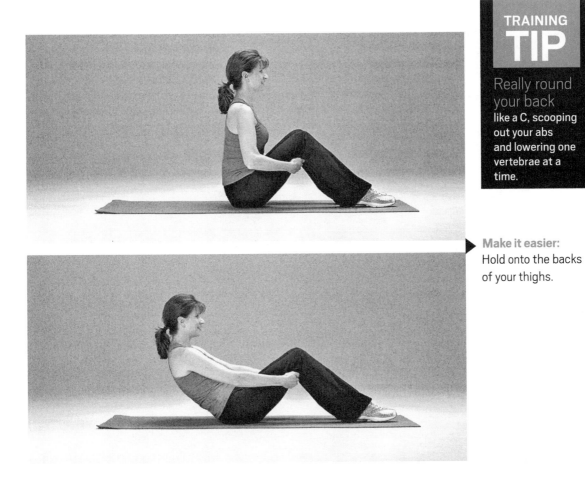

TRAINING TIP

Really round your back like a C, scooping out your abs and lowering one vertebrae at a time.

▶ **Make it easier:** Hold onto the backs of your thighs.

Make it harder: Hold your left foot off the floor as you do half of the reps, then switch legs.

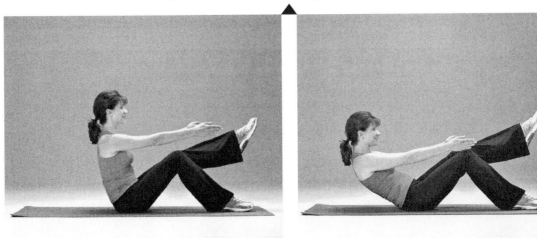

Bicycle
(targets front and side abs and quads)

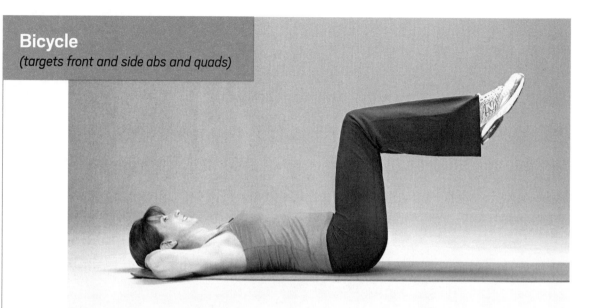

▼

MAIN MOVE

Lie on your back and pull your knees in toward your chest so that both your hips and knees are bent 90 degrees. Place your hands behind your head. Exhale as you curl your head and shoulders off the floor and twist your torso to the right. At the same time, pull your right knee in toward your chest and extend your left leg so that it's at about a 45-degree angle to the floor. Crunch, bringing your left shoulder toward your right knee. Inhale as you slowly lower. Repeat, twisting to the left. Continue alternating sides for 10 to 20 total reps.

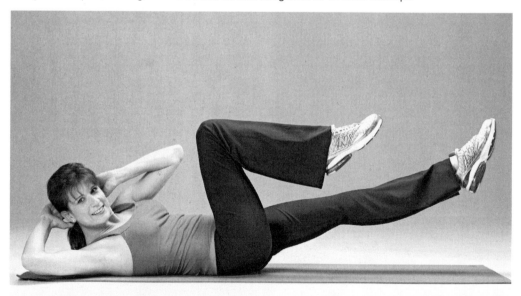

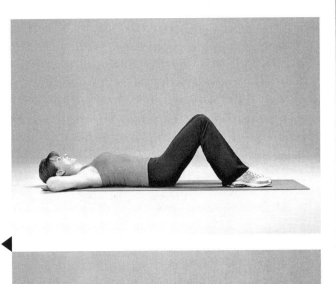

TRAINING
TIP

To fully
engage your
oblique
(side ab) mus-
cles, focus on
pulling your
shoulder—instead
of your elbow—
toward the oppo-
site knee. This
ensures that
you're twisting
from your torso
and prevents
you from pulling
on your head,
which could
strain your neck.

Make it easier:
Keep your feet on the
floor and lift one leg at
a time, bringing your
shoulder toward the
opposite knee.

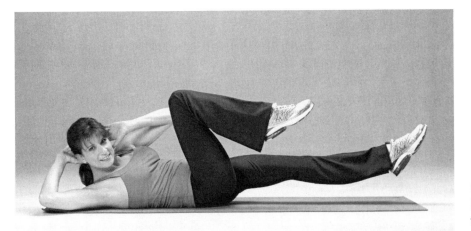

Make it harder:
Lower the ex-
tended leg closer
to the floor without
touching it.

☞ Never skip your warm-up, cool-down, and stretches. *See page 54 for more details about when and how to do them.*

RIGHT NOW, YOU'RE PROBABLY EXCITED, but a little nervous, too. That's understandable. The WOW program is all new to you, so you don't know what to expect. But by this time next week, it will be familiar. In the meantime, don't worry if you can't do everything perfectly. It's okay. We're after progress, not perfection. Take a deep breath, relax, and just get started.

YOUR WORKOUT AT A GLANCE

DAY	ACTIVITY//WORKOUT	TOTAL
1	Basic Interval Walk I (30 min) // Lower-Body Strength Workout (15 min)	45 min
2	Toning Walk I (20 min)	20 min
3	Basic Interval Walk I (30 min) // Core Strength Workout (15 min)	45 min
4	Toning Walk I (20 min)	20 min
5	Basic Interval Walk I (30 min) // Lower-Body Strength Workout (15 min)	45 min
6	Long Walk I (45 min) // Core Strength Workout (15 min)	60 min
7	Rest	

||||||||||||||||||||||||||||||||||||||||||||||||||||||||||||||||||||||||||||||||||

WHAT YOU'LL **DO THIS WEEK**

3 x Basic Interval Walk I   2 x Toning Walk I   2 x Lower-Body Strength Workout

2 x Core Strength Workout   1 x Long Walk I

||||||||||||||||||||||||||||||||||||||||||||||||||||||||||||||||||||||||||||||||||

" Do not look behind you; look ahead. There is a whole new world waiting for a thinner and fitter you.

—KATHY ASHENFELTER, LOST 22½ POUNDS AND 12¾ INCHES ON THE WOW PROGRAM

Workout Summary

THE DETAILS OF THE WALKING ROUTINES follow. See Toning Exercises on page 90 for descriptions of the Toning Walk moves.

LOWER-BODY STRENGTH WORKOUT
(page 81)
Do 6–8 reps of the following exercises:
>> **Cross Leg Swing**
>> **One-Leg Squat**
>> **Rear Kick**
>> **Reverse Lunge**
>> **Moving Squat**

CORE STRENGTH WORKOUT
(page 97)
>> **Plank** *(Hold once for 15 seconds)*
Do 6–8 reps of the following exercises:
>> **Tabletop Balance**
>> **Side Plank**
>> **Roll Down**
>> **Bicycle**

Believe in Yourself—You *Can* Do This!

I'VE ALWAYS BEEN A BIG BELIEVER that your attitude can make or break your efforts to become more active. A recent study confirmed my suspicion, finding that high self-efficacy—in other words, an I-can-do-it mind-set—is the single biggest predictor of sticking with an exercise program. When experts tracked 200 new exercisers, they found that those who believed in themselves were 139 percent more likely to be active a year later, compared with less-confident types.[4]

Our minds are powerful tools! Unfortunately, most of us women aren't hardwired to think this way, especially if we weren't athletic as kids or we have bad memories of gym class. But that's all about to change; you are taking your first steps to thinking and acting like an athlete. (Yes, walkers are athletes, too!) Just as you build up your muscles, let's build up that can-do attitude!

Start with what you know. The biggest indicator of self-efficacy is past performance. You're starting out with high marks in this area because you know how to walk. You do it every day! Unlike signing up for a kickboxing class or taking up tennis, starting with an activity for which you already have the necessary skills makes believing in your ability to do it a whole lot easier.

Seek out role models. This is another way to bolster your confidence. So read all the profiles of our WOW test panelists, as well as the success stories in *Prevention* and other magazines and online. Go to charity walks or races, even marathons, and notice all the different sizes and shapes of the people who cross the finish line. Anyone can achieve success if they put their minds to it. That includes you!

Stop putting yourself down. We all do a lot of self-talk; unfortunately, most of it tends to be the negative kind. In order to succeed, you need to turn off self-defeating thoughts as soon as they pop into your head. It may sound simple, but it takes practice. Every time you start to criticize or doubt yourself, talk back. Simply say, *"Stop! I can do whatever I put my mind to."*

Acknowledge your successes, even the small ones. Even if you're so busy that you have only enough time for a 10-minute workout, you should pat yourself on the back. It may not seem like much, but avoiding the common trap of saying *"I'll do it tomorrow"* and not getting stuck on the idea that it's all or nothing is a huge achievement. Recognizing these types of successes instead of just focusing on the scale will go a long way toward keeping you on track.

Get support. Having others to cheer you on can give you the boost you need to keep believing in yourself when the going gets tough. I've experienced this myself, and I've heard it from many of our walkers who've completed half and full marathons. Even when they feel as if they can't take another step, encouraging words such as "You can do it!"— even from total strangers—help them to dig deep and push on.

Eyes Up
One of the quickest ways to stand more erect is to simply look up and keep your eyes on the horizon.

Arms Up
Bend your elbows 90 degrees and swing your arms forward and back. Keep your elbows in and your hands close to your body, so they're almost skimming your sides. On the back motion, bring your hand just past your hip. As your hand comes forward, let it swing to about chest height, but don't allow it to pass the midline of your body.

BASIC INTERVAL WALK I

During this workout, focus on pushing yourself out of your comfort zone for the fast intervals. They should feel hard; remember, this isn't supposed to be a walk in the park! Refer back to the chart on page 67 for a guide on how to gauge your intensity.

TIME	ACTIVITY	INTENSITY
0:00–5:00	Warm-Up (5 min)	3→5
5:00–6:00	Moderate (1 min)	5–6
6:00–6:30	Fast (30 sec)	7–8
6:30–7:30	Moderate (1 min)	5–6
7:30–8:00	Fast (30 sec)	7–8
8:00–9:00	Moderate (1 min)	5–6
9:00–9:30	Fast (30 sec)	7–8
9:30–10:30	Moderate (1 min)	5–6
10:30–11:00	Fast (30 sec)	7–8
11:00–12:00	Moderate (1 min)	5–6
12:00–12:30	Fast (30 sec)	7–8
12:30–13:30	Moderate (1 min)	5–6
13:30–14:00	Fast (30 sec)	7–8
14:00–15:00	Moderate (1 min)	5–6
15:00–15:30	Fast (30 sec)	7–8
15:30–16:30	Moderate (1 min)	5–6
16:30–17:00	Fast (30 sec)	7–8
17:00–18:00	Moderate (1 min)	5–6
18:00–18:30	Fast (30 sec)	7–8
18:30–19:30	Moderate (1 min)	5–6
19:30–20:00	Fast (30 sec)	7–8
20:00–21:00	Moderate (1 min)	5–6
21:00–21:30	Fast (30 sec)	7–8
21:30–22:30	Moderate (1 min)	5–6
22:30–23:00	Fast (30 sec)	7–8
23:00–24:00	Moderate (1 min)	5–6
24:00–24:30	Fast (30 sec)	7–8
24:30–25:30	Moderate (1 min)	5–6
25:30–30:00	Cool-Down (4.5 min)	5→3

TONING WALK I

Between bouts of brisk walking, you'll slow your pace slightly and do upper-body exercises to firm up your arms, shoulders, back, and chest while you walk off fat with this double-duty routine. Refer to pages 90 to 96 to refresh your memory on how to do the toning exercises.

TIME	ACTIVITY	INTENSITY
0:00–4:00	Warm-Up (4 min)	3→5
4:00–4:45	Pull-Down, right arm (45 sec; 20 reps)	5–6
4:45–5:45	Brisk Walk (1 min)	6–7
5:45–6:30	Pull-Down, left arm (45 sec; 20 reps)	5–6
6:30–7:30	Brisk Walk (1 min)	6–7
7:30–8:15	Front Press (45 sec; 20 reps)	5–6
8:15–9:15	Brisk Walk (1 min)	6–7
9:15–10:00	Row, right arm (45 sec; 20 reps)	5–6
10:00–11:00	Brisk Walk (1 min)	6–7
11:00–11:45	Row, left arm (45 sec; 20 reps)	5–6
11:45–12:45	Brisk Walk (1 min)	6–7
12:45–13:30	Overhead Press (45 sec; 20 reps)	5–6
13:30–14:30	Brisk Walk (1 min)	6–7
14:30–15:15	Front Pull (45 sec; 20 reps)	5–6
15:15–16:15	Brisk Walk (1 min)	6–7
16:15–17:00	Arm Pull (45 sec; 20 reps)	5–6
17:00–18:00	Brisk Walk (1 min)	6–7
18:00–20:00	Cool-Down (2 min)	5→3

LONG WALK I

The focus of this walk is duration, not speed. Choose a pace that is comfortable and that you feel confident in maintaining for the recommended time. By all means, walk longer if you feel good.

0:00–5:00	Warm-Up (5 min)	3→5
5:00–40:00	Easy to Moderate Walk (35 min)	4–6
40:00–45:00	Cool-Down (5 min)	5→3

> **Changes don't happen as quickly as we might want, but they do come when we persevere.**
>
> —YVONNE SHORB,
> **LOST 14 POUNDS AND 6½ INCHES ON THE WOW PROGRAM**

CONGRATULATIONS! YOU MADE IT through the hardest part of any weight loss program—getting started! And I bet you're already standing taller. Now that you know what to expect, this week should feel a little easier. You'll be repeating Week 1 almost exactly. The only changes are to increase your Long Walk from 45 minutes to 60 minutes and to increase the number of repetitions for the lower-body and core exercises. Go for it!

YOUR WORKOUT AT A GLANCE

DAY	ACTIVITY//WORKOUT	TOTAL
1	Basic Interval Walk I (30 min) // Lower-Body Strength Workout (15 min)	45 min
2	Toning Walk I (20 min)	20 min
3	Basic Interval Walk I (30 min) // Core Strength Workout (15 min)	45 min
4	Toning Walk I (20 min)	20 min
5	Basic Interval Walk I (30 min) // Lower-Body Strength Workout (15 min)	45 min
6	Long Walk II (60 min) // Core Strength Workout (15 min)	75 min
7	Rest	

WHAT YOU'LL **DO THIS WEEK**

3 x Basic Interval Walk I   2 x Toning Walk I   2 x Lower-Body Strength Workout

2 x Core Strength Workout   1 x Long Walk II

Workout Summary

THE DETAILS OF THE WALKING ROUTINES follow. See Toning Exercises on page 90 for descriptions of the Toning Walk moves.

LOWER-BODY STRENGTH WORKOUT
(page 81)

Do 8-10 reps of the following exercises:
- >> **Cross Leg Swing**
- >> **One-Leg Squat**
- >> **Rear Kick**
- >> **Reverse Lunge**
- >> **Moving Squat**

CORE ROUTINE STRENGTH WORKOUT
(page 97)

- >> **Plank** *(Hold once for 30 seconds)*

Do 8-10 reps of the following exercises:
- >> **Tabletop Balance**
- >> **Side Plank**
- >> **Roll Down**
- >> **Bicycle**

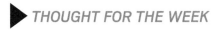
Don't Ignore Your Diet

ONE OF THE BIGGEST MISTAKES that I've seen people make when they start exercising is to increase their eating. In fact, a study published in the *International Journal of Obesity* found that when 35 overweight women and men started exercising, some of them compensated for their workouts by taking in as many as 270 extra calories a day—negating more than half of the calories they burned.[5] Some research shows that regular exercise can increase levels of ghrelin, an appetite-stimulating hormone, in an effort to protect the body from losing too much weight too quickly.[6]

But that's probably not the whole story. Many foods today contain loads of calories due to either lots of added fat and sugar or simply larger serving sizes. And it's all too easy to eat back the calories that you just burned off with exercise. A typical moderate 45-minute jaunt burns about 225 calories. Just having a glass of wine and a few crackers with brie is more than enough to wipe out the calorie deficit from your workout. Now you see why the scale might not budge. It's the last thing I want to happen to you when you're putting so much effort into your workouts. That's why I asked nutritionist Heidi McIndoo, RD, to design a delicious, easy-to-follow eating plan to accompany the Walk Off Weight program.

One of the best ways to avoid this weight loss saboteur is to pay attention to what you're eating when you start an exercise program. The Walk Off Weight eating plan in Chapter 7 makes it simple to do. Stick to the meal plans and guidelines, and you'll keep your appetite and calories under control, be properly fueled for your workouts—and lose more weight. Our WOW test panelists who followed both the diet and exercise plans lost nearly three times as many pounds as those who followed only the exercise program. And when one of our exercise-only participants, Laura Chiles, started the diet after completing the 8-week walking program, she lost an additional 13 pounds in just 4 weeks—four times more than she lost on the exercise plan alone. (See her story on page 176.)

Even if you don't want to follow a specific diet plan, if there's any chance that your eating habits may be an issue for you, I recommend that you start tracking your food intake. It's easier to say no to seconds, big portions, and high-calorie treats if you know you have to write them down. In one study, dieters who regularly recorded what they ate and when they exercised lost nearly twice as much weight as those who didn't keep track.[7] You can do this online at prevention.com/healthtracker or use the Walk Off Weight journal that starts on page 303.

**technique
FOCUS**

Up, Roll, Push

The heel-to-toe roll is key to powering a strong, quick stride.
1. As you step, focus on landing on your heel with your toes up in the air. If you hear slapping as you walk, that means you're landing flat-footed.
2. The next phase of the action is rolling from your heel to your toes as smoothly as possible.
3. Finally, push off with your toes as if you're kicking sand behind you.

BASIC INTERVAL WALK I

TIME	ACTIVITY	INTENSITY
0:00–5:00	Warm-Up (5 min)	3→5
5:00–6:00	Moderate (1 min)	5–6
6:00–6:30	Fast (30 sec)	7–8
6:30–7:30	Moderate (1 min)	5–6
7:30–8:00	Fast (30 sec)	7–8
8:00–9:00	Moderate (1 min)	5–6
9:00–9:30	Fast (30 sec)	7–8
9:30–10:30	Moderate (1 min)	5–6
10:30–11:00	Fast (30 sec)	7–8
11:00–12:00	Moderate (1 min)	5–6
12:00–12:30	Fast (30 sec)	7–8
12:30–13:30	Moderate (1 min)	5–6
13:30–14:00	Fast (30 sec)	7–8
14:00–15:00	Moderate (1 min)	5–6
15:00–15:30	Fast (30 sec)	7–8
15:30–16:30	Moderate (1 min)	5–6
16:30–17:00	Fast (30 sec)	7–8
17:00–18:00	Moderate (1 min)	5–6
18:00–18:30	Fast (30 sec)	7–8
18:30–19:30	Moderate (1 min)	5–6
19:30–20:00	Fast (30 sec)	7–8
20:00–21:00	Moderate (1 min)	5–6
21:00–21:30	Fast (30 sec)	7–8
21:30–22:30	Moderate (1 min)	5–6
22:30–23:00	Fast (30 sec)	7–8
23:00–24:00	Moderate (1 min)	5–6
24:00–24:30	Fast (30 sec)	7–8
24:30–25:30	Moderate (1 min)	5–6
25:30–30:00	Cool-Down (4.5 min)	5→3

TONING WALK I

TIME	ACTIVITY	INTENSITY
0:00–4:00	Warm-Up (4 min)	3→5
4:00–4:45	Pull-Down, right arm (45 sec; 20 reps)	5–6
4:45–5:45	Brisk Walk (1 min)	6–7
5:45–6:30	Pull-Down, left arm (45 sec; 20 reps)	5–6
6:30–7:30	Brisk Walk (1 min)	6–7
7:30–8:15	Front Press (45 sec; 20 reps)	5–6
8:15–9:15	Brisk Walk (1 min)	6–7
9:15–10:00	Row, right arm (45 sec; 20 reps)	5–6
10:00–11:00	Brisk Walk (1 min)	6–7
11:00–11:45	Row, left arm (45 sec; 20 reps)	5–6
11:45–12:45	Brisk Walk (1 min)	6–7
12:45–13:30	Overhead Press (45 sec; 20 reps)	5–6
13:30–14:30	Brisk Walk (1 min)	6–7
14:30–15:15	Front Pull (45 sec; 20 reps)	5–6
15:15–16:15	Brisk Walk (1 min)	6–7
16:15–17:00	Arm Pull (45 sec; 20 reps)	5–6
17:00–18:00	Brisk Walk (1 min)	6–7
18:00–20:00	Cool-Down (2 min)	5→3

LONG WALK II

0:00–5:00	Warm-Up (5 min)	3→5
5:00–55:00	Easy to Moderate Walk (50 min)	4–6
55:00–60:00	Cool-Down (5 min)	5→3

THAT INITAL BURST OF EXCITEMENT may be fading, but stay strong. Focus on all of the benefits that you're getting, like more energy. For this week's workouts, there are lots of changes. But you're ready for them! First, you'll increase the Interval Walk to 45 minutes. Next, you'll do about 30 reps of each of the band exercises in the Toning Walk, and you'll up the count for the other strength routines, too. Finally, you'll aim to add another 15 minutes to your Long Walk. If you can't do it all, that's okay. Just make progress, and you'll see changes.

YOUR WORKOUT AT A GLANCE

DAY	ACTIVITY//WORKOUT	TOTAL
1	Basic Interval Walk II (45 min) // Lower-Body Strength Workout (15 min)	60 min
2	Toning Walk II (25 min)	25 min
3	Basic Interval Walk II (45 min)// Core Strength Workout (15 min)	60 min
4	Toning Walk II (25 min)	25 min
5	Basic Interval Walk II (45 min) // Lower-Body Strength Workout (15 min)	60 min
6	Long Walk III (75 min) // Core Strength Workout (15 min)	90 min
7	Rest	

WHAT YOU'LL **DO THIS WEEK**

**3 x Basic Interval Walk II   2 x Toning Walk II   2 x Lower-Body Strength Workout
2 x Core Strength Workout   1 x Long Walk III**

Workout Summary

THE DETAILS OF THE WALKING ROUTINES follow. See Toning Exercises on page 90 for descriptions of the Toning Walk moves.

LOWER-BODY STRENGTH WORKOUT
(page 81)
Do 10-12 reps of the following exercises:
>> **Cross Leg Swing**
>> **One-Leg Squat**
>> **Rear Kicks**
>> **Reverse Lunge**
>> **Moving Squats**

CORE STRENGTH WORKOUT
(page 97)
>> **Plank** *(Hold once for 45 seconds)*
Do 10-12 reps of the following exercises:
>> **Tabletop Balance**
>> **Side Plank**
>> **Roll Down**
>> **Bicycle**

The Right Way to Use the Scale

IF YOU'VE BEEN CONSISTENTLY LOSING WEIGHT, good for you! But maybe you're not losing as fast as you'd like, or you're seeing a change in inches but not on the scale. Then again, you might still be waiting for those pounds to budge. They will, if you stick with it. After all, it's been only 3 weeks!

Don't let the number on the scale slow you down or make you start doubting yourself. Focus on where you're seeing the positive results—whether it's better-fitting clothes, a stronger body, lost inches, or more energy. Be proud of yourself for sticking with the program for 3 weeks. That's a huge accomplishment that many people never get to! In fact, I recently saw a survey in which people cited not seeing results fast enough as the number one reason for giving up on exercise. We are a society that wants quick fixes. The thing is, if you quit, you'll never see any results.

Besides, the scale is incredibly fickle, especially for women! It can fluctuate 5 or so pounds, depending on your menstrual cycle—and even more than that if you're peri-menopausal, when you may not have any idea where you are in your cycle. A super-sweaty workout can take off a pound or more—but drink some water, and you're right back to where you were (but don't let that discourage you from drinking plenty of water—in the long run, water will help you lose weight, I promise!). Load up on the sodium and watch the number rise (water can help counteract this effect). Weigh yourself right after a meal and then an hour or two later, and you'll get different numbers. I've seen a difference of up to 4 pounds just from morning to night; by the next morning, I was back to where I had been 24 hours earlier.

My point is that your body weight naturally fluctuates. That's why you shouldn't give the number on the scale the power to determine whether or not you're going to have a good day or a bad one, be in a good mood or a bad one, or succeed or fail. Other people don't see the number on the scale; they see how tall and confident you stand, how much energy you have, how strong and toned you are, and how much younger you're acting.

The weight didn't come on overnight, and it won't go away overnight, either. You're not going to get the kinds of numbers that you see on *The Biggest Loser* every week. That's just not the way it works in the real world. With a workout-focused program, a loss of $1/2$ pound a week is typical; 1 to 2 pounds a week is fabulous—and losing slow and steady may help you to keep those pounds off for good.

What's most important is the big picture—that over time, the number is headed in the right direction. But the path isn't going to be a straight line; it's going to be wavy.

Inch measurements and the fit of your clothes are much better indicators of how you're doing. So try to focus on those more and the scale less. And give it time. You're setting yourself up for long-term success—and you're getting loads of other health benefits along the way.

technique
FOCUS

Strong
Push-Off

The key to getting maximum acceleration from your push-off is to wait until your foot is behind you. You should have a longer stride behind you than in front of you. Then think of lifting your heel as you push off so that someone who is walking behind you could see the sole of your shoe.

BASIC INTERVAL WALK II

TIME	ACTIVITY	INTENSITY
0:00–5:00	Warm-Up (5 min)	3→5
5:00–6:00	Moderate (1 min)	5–6
6:00–6:30	Fast (30 sec)	7–8
6:30–7:30	Moderate (1 min)	5–6
7:30–8:00	Fast (30 sec)	7–8
8:00–9:00	Moderate (1 min)	5–6
9:00–9:30	Fast (30 sec)	7–8
9:30–10:30	Moderate (1 min)	5–6
10:30–11:00	Fast (30 sec)	7–8
11:00–12:00	Moderate (1 min)	5–6
12:00–12:30	Fast (30 sec)	7–8
12:30–13:30	Moderate (1 min)	5–6
13:30–14:00	Fast (30 sec)	7–8
14:00–15:00	Moderate (1 min)	5–6
15:00–15:30	Fast (30 sec)	7–8
15:30–16:30	Moderate (1 min)	5–6
16:30–17:00	Fast (30 sec)	7–8
17:00–18:00	Moderate (1 min)	5–6
18:00–18:30	Fast (30 sec)	7–8
18:30–19:30	Moderate (1 min)	5–6
19:30–20:00	Fast (30 sec)	7–8
20:00–21:00	Moderate (1 min)	5–6
21:00–21:30	Fast (30 sec)	7–8
21:30–22:30	Moderate (1 min)	5–6

TIME	ACTIVITY	INTENSITY
22:30–23:00	Fast (30 sec)	7–8
23:00–24:00	Moderate (1 min)	5–6
24:00–24:30	Fast (30 sec)	7–8
24:30–25:30	Moderate (1 min)	5–6
25:30–26:00	Fast (30 sec)	7–8
26:00–27:00	Moderate (1 min)	5–6
27:00–27:30	Fast (30 sec)	7–8
27:30–28:30	Moderate (1 min)	5–6
28:30–29:00	Fast (30 sec)	7–8
29:00–30:00	Moderate (1 min)	5–6
30:00–30:30	Fast (30 sec)	7–8
30:30–31:30	Moderate (1 min)	5–6
31:30–32:00	Fast (30 sec)	7–8
32:00–33:00	Moderate (1 min)	5–6
33:00–33:30	Fast (30 sec)	7–8
33:30–34:30	Moderate (1 min)	5–6
34:30–35:00	Fast (30 sec)	7–8
35:00–36:00	Moderate (1 min)	5–6
36:00–36:30	Fast (30 sec)	7–8
36:30–37:30	Moderate (1 min)	5–6
37:30–38:00	Fast (30 sec)	7–8
38:00–39:00	Moderate (1 min)	5–6
39:00–39:30	Fast (30 sec)	7–8
39:30–40:30	Moderate (1 min)	5–6
40:30–45:00	Cool-Down (4.5 min)	5→3

TONING WALK II

TIME	ACTIVITY	INTENSITY
0:00–5:00	Warm-Up (5 min)	3→5
5:00–6:00	Pull-Down, right arm (1 min; 30 reps)	5–6
6:00–7:00	Brisk Walk (1 min)	6–7
7:00–8:00	Pull-Down, left arm (1 min; 30 reps)	5–6
8:00–9:00	Brisk Walk (1 min)	6–7
9:00–10:00	Front Press (1 min; 30 reps)	5–6
10:00–11:00	Brisk Walk (1 min)	6–7
11:00–12:00	Row, right arm (1 min; 30 reps)	5–6
12:00–13:00	Brisk Walk (1 min)	6–7
13:00–14:00	Row, left arm (1 min; 30 reps)	5–6
14:00–15:00	Brisk Walk (1 min)	6–7
15:00–16:00	Overhead Press (1 min; 30 reps)	5–6
16:00–17:00	Brisk Walk (1 min)	6–7
17:00–18:00	Front Pull (1 min; 30 reps)	5–6
18:00–19:00	Brisk Walk (1 min)	6–7
19:00–20:00	Arm Pull (1 min; 30 reps)	5–6
20:00–21:00	Brisk Walk (1 min)	6–7
21:00–25:00	Cool-Down (4 min)	5→3

LONG WALK III

TIME	ACTIVITY	INTENSITY
0:00–5:00	Warm-Up (5 min)	3→5
5:00–70:00	Easy to Moderate Walk (65 min)	4–6
70:00–75:00	Cool-Down (5 min)	5→3

YOU'RE JUST ABOUT READY FOR Phase 2; way to go! Keep up the good work. You'll be rewarded with shorter workouts next week. But for now, let's focus on this week. The workout schedule is almost identical to Week 3. Just add some more reps to your strength workouts, and try to hit 90 minutes for your Long Walk. You can go even longer, if you feel good and have the time. You might be amazed by what your body is capable of doing!

YOUR WORKOUT AT A GLANCE

DAY	ACTIVITY//WORKOUT	TOTAL
1	Basic Interval Walk II (45 min) // Lower-Body Strength Workout (15 min)	60 min
2	Toning Walk II (25 min)	25 min
3	Basic Interval Walk II (45 min)// Core Strength Workout (15 min)	60 min
4	Toning Walk II (25 min)	25 min
5	Basic Interval Walk II (45 min) // Lower-Body Strength Workout (15 min)	60 min
6	Long Walk IV (90 min) // Core Strength Workout (15 min)	105 min
7	Rest	

WHAT YOU'LL **DO THIS WEEK**

**3 x Basic Interval Walk II   2 x Toning Walk II   2 x Lower-Body Strength Workout
2 x Core Strength Workout   1 x Long Walk IV**

Workout Summary

THE DETAILS OF THE WALKING ROUTINES follow. See Toning Exercises on page 90 for descriptions of the Toning Walk moves.

LOWER-BODY STRENGTH WORKOUT
(page 81)
Do 12–15 reps of the following exercises:
>> **Cross Leg Swing**
>> **One-Leg Squat**
>> **Rear Kick**
>> **Reverse Lunge**
>> **Moving Squat**

CORE STRENGTH WORKOUT
(page 97)
>> **Plank** *(Hold once for 1 minute)*
Do 12–15 reps of the following exercises:
>> **Tabletop Balance**
>> **Side Plank**
>> **Roll Down**
>> **Bicycle**

Move All Day Long

IF YOU'RE STICKING WITH THE WOW PROGRAM, you've been exercising about an hour almost every day of the week. That is a huge accomplishment! But what are you doing the other 23 hours a day? Hopefully, you're sleeping for 7 to 8 of them. That leaves about 15 hours.

For most Americans, too many of those hours are spent sitting in front of a computer, in a car, or on the sofa. And surprisingly, you may be doing more of that since you started exercising. In a study from the Netherlands, researchers found that when a group of women and men—average age 59—started working out twice a week, their everyday activity level decreased by 22 percent.[8]

Scientists don't know exactly why some people slow down when they start an exercise program; for others, in fact, working out can have the exact opposite effect. Our WOW test panelists regularly reported having so much more energy that they were going on bike rides, swimming with their kids, mowing the lawn, taking extra walks with friends, and even cleaning out their garages—all on top of their workouts. If that sounds like you, awesome! Keep it up! All that extra activity will only help you to become fitter, healthier, and slimmer over time.

On the other hand, if you're not seeing an uptick in your everyday activity—and especially if you haven't really lost any weight to this point—it's time to get moving. One of the reasons for the slowdown may be postworkout fatigue. You can avoid this by making sure that you're getting enough sleep at night and that you're eating properly—choosing foods such as whole grains, fruits, vegetables, lean proteins, and healthy fats that provide all-day energy. Refined foods such as white bread, white pasta, and processed foods loaded with sugar will give you quick bursts of energy, but they won't keep you going hour after hour.

Next, make sure that you're moving throughout the day. A simple pedometer can help you keep tabs on this type of activity (see page 42). For a more detailed assessment, especially of things such as fidgeting or standing instead of sitting (yes, all these little actions add up!), try a device such as the BodyBugg, which monitors all types of activity, not just walking. While these actions may seem insignificant, they can have a big impact on your ability to lose weight. Over the course of a day, they can add up to an extra 350 calories burned, according to Mayo Clinic studies.[9]

Moving throughout the day, not just during workouts, is essential to maximize your body's fat-burning ability and make weight loss easier. Research has shown that a decrease in everyday activities may shut down an enzyme that controls fat metabolism.[10] And even a half hour or an hour workout a day isn't enough to turn it back on. You need regular activity throughout the day.

technique
FOCUS

Quicker, Shorter Steps
One of the most common mistakes people make when they try to walk faster is that they take steps that are too long. The secret to speed is taking more, quicker steps, not excessively long ones. Think short as you step forward, keeping your stride more underneath and behind you. A great way to push yourself to take quicker, shorter steps is to track your number of steps and then aim to increase it over the course of the program.

CHAPTER 5 WOW PHASE 1: WEEKS 1–4

BASIC INTERVAL WALK II

TIME	ACTIVITY	INTENSITY
0:00–5:00	Warm-Up (5 min)	3→5
5:00–6:00	Moderate (1 min)	5–6
6:00–6:30	Fast (30 sec)	7–8
6:30–7:30	Moderate (1 min)	5–6
7:30–8:00	Fast (30 sec)	7–8
8:00–9:00	Moderate (1 min)	5–6
9:00–9:30	Fast (30 sec)	7–8
9:30–10:30	Moderate (1 min)	5–6
10:30–11:00	Fast (30 sec)	7–8
11:00–12:00	Moderate (1 min)	5–6
12:00–12:30	Fast (30 sec)	7–8
12:30–13:30	Moderate (1 min)	5–6
13:30–14:00	Fast (30 sec)	7–8
14:00–15:00	Moderate (1 min)	5–6
15:00–15:30	Fast (30 sec)	7–8
15:30–16:30	Moderate (1 min)	5–6
16:30–17:00	Fast (30 sec)	7–8
17:00–18:00	Moderate (1 min)	5–6
18:00–18:30	Fast (30 sec)	7–8
18:30–19:30	Moderate (1 min)	5–6
19:30–20:00	Fast (30 sec)	7–8
20:00–21:00	Moderate (1 min)	5–6
21:00–21:30	Fast (30 sec)	7–8
21:30–22:30	Moderate (1 min)	5–6

TIME	ACTIVITY	INTENSITY
22:30–23:00	Fast (30 sec)	7–8
23:00–24:00	Moderate (1 min)	5–6
24:00–24:30	Fast (30 sec)	7–8
24:30–25:30	Moderate (1 min)	5–6
25:30–26:00	Fast (30 sec)	7–8
26:00–27:00	Moderate (1 min)	5–6
27:00–27:30	Fast (30 sec)	7–8
27:30–28:30	Moderate (1 min)	5–6
28:30–29:00	Fast (30 sec)	7–8
29:00–30:00	Moderate (1 min)	5–6
30:00–30:30	Fast (30 sec)	7–8
30:30–31:30	Moderate (1 min)	5–6
31:30–32:00	Fast (30 sec)	7–8
32:00–33:00	Moderate (1 min)	5–6
33:00–33:30	Fast (30 sec)	7–8
33:30–34:30	Moderate (1 min)	5–6
34:30–35:00	Fast (30 sec)	7–8
35:00–36:00	Moderate (1 min)	5–6
36:00–36:30	Fast (30 sec)	7–8
36:30–37:30	Moderate (1 min)	5–6
37:30–38:00	Fast (30 sec)	7–8
38:00–39:00	Moderate (1 min)	5–6
39:00–39:30	Fast (30 sec)	7–8
39:30–40:30	Moderate (1 min)	5–6
40:30–45:00	Cool-Down (4.5 min)	5→3

TONING WALK II

TIME	ACTIVITY	INTENSITY
0:00–5:00	Warm-Up (5 min)	3→5
5:00–6:00	Pull-Down, right arm (1 min; 30 reps)	5–6
6:00–7:00	Brisk Walk (1 min)	6–7
7:00–8:00	Pull-Down, left arm (1 min; 30 reps)	5–6
8:00–9:00	Brisk Walk (1 min)	6–7
9:00–10:00	Front Press (1 min; 30 reps)	5–6
10:00–11:00	Brisk Walk (1 min)	6–7
11:00–12:00	Row, right arm (1 min; 30 reps)	5–6
12:00–13:00	Brisk Walk (1 min)	6–7
13:00–14:00	Row, left arm (1 min; 30 reps)	5–6
14:00–15:00	Brisk Walk (1 min)	6–7
15:00–16:00	Overhead Press (1 min; 30 reps)	5–6
16:00–17:00	Brisk Walk (1 min)	6–7
17:00–18:00	Front Pull (1 min; 30 reps)	5–6
18:00–19:00	Brisk Walk (1 min)	6–7
19:00–20:00	Arm Pull (1 min; 30 reps)	5–6
20:00–21:00	Brisk Walk (1 min)	6–7
21:00–25:00	Cool-Down (4 min)	5→3

LONG WALK IV

0:00–5:00	Warm-Up (5 min)	3→5
5:00–85:00	Easy to Moderate Walk (80 min)	4–6
85:00–90:00	Cool-Down (5 min)	5→3

AGE: 50 HEIGHT: 5'7"
POUNDS LOST: $10^{3}/_{4}$
INCHES LOST: $9^{1}/_{2}$ overall, including 3 from her waist
MAJOR ACCOMPLISHMENT: Lowered her total cholesterol by 51 points and her LDL cholesterol by 44 points

A Workout Change Jump-Starts Results

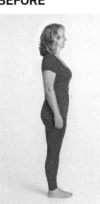

BEFORE

AFTER

DENISE JENNINGS had been following the same routine for years, reluctantly rising in the dark three times a week to head to a gloomy gym for an early-morning workout and doing her best to stick to a low-fat diet. But it wasn't working. Not only was she bored out of her mind, but her weight had been steadily rising over the last decade.

The WOW program changed all of that. "I knew that the food logging would keep me accountable, and the exercise schedule seemed more realistic for my changing lifestyle," Denise explained.

As fate would have it, just a few days after starting WOW, Denise was off to Rome for a family vacation. She seized the opportunity to learn to shop for food in an entirely new culture—not to mention language! "It was a lot easier than I'd imagined," Denise said, thanks to smaller portions. "Italian bread is sliced small and thin, not the giant slices we're used to in the United States." She could even treat herself, thanks to the inch-long cannolis she discovered. "At home, cannolis are more than double that!"

WOW also changed Denise's perspective on exercise.

"In the past, I thought that I had to run or do some other vigorous gym-type exercise to get noticeable results, but I'd been doing that for years without getting anywhere," Denise added. By not having to drive to and from the gym, Denise was actually spending less time on exercise. Even the workouts were shorter than the ones she got from a personal trainer, yet she was seeing better results. A few weeks into the program, she reported, "I love that my short-sleeve tops are not as tight around my arms."

At the gym, Denise said, she always felt like a hamster on a wheel: "Why go faster if you're going nowhere?" But walking outdoors helped her shave 1 minute and 20 seconds off her time when we tested how quickly she could complete a mile.

Denise is also more consistent with her training now. "Before, if I missed a morning gym workout, I would never work out at night. Now, I'd go in the afternoon or evening. That's how much I love it!"

And she loves the results. "The other night, my daughter and I were walking to the car, and she said, 'So, Mom, is this how fast you're going to walk everywhere you go now?'" laughed Denise. "I didn't even know I was being speedy. It just feels easier because I'm stronger now."

P.S. *Three months after the official end of the program, Denise recorded an additional $2^{1}/_{2}$-pound weight loss and shaved another $3^{1}/_{2}$ inches off her figure, for a grand total of $13^{1}/_{4}$ pounds and 13 inches lost in 5 months.*

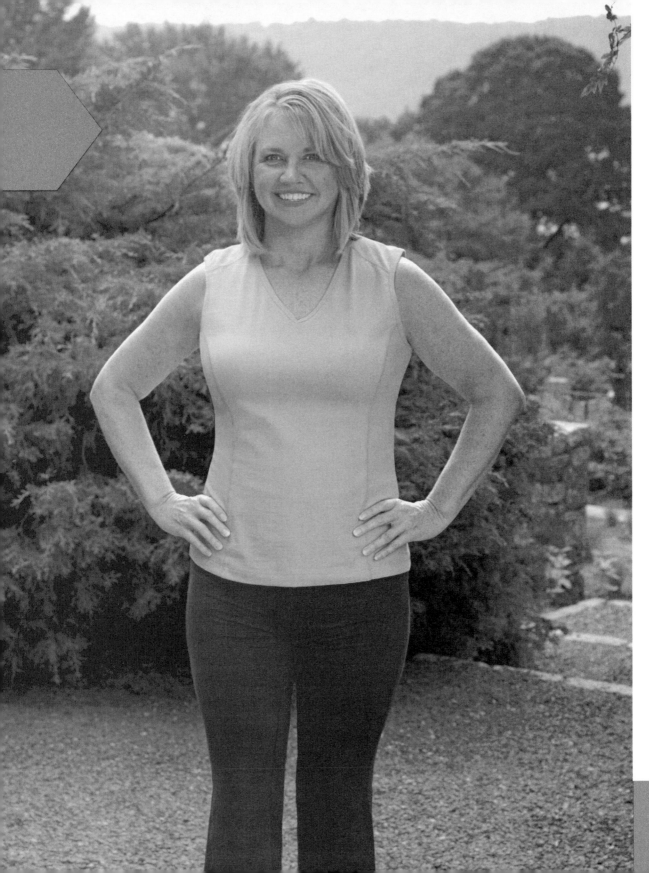

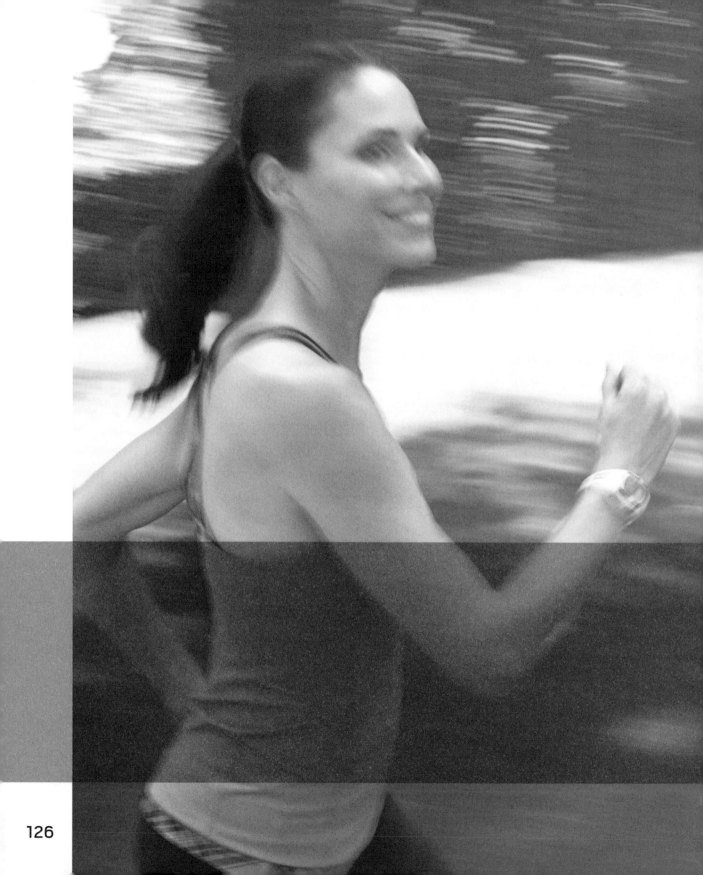

6

WOW PHASE 2:
WEEKS 5–8

WOO-HOO! YOU'RE HALFWAY THROUGH THE WOW PROGRAM. Congratulations! According to one survey, nearly a quarter of the people who start an exercise program drop out after just 2 weeks. But not you! You've hung in there, making yours a true success story already. And the best is yet to come!

Phase 2 of the WOW program challenges your body in new ways with fresh workouts to keep those fabulous results coming! The focus is on shorter, more vigorous bouts of exercise, which means turning up the speed. Your interval workouts will be just 20 or 30 minutes, with shorter but more intense bouts of very fast walking. And each week, you'll challenge yourself to cover a mile as fast as possible.

For the strength workouts, you'll be doing one total-body routine, instead of isolating body parts and doing multiple moves for each.

Now ready, set . . . let's go!

Phase 2: AT A GLANCE

HIGHER-INTENSITY, SHORTER-DURATION TRAINING

WEEK	DAY 1	DAY 2	DAY 3	DAY 4	DAY 5	DAY 6	DAY 7
5	Supercharged Interval Walk I **20 MIN TOTAL**	Recovery Walk 20 min **Total-Body Strength Workout** 20 min **40 MIN TOTAL**	Supercharged Interval Walk I **20 MIN TOTAL**	Recovery Walk 20 min **Total-Body Strength Workout** 20 min **40 MIN TOTAL**	Supercharged Interval Walk I **20 MIN TOTAL**	Speed Walk **<30 MIN TOTAL**	Rest
6	Supercharged Interval Walk I **20 MIN TOTAL**	Recovery Walk 20 min **Total-Body Strength Workout** 20 min **40 MIN TOTAL**	Supercharged Interval Walk I **20 MIN TOTAL**	Recovery Walk 20 min **Total-Body Strength Workout** 20 min **40 MIN TOTAL**	Supercharged Interval Walk I **20 MIN TOTAL**	Speed Walk **<30 MIN TOTAL**	Rest
7	Supercharged Interval Walk II **30 MIN TOTAL**	Recovery Walk 25 min **Total-Body Strength Workout** 20 min **45 MIN TOTAL**	Supercharged Interval Walk II **30 MIN TOTAL**	Recovery Walk 25 min **Total-Body Strength Workout** 20 min **45 MIN TOTAL**	Supercharged Interval Walk II **30 MIN TOTAL**	Speed Walk **<30 MIN TOTAL**	Rest
8	Supercharged Interval Walk II **30 MIN TOTAL**	Recovery Walk 25 min **Total-Body Strength Workout** 20 min **45 MIN TOTAL**	Supercharged Interval Walk II **30 MIN TOTAL**	Recovery Walk 25 min **Total-Body Strength Workout** 20 min **45 MIN TOTAL**	Supercharged Interval Walk II **30 MIN TOTAL**	Speed Walk **<30 MIN TOTAL**	Rest

TOTAL-BODY STRENGTH WORKOUT

THESE MOVES WORK YOUR UPPER AND LOWER BODY at the same time. Do this routine two or three times a week, taking a 30- to 60-second break between moves. Each week, you'll be increasing the number of repetitions. Here's what you should try to aim for, repeating on each side when appropriate:

WEEK 5: 8–10 reps
WEEK 6: 10–12 reps
WEEK 7: 15–17 reps
WEEK 8: 18–20 reps

If you find that you're wobbly when doing any of these moves, lightly hold onto something sturdy such as the back of a chair or the wall to help maintain your balance, at least to start out.

If you're doing this workout separate from your walks, warm up first by walking at an easy pace for about 5 minutes. Then do these moves to prepare your torso muscles for their workout: Roll your shoulders forward and back; twist your torso to the left and right, reaching the opposite arm across your chest; and reach each arm overhead, stretching to the opposite side.

How to Use the Resistance Band

For some of the moves, you'll need a sturdy place to hold the center or one end of your band. For a floor-level anchor, slide the band under a heavy piece of furniture, or loop or tie it around a sturdy object such as a railing or sofa leg. For a waist-level anchor, loop or tie the band to a railing or doorknob (stand so that the door swings away from you, then close it). You can also put a knot in the band and pinch it in a door or window, or purchase a door anchor to attach it (see Resources on page 320 for more information). No matter where you anchor the band, always check that it is secure before beginning an exercise. I can tell you from personal experience that a band snapping off an anchor point really hurts.

Stretching and releasing the band's resistance with control is key to maximizing toning and avoiding injury. Don't let the band snap back once you've reached the top of a move; pause, then slowly release, resisting against the band's pull as you do. To increase resistance, shorten the band by folding it lengthwise, adjusting your hand position to choke up on it, or wrapping it around your hands. To reduce resistance, give yourself more slack by moving your hands farther apart or farther away from the anchor point.

Balancing Deadlift with Arm Raise
(targets glutes, legs, abs, and shoulders)

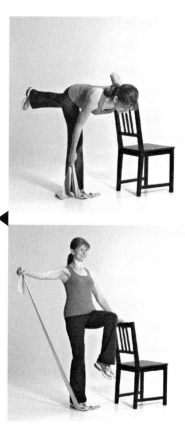

MAIN MOVE
Stand with one end of a resistance band under your right foot and hold the other end in your right hand. With your left hand, lightly hold onto a chair for balance. Slowly hinge forward from your hips, lowering your torso toward the floor as your left leg rises behind you, as far as comfortable or until your body and leg are parallel to the floor. Choke up on the band as you lower. Squeeze your glutes and stand back up, raising your left knee in front of you. Release a little of the band, then raise your right arm out to the side up to shoulder height. Hold, then slowly lower and repeat.

Make it easier: When you stand back up, lower your foot to the floor instead of lifting your knee in front of you.

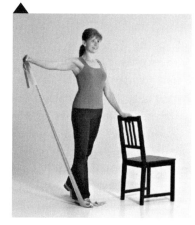

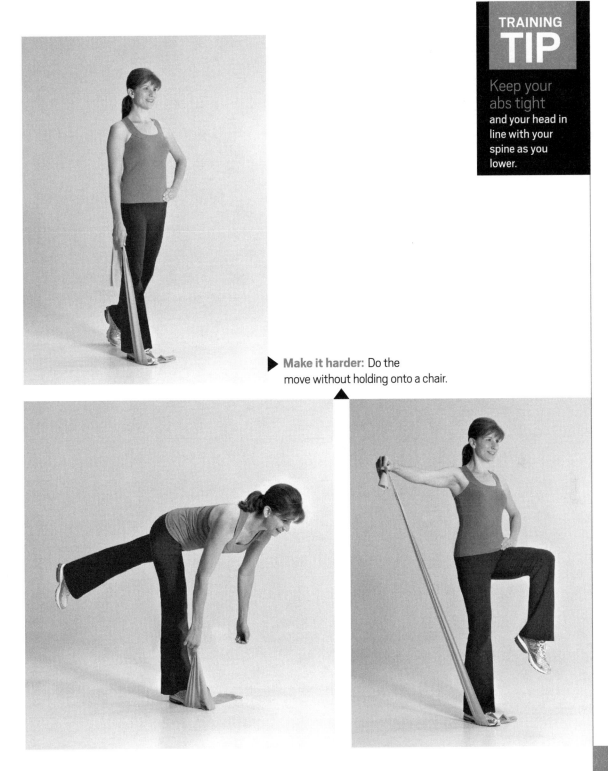

TRAINING
TIP

Keep your
abs tight
and your head in
line with your
spine as you
lower.

▶ **Make it harder:** Do the
move without holding onto a chair.

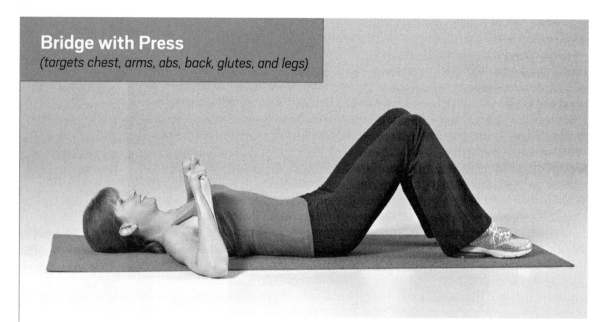

Bridge with Press
(targets chest, arms, abs, back, glutes, and legs)

MAIN MOVE

Sit on the floor and loop a resistance band around your upper back so that it's under your armpits. Lie on your back with your knees bent and your feet about a foot from your butt. Grasp each end of the band with your hands near your chest, palms facing forward, with your elbows pointing out. Contract your abs and glutes and lift your butt off the floor so that your body forms a straight line from your shoulders to your knees. At the same time, straighten your arms, pressing your hands toward the ceiling. Hold for a second before lowering your arms, then your body.

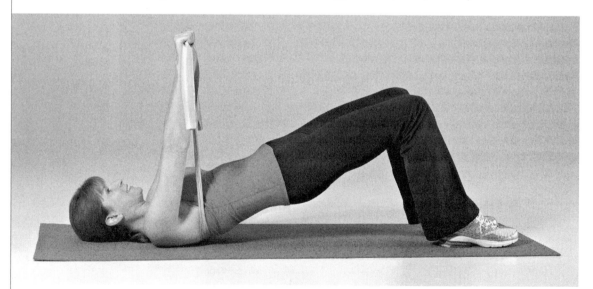

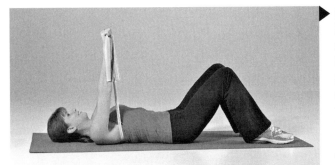

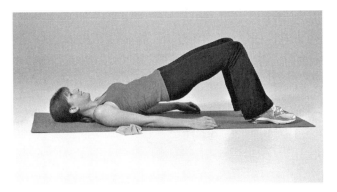

Make it easier:
Do the moves separately. Keeping your butt on the floor, press your arms straight up toward the ceiling and then lower. Perform all the reps with your arms, then relax your arms at your sides and switch to the butt lifts. Contracting your abs and glutes, lift your butt off the floor and then lower. Perform all the reps.

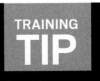
Make it harder:
Raise your right foot off the floor, extending your leg, and perform the exercise. Switch legs halfway through the reps.

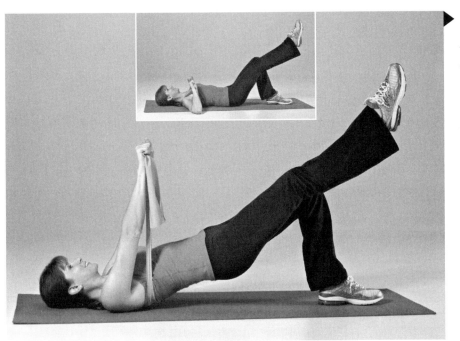

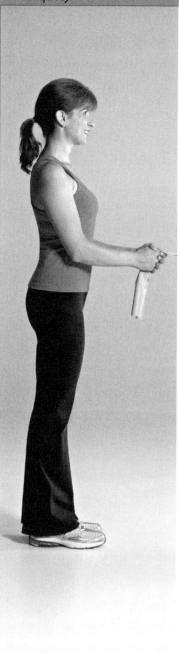

Rotating Lunge
(targets legs, glutes, and obliques)

MAIN MOVE

Anchor the center of a resistance band at about waist level by tying it to a door handle or putting a knot in the band and pinching it in a door (check that it's secure before you begin). Stand facing the band, holding the ends with both hands so the band is taut. Your feet should be together, your arms out in front at about waist height, and your elbows bent. Step your left foot behind you 2 to 3 feet, with your toes pointing forward. Bend your knees and lower until your right knee is bent 90 degrees, keeping your knee over your ankle. At the same time, rotate your torso to the right. Hold, then press into your right foot to stand back up and rotate back to center.

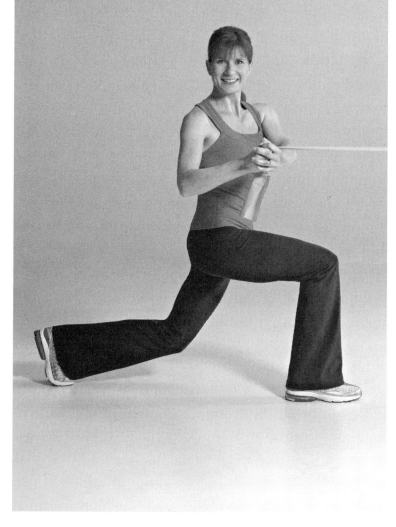

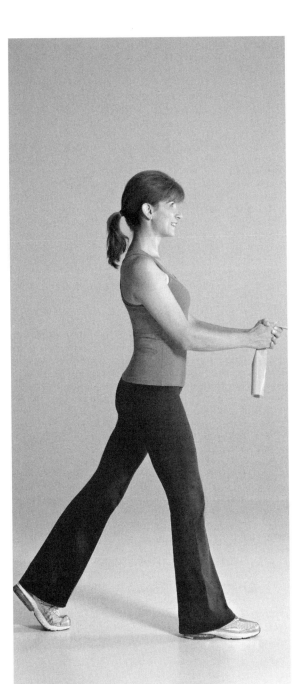

TRAINING
TIP

Don't lean forward as you lower toward the floor. Your torso should stay straight, with your ears over your shoulders, your shoulders over your hips, and the knee of your back leg under your hips or slightly behind them.

Make it easier: Do the move with your feet stationary, one in front of the other, 2 to 3 feet apart.

Make it harder: As you stand back up, raise your left knee in front of you before stepping back into the next lunge.

Row with Leg Swing
(targets upper back, hips, and glutes)

MAIN MOVE ◀

Anchor a resistance band at about waist level. Stand facing the band, holding an end in each hand, with your feet together and your arms extended in front of you. Bend your elbows and pull your arms back, squeezing your shoulder blades together and keeping your arms close to your body, until your hands are near your hips and elbows are pointing behind you. At the same time, raise your left knee in front of you to hip height. Extend your arms back out in front of you and swing your left leg behind you, flexing your foot and squeezing your glutes as you do. Continue without lowering your left foot to the floor.

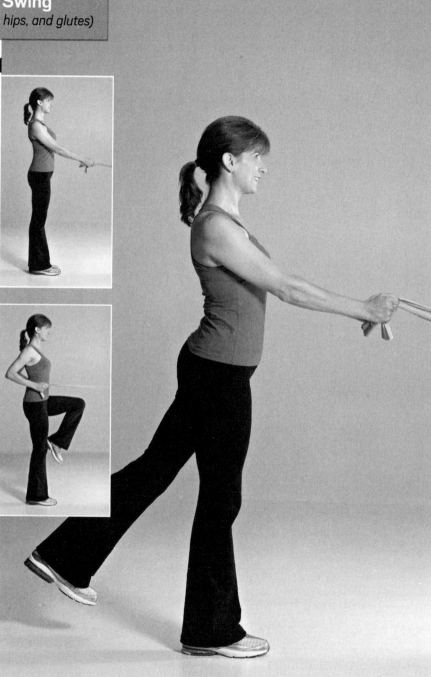

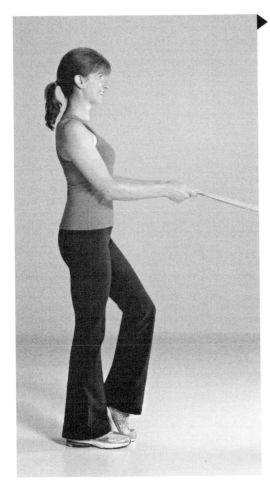

Make it easier: Skip the backward leg swing and instead lower your foot to the floor after each knee lift. Or, keep doing the backward leg swing, but touch your foot to the floor in between the knee lift and the leg swing to help stabilize you.

TRAINING TIP

Keep your abs tight and don't lean forward, especially as you raise your leg behind you. If you're having trouble balancing, hold onto something sturdy with one hand and do single arm rows for half the reps, then switch sides.

Make it harder: When your leg is extended behind you, pulse it three times, raising and lowering it an inch or so, before bringing it forward into the knee lift.

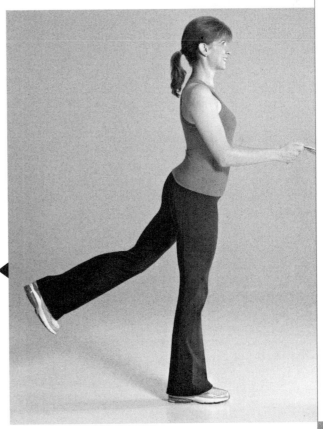

Crunch and Extend
(targets abs and arms)

MAIN MOVE

Anchor the center of a resistance band near the floor and lie so that it's behind your head. Grasp each end with your hands and bend your arms so that your elbows point up and your hands are on either side of your head. Contract your abs and curl your head and shoulders off the floor, keeping your arms stationary. Hold the crunch position and extend your arms. Hold, then slowly bend your arms and lower your head.

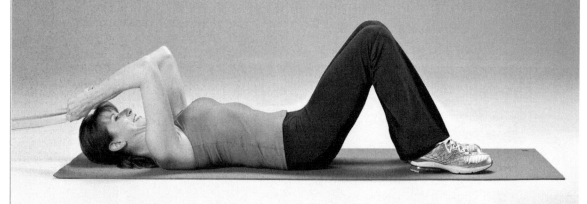

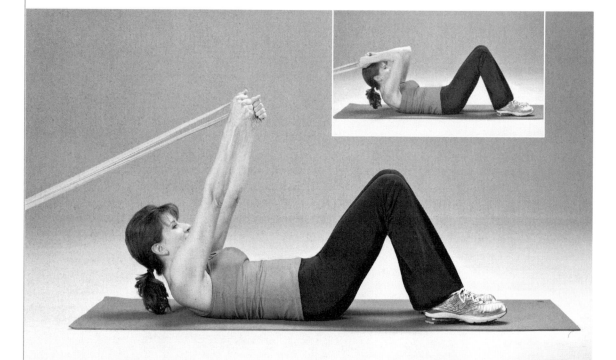

Make it easier:
Do the moves separately. Keeping your head on the floor, extend and bend your arms. Perform all the reps with your arms, then drop the band and switch to the crunches. Place your fingertips behind your head with your elbows out. Contracting your abs, curl your head and shoulders off the floor and then lower, performing all the reps.

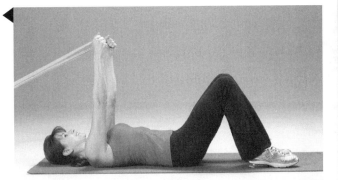

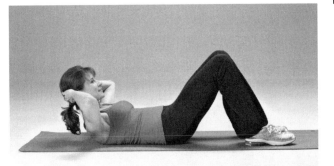

TRAINING TIP

Don't pull your chin down toward your chest. You should be able to fit your fist between your chin and chest at all times to avoid straining your neck.

Make it harder:
Extend your legs up toward the ceiling, keeping them raised throughout all the movements and all the reps.

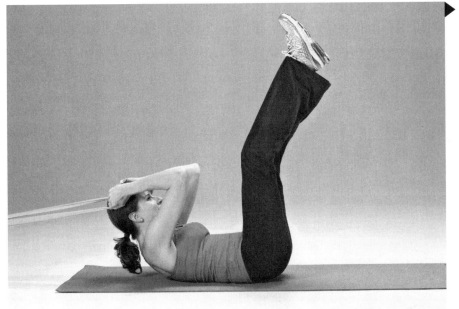

Elevated Squat with Curl
(targets legs, butt, and arms)

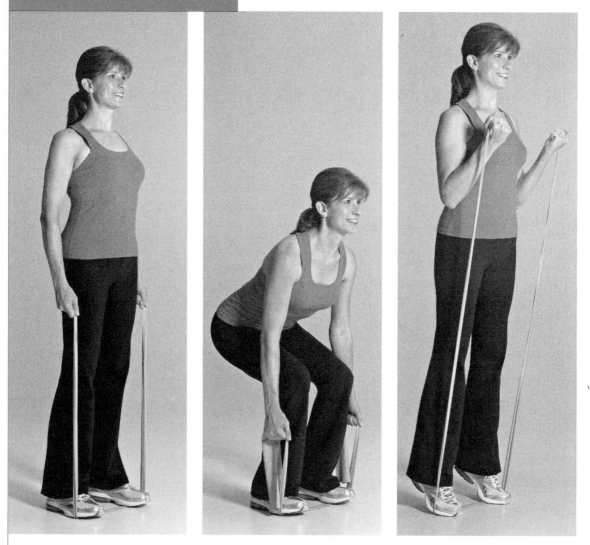

MAIN MOVE

Stand with a resistance band under the balls of your feet, with your feet about shoulder-width apart, your toes pointing forward, and your arms at your sides. Holding one end of the band in each hand, bend your hips and knees, sitting back as if you were lowering into a chair. Choke up on the band for resistance, then stand up. Release some of the band to bend your elbows and raise your hands toward your shoulders. Finally, lift your heels off the floor so that you're balancing on your toes. Lower your heels, then your arms.

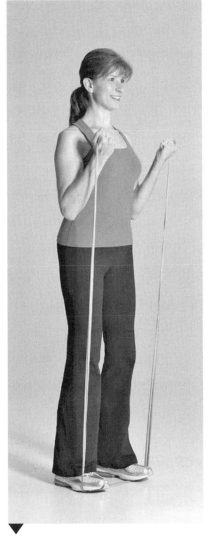

Make it easier: Skip the heel lift, keeping your feet flat on the floor the entire time.

Make it harder: In the squat position, raise your heels off the floor (your knees will be past your toes, it's okay); then stand up while balancing on your toes.

☞ **Never skip your warm-up, cool-down, and stretches.** *See page 54 for more details about when and how to do them.*

THIS WEEK, YOUR WORKOUTS SHRINK, but that doesn't mean they're less effective. The focus for this phase of the WOW program is quality, not quantity. You'll make up for fewer minutes by pushing yourself harder. But don't panic; I know you can do it.

For your Speed Walk, you'll need to map out a 1-mile route that's relatively flat. (You'll be using the same route every week, so keep that in mind.) You can go to a track (most are ¼ mile, so four laps will do it) or a marked path; use a GPS device (page 42); or premeasure a route in your car, on a bike with an odometer, or at mapmywalk.com. Another option: Do your Speed Walk on a treadmill.

YOUR WORKOUT AT A GLANCE

DAY	ACTIVITY//WORKOUT	TOTAL
1	Supercharged Interval Walk I (20 min)	20 min
2	Recovery Walk (20 min) // Total-Body Strength Workout (20 min)	40 min
3	Supercharged Interval Walk I (20 min)	20 min
4	Recovery Walk (20 min) // Total-Body Strength Workout (20 min)	40 min
5	Supercharged Interval Walk I (20 min)	20 min
6	Speed Walk (<30 min) // Total-Body Strength Workout (20 min, optional)	about 50 min
7	Rest	

WHAT YOU'LL **DO THIS WEEK**

3 x Supercharged Interval Walk I ○ 2 x or 3 x Total-Body Strength Workout
2 x Recovery Walk ○ 1 x Speed Walk

Workout Summary

THE DETAILS OF THE WALKING ROUTINES follow.

TOTAL-BODY STRENGTH WORKOUT (page 129)
Do 8-10 reps of the following exercises:
>> **Balancing Deadlift with Arm Raise**
>> **Bridge with Press**
>> **Rotating Lunge**
>> **Row with Leg Swing**
>> **Crunch and Extend**
>> **Elevated Squat with Curl**

You Can Survive Slipups

IT HAPPENS TO THE BEST OF US. Whether you're starting an exercise program, trying to improve your eating habits, or making some other healthy behavior change, you usually start out strong. For the first few weeks or even months, you're right on track. And then . . . you slip!

It might be a week of missed workouts because of a big project at work or a one-night binge after a fight with your spouse. The details don't matter. What's most important is that as soon as you realize what's happened, you skip the guilt, pick yourself up, and immediately—I mean immediately, not after one more spoonful of ice cream or another night of channel surfing—get back on track. That very moment, brush your teeth so you don't eat anymore, drink a tall glass of icy cold water, munch on some crunchy carrots, put on your sneakers and take a walk, turn on some music and dance around your living room, pump out some crunches and push-ups, or simply go to bed—whatever is necessary to catch yourself and prevent a slip from becoming a fall and spiralling out of control.

I was so proud of Susan Moyer, one of our test panelists, when she did exactly this. Here's what she wrote in her weekly log:

"One night, I fell back into my old bad habit of destressing after work by eating. I ate a medium-size bag of hard pretzels and frozen yogurt right from the container while sitting in front of the TV. When I stopped and recognized what I was doing, I realized that I don't have to mindlessly eat to destress. Walking or calling a friend or getting outside—anything else—is better than watching TV and mindlessly channel surfing and eating."

She's absolutely correct. And because she didn't let this one slip—or any of the others that she's had since completing the program—trip her up, Susan shed an additional $7\frac{1}{2}$ pounds when we did a 3-month follow-up for a total weight loss of $24\frac{3}{4}$ pounds.

Research supports that you don't have to be perfect to succeed at weight loss. At Brown University, researchers put 142 overweight people on the same weight loss program. The key difference: One group followed the plan for 14 straight weeks; another took a 6-week hiatus at the midpoint; and the third group took a 2-week break every few weeks. Eleven months later, everybody had lost an average of 16 pounds.[1] The lesson here is to not beat yourself up for slipping but instead get back on track. You'll still see great results.

---

technique FOCUS

Pull
Instead of letting momentum direct your arm swing, take control and put some power into it. Focus on the muscles in the middle of your upper back, pulling each arm back toward your hip.

Squeeze
Each time your heel strikes the ground, your glutes should contract. Pay attention to it. Put your hand on your butt and feel it. Use these powerful muscles to pull your body over your front leg and propel you forward.

SUPERCHARGED INTERVAL WALK I

During this workout, you'll be doing 15-second high-intensity speed bursts. The intervals are super-short so that you can really push yourself to the max. Then, you'll recover for 30 seconds.

TIME	ACTIVITY	INTENSITY
0:00–5:00	Warm-Up (5 min)	3→5
5:00–6:00	Moderate (1 min)	5–6
6:00–6:15	Very Fast (15 sec)	8–9
6:15–6:45	Easy to Moderate (30 sec)	4–6
6:45–7:00	Very Fast (15 sec)	8–9
7:00–7:30	Easy to Moderate (30 sec)	4–6
7:30–7:45	Very Fast (15 sec)	8–9
7:45–8:15	Easy to Moderate (30 sec)	4–6
8:15–8:30	Very Fast (15 sec)	8–9
8:30–9:00	Easy to Moderate (30 sec)	4–6
9:00–9:15	Very Fast (15 sec)	8–9
9:15–9:45	Easy to Moderate (30 sec)	4–6
9:45–10:00	Very Fast (15 sec)	8–9
10:00–10:30	Easy to Moderate (30 sec)	4–6
10:30–10:45	Very Fast (15 sec)	8–9
10:45–11:15	Easy to Moderate (30 sec)	4–6
11:15–11:30	Very Fast (15 sec)	8–9
11:30–12:00	Easy to Moderate (30 sec)	4–6
12:00–12:15	Very Fast (15 sec)	8–9
12:15–12:45	Easy to Moderate (30 sec)	4–6
12:45–13:00	Very Fast (15 sec)	8–9
13:00–13:30	Easy to Moderate (30 sec)	4–6
13:30–13:45	Very Fast (15 sec)	8–9
13:45–14:15	Easy to Moderate (30 sec)	4–6
14:15–14:30	Very Fast (15 sec)	8–9
14:30–15:00	Easy to Moderate (30 sec)	4–6
15:00–15:15	Very Fast (15 sec)	8–9
15:15–15:45	Easy to Moderate (30 sec)	4–6
15:45–16:00	Very Fast (15 sec)	8–9
16:00–16:30	Easy to Moderate (30 sec)	4–6
16:30–20:00	Cool-Down (3.5 min)	5→3

RECOVERY WALK

The purpose of this walk is to get your body moving a little to recover from the previous day's high-intensity workout. It's also an opportunity to take advantage of the fat-burning boost and appetite-suppressing bonus that research has shown you get when you do both cardio and strength training on the same day. If you feel good and want to go longer, be my guest! Just keep the intensity in the easy to moderate range.

TIME	ACTIVITY	INTENSITY
0:00–3:00	Warm-Up (3 min)	3→5
3:00–18:00	Moderate Walk (15 min)	5–6
18:00–20:00	Cool-Down (2 min)	5→3

SPEED WALK

During this walk, you want to push yourself to go faster. Map out a 1-mile route. You'll do your warm-up and cool-down separately, so, in total, you'll be covering a little more than a mile.

Walk your mile at a pace that you feel you can maintain for the entire distance. You should be breathing heavily (a 6 to 8 effort level), but not panting. Make note of your time on the logs provided in the Walk Off Weight journal starting on page 304.

ACTIVITY	INTENSITY
Warm-Up (5 min)	3→5
Brisk to Very Fast Walk (times will vary)	6–8
Cool-Down (5 min)	5→3

BECAUSE THE WORKOUTS ARE SHORTER in this phase of WOW, you might be feeling as if you should do more. If you're really up for it, go ahead and extend your walks a bit—but don't sacrifice the intensity of your intervals. Remember, it's about quality, not quantity.

The only thing that's changing for this week's workout schedule is the number of reps you'll be doing when strength training. And maybe you'll finish that mile-long Speed Walk a little faster this week. Good luck!

YOUR WORKOUT AT A GLANCE

DAY	ACTIVITY//WORKOUT	TOTAL
1	Supercharged Interval Walk I (20 min)	20 min
2	Recovery Walk (20 min) // Total-Body Strength Workout (20 min)	40 min
3	Supercharged Interval Walk I (20 min)	20 min
4	Recovery Walk (20 min) // Total-Body Strength Workout (20 min)	40 min
5	Supercharged Interval Walk I (20 min)	20 min
6	Speed Walk (<30 min) // Total-Body Strength Workout (20 min, optional)	50 min
7	Rest	

WHAT YOU'LL **DO THIS WEEK**

3 x Supercharged Interval Walk I ○ 2 x or 3 x Total-Body Strength Workout
2 x Recovery Walks ○ 1 x Speed Walk

Workout Summary

THE DETAILS OF THE WALKING ROUTINES follow.

TOTAL-BODY STRENGTH
WORKOUT (page 129)
Do 10-12 reps of the following exercises:
>> **Balancing Deadlift with Arm Raise**
>> **Bridge with Press**
>> **Rotating Lunge**
>> **Row with Leg Swing**
>> **Crunch and Extend**
>> **Elevated Squat with Curl**

You Deserve This!

WE ALL KNOW IT'S IMPORTANT to take care of ourselves. But there must be something in the female genes that drives us to always put the needs of everyone else—our kids, spouses, families, bosses, co-workers, friends, neighbors, churches, schools, community organizations, cats, dogs, the list goes on—ahead of our own. We promise ourselves that once the kids are in school, a big work project is turned in, the home improvements are complete, a sick relative is feeling better, vacation is over, the kids leave for college—and that list goes on, too—we'll start.

There is never going to be a perfect time to start taking care of yourself. That's why I'm so proud of you for coming this far. By starting the WOW program, you've taken the first step to making yourself a priority. Now you just need to keep it up!

Of course, there will be times when you have to make adjustments when a family member is sick, for example, or when you're working long hours. But now that you know how much better you can feel and perform, keep that at the forefront of your mind. Then sneak in little good-for-you moments, such as going for a quick 10-minute walk (or even 5 minutes, if that's all you can manage) or closing your eyes and sipping a hot cup of green tea. And make sure that you get back to your good-for-me routine of eating right and exercising regularly as soon as you can.

While these things may appear to be indulgent or selfish, they're not. They are essential to your well-being and ability to take care of others. This was a sentiment I heard over and over again from our test panelists once they completed the program:

"It is now time—you have already paid your dues—to do something for you. This is not selfish, but practical. If you want to continue to nurture others, you have to nurture yourself!" —Mary Lou Phillips

"Do something, even if it's only 10 minutes . . . Just start, even though the dishes are piling up in the sink, even though you really should vacuum your living room, even though you have a ton of work to do . . . It will all be there when you get back, and you will probably be able to do it more quickly and efficiently, since your energy level will increase. It's such a small investment—you are worth it!" —Deb Baer

technique FOCUS

Swivel Hips
The hip action you want is forward and back, not side to side. To loosen up your hips so that they move more freely, walk like a model, allowing your feet to cross over the midline of your body as you step. Do this for a few minutes during your warm-up.

SUPERCHARGED INTERVAL WALK I

TIME	ACTIVITY	INTENSITY
0:00–5:00	Warm-Up (5 min)	3→5
5:00–6:00	Moderate (1 min)	5–6
6:00–6:15	Very Fast (15 sec)	8–9
6:15–6:45	Easy to Moderate (30 sec)	4–6
6:45–7:00	Very Fast (15 sec)	8–9
7:00–7:30	Easy to Moderate (30 sec)	4–6
7:30–7:45	Very Fast (15 sec)	8–9
7:45–8:15	Easy to Moderate (30 sec)	4–6
8:15–8:30	Very Fast (15 sec)	8–9
8:30–9:00	Easy to Moderate (30 sec)	4–6
9:00–9:15	Very Fast (15 sec)	8–9
9:15–9:45	Easy to Moderate (30 sec)	4–6
9:45–10:00	Very Fast (15 sec)	8–9
10:00–10:30	Easy to Moderate (30 sec)	4–6
10:30–10:45	Very Fast (15 sec)	8–9
10:45–11:15	Easy to Moderate (30 sec)	4–6
11:15–11:30	Very Fast (15 sec)	8–9
11:30–12:00	Easy to Moderate (30 sec)	4–6
12:00–12:15	Very Fast (15 sec)	8–9
12:15–12:45	Easy to Moderate (30 sec)	4–6
12:45–13:00	Very Fast (15 sec)	8–9
13:00–13:30	Easy to Moderate (30 sec)	4–6
13:30–13:45	Very Fast (15 sec)	8–9
13:45–14:15	Easy to Moderate (30 sec)	4–6
14:15–14:30	Very Fast (15 sec)	8–9
14:30–15:00	Easy to Moderate (30 sec)	4–6
15:00–15:15	Very Fast (15 sec)	8–9
15:15–15:45	Easy to Moderate (30 sec)	4–6
15:45–16:00	Very Fast (15 sec)	8–9
16:00–16:30	Easy to Moderate (30 sec)	4–6
16:30–20:00	Cool-Down (3.5 min)	5→3

RECOVERY WALK

TIME	ACTIVITY	INTENSITY
0:00–3:00	Warm-Up (3 min)	3→5
3:00–18:00	Moderate Walk (15 min)	5–6
18:00–20:00	Cool-Down (2 min)	5→3

SPEED WALK

ACTIVITY	INTENSITY
Warm-Up (5 min)	3→5
Brisk to Very Fast Walk (times will vary)	6–8
Cool-Down (5 min)	5→3

YOU HAVE COME SO FAR IN JUST 6 WEEKS. If you haven't already, reward yourself for all your hard work. Get a pedicure (your feet certainly deserve it!), buy a new pair of earrings, or curl up with a favorite book.

Along with another increase in the number of reps for the Total-Body Strength Workout (hello, shapelier muscles!), you'll be extending your Recovery Walks by 5 minutes and your Supercharged Interval Walks by 10 minutes to really maximize your fat burn. Faster, faster, faster! I know you can do it!

YOUR WORKOUT AT A GLANCE

DAY	ACTIVITY//WORKOUT	TOTAL
1	Supercharged Interval Walk II (30 min)	30 min
2	Recovery Walk (25 min) // Total-Body Strength Workout (20 min)	45 min
3	Supercharged Interval Walk II (30 min)	30 min
4	Recovery Walk (25 min) // Total-Body Strength Workout (20 min)	45 min
5	Supercharged Interval Walk II (30 min)	30 min
6	Speed Walk (<30 min) // Total-Body Strength Workout (20 min, optional)	<50 min
7	Rest	

||||||||||||||||||||||||||||||||||||||||||||||||||||||||||||||||||||||||||||||||||||

WHAT YOU'LL **DO THIS WEEK**

3 x Supercharged Interval Walk II ○ 2 x or 3 x Total-Body Strength Workout
2 x Recovery Walk ○ 1 x Speed Walk

||||||||||||||||||||||||||||||||||||||||||||||||||||||||||||||||||||||||||||||||||||

Workout Summary

THE DETAILS OF THE WALKING ROUTINES follow.

TOTAL-BODY STRENGTH WORKOUT

(page 129)
Do 15–17 reps of the following exercises:
>> **Balancing Deadlift with Arm Raise**
>> **Bridge with Press**

>> **Rotating Lunge**
>> **Row with Leg Swing**
>> **Crunch and Extend**
>> **Elevated Squat with Curl**

Sleep Makes Weight Loss Easier

OKAY, THIS WEEK'S ADVICE IS as much for me as it is for you: Make sure that you're getting enough sleep! (I'm really bad about this too, especially when I'm juggling a lot of responsibilities.) In addition to affecting your health—research has linked inadequate shut-eye with heart disease, high blood pressure, diabetes, and depression—a lack of sleep can make losing weight a lot harder. Studies have shown that getting too little sleep can alter hunger hormone levels, priming you to overeat and crave sugary, fatty foods such as candy, cookies, and cake.[2] Just what you need when you're trying to get in shape!

To make matters worse, too little snoozing also elevates stress hormones that direct fat right to your belly. It also decreases levels of growth hormone, which is important to maintaining your body's metabolism-revving muscle.

So how much is enough? Based on studies, 7 to 8 hours is a good goal to shoot for, though what's best for each person varies. According to the Better Sleep Council, a nonprofit organization in Alexandria, Virginia, 20 percent of women ages 40 to 60 clock in fewer than 5 hours a night—which could be having a big impact on their health.

Thankfully, exercise can help you get the rest your body needs. Many of our test panelists reported sleeping better once they started the WOW program. And, of course, there are other easy steps you can take to improve your sleep, such as cutting back on caffeine (you may want to switch to decaf green tea if you're following the WOW eating plan), keeping a regular sleep schedule, limiting alcohol intake, creating a cool and dark sleep environment, and using your bedroom only for sleeping—not for reading, eating, or watching TV.

Some people should see their doctors for conditions that may be keeping them awake at night, such as sleep apnea or unrelenting hot flashes. But I suspect that most of us could get a good night's sleep if we'd just get into bed and shut off our brains. We go-go-go all day, taking care of our families, homes, jobs, social networks, and occasionally ourselves. We stay up late or roll out of bed early to get everything done. And when we finally crawl under the covers, we think about everything else we need to do, or we problem-solve some issue that's affecting our lives. If this sounds like you, try powering down before bedtime with these tips.

Dim all the lights. After dinner, turn off as many lights as possible—especially bright overhead ones—and use smaller, dimmer ones instead. (It'll save on your electric bill, and it's good for the environment, too!) Bright lights signal your body that it's time to wake up, when you should be winding down.

Unplug technology an hour before bed. The glow from the TV or computer can act just like bright lights. And news of the latest economic turmoil or e-mails from your boss are even more likely to keep you up at night.

Unwind. Choose an activity that works for you. Listen to music, read a book, talk with your spouse, stretch, meditate, write in a journal—whatever works to relax your mind.

technique
FOCUS

Put It All
Together
You have every-
thing you need,
so give it your all
this week!

SUPERCHARGED INTERVAL WALK II

TIME	ACTIVITY	INTENSITY	TIME	ACTIVITY	INTENSITY
0:00–5:00	Warm-Up (5 min)	3→5	15:15–15:45	Easy to Moderate (30 sec)	4–6
5:00–6:00	Moderate (1 min)	5–6	15:45–16:00	Very Fast (15 sec)	8–9
6:00–6:15	Very Fast (15 sec)	8–9	16:00–16:30	Easy to Moderate (30 sec)	4–6
6:15–6:45	Easy to Moderate (30 sec)	4–6	16:30–16:45	Very Fast (15 sec)	8–9
6:45–7:00	Very Fast (15 sec)	8–9	16:45–17:15	Easy to Moderate (30 sec)	4–6
7:00–7:30	Easy to Moderate (30 sec)	4–6	17:15–17:30	Very Fast (15 sec)	8–9
7:30–7:45	Very Fast (15 sec)	8–9	17:30–18:00	Easy to Moderate (30 sec)	4–6
7:45–8:15	Easy to Moderate (30 sec)	4–6	18:00–18:15	Very Fast (15 sec)	8–9
8:15–8:30	Very Fast (15 sec)	8–9	18:15–18:45	Easy to Moderate (30 sec)	4–6
8:30–9:00	Easy to Moderate (30 sec)	4–6	18:45–19:00	Very Fast (15 sec)	8–9
9:00–9:15	Very Fast (15 sec)	8–9	19:00–19:30	Easy to Moderate (30 sec)	4–6
9:15–9:45	Easy to Moderate (30 sec)	4–6	19:30–19:45	Very Fast (15 sec)	8–9
9:45–10:00	Very Fast (15 sec)	8–9	19:45–20:15	Easy to Moderate (30 sec)	4–6
10:00–10:30	Easy to Moderate (30 sec)	4–6	20:15–20:30	Very Fast (15 sec)	8–9
10:30–10:45	Very Fast (15 sec)	8–9	20:30–21:00	Easy to Moderate (30 sec)	4–6
10:45–11:15	Easy to Moderate (30 sec)	4–6	21:00–21:15	Very Fast (15 sec)	8–9
11:15–11:30	Very Fast (15 sec)	8–9	21:15–21:45	Easy to Moderate (30 sec)	4–6
11:30–12:00	Easy to Moderate (30 sec)	4–6	21:45–22:00	Very Fast (15 sec)	8–9
12:00–12:15	Very Fast (15 sec)	8–9	22:00–22:30	Easy to Moderate (30 sec)	4–6
12:15–12:45	Easy to Moderate (30 sec)	4–6	22:30–22:45	Very Fast (15 sec)	8–9
12:45–13:00	Very Fast (15 sec)	8–9	22:45–23:15	Easy to Moderate (30 sec)	4–6
13:00–13:30	Easy to Moderate (30 sec)	4–6	23:15–23:30	Very Fast (15 sec)	8–9
13:30–13:45	Very Fast (15 sec)	8–9	23:30–24:00	Easy to Moderate (30 sec)	4–6
13:45–14:15	Easy to Moderate (30 sec)	4–6	24:00–24:15	Very Fast (15 sec)	8–9
14:15–14:30	Very Fast (15 sec)	8–9	24:15–24:45	Easy to Moderate (30 sec)	4–6
14:30–15:00	Easy to Moderate (30 sec)	4–6	24:45–25:00	Very Fast (15 sec)	8–9
15:00–15:15	Very Fast (15 sec)	8–9	25:00–25:30	Easy to Moderate (30 sec)	4–6
			25:30–30:00	Cool-Down (4.5 min)	5→3

RECOVERY WALK

TIME	ACTIVITY	INTENSITY
0:00–3:00	Warm-Up (3 min)	3→5
3:00–23:00	Moderate Walk (20 min)	5–6
23:00–25:00	Cool-Down (2 min)	5→3

SPEED WALK

ACTIVITY	INTENSITY
Warm-Up (5 min)	3→5
Brisk to Very Fast Walk (times will vary)	6–8
Cool-Down (5 min)	5→3

YOU'RE IN THE HOMESTRETCH! You should be so proud of yourself. I'm certainly proud of you! This week just up those toning reps a bit more and keep walking strong. Go, go, go! And don't forget to treat yourself at the end of the week—perhaps a massage, a facial, a new outfit, or a new pair of shoes—for a job well done.

> Walk, and then walk some more. Your body needs to move.

—*DEBBIE ADIE,*
LOST 15 POUNDS AND 11 INCHES ON THE WOW PROGRAM

YOUR WORKOUT AT A GLANCE

DAY	ACTIVITY//WORKOUT	TOTAL
1	Supercharged Interval Walk II (30 min)	30 min
2	Recovery Walk (25 min) // Total-Body Strength Workout (20 min)	45 min
3	Supercharged Interval Walk II (30 min)	30 min
4	Recovery Walk (25 min) // Total-Body Strength Workout (20 min)	45 min
5	Supercharged Interval Walk II (30 min)	30 min
6	Speed Walk (<30 min) // Total-Body Strength Workout (20 min, optional)	<50 min
7	Rest	

WHAT YOU'LL **DO THIS WEEK**

3 x Supercharged Interval Walk II ○ 2 x or 3 x Total-Body Strength Workout
2 x Recovery Walk ○ 1 x Speed Walk

Workout Summary

THE DETAILS OF THE WALKING ROUTINES follow.

TOTAL-BODY STRENGTH WORKOUT (page 129)
Do 18–20 reps of the following exercises:
>> **Balancing Deadlift with Arm Raise**
>> **Bridge with Press**

>> **Rotating Lunge**
>> **Row with Leg Swing**
>> **Crunch and Extend**
>> **Elevated Squat with Curl**

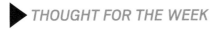

What's Next?

YOU DID IT! As you complete this final week of the WOW program, notice how far you have come. Feel those muscles in your legs; hopefully you're seeing them, too. And no more shin pain! Smile when you're getting dressed because your clothes fit better. Enjoy all the energy, good moods, and confidence you now have. Rejoice when you do your Speed Walk and you clock a faster time than you did 4 weeks ago.

You've come a long way, but this isn't the end. With your new fitter, stronger, healthier body and mind, there is nothing that you can't do. You can lose more weight. You can walk a marathon. You can find a new relationship. You can take on a triathlon. You can get that promotion. You can start your own business. You can go on a cycling vacation. Anything you put your mind to, you can accomplish! (To help you along the way, check out Chapter 9 for ways to continue the WOW program and achieve your goals.)

Now go out there and enjoy your slimmer, firmer, younger body. Take dancing lessons with your spouse, coach your kid's (or grandkid's) soccer team, or go hiking with friends. Life is more fun when you're fit and strong!

technique
FOCUS

Keep It Up
Eyes up, arms bent, fast steps! You know what to do, so get out there and do it!

SUPERCHARGED INTERVAL WALK II

TIME	ACTIVITY	INTENSITY	TIME	ACTIVITY	INTENSITY
0:00–5:00	Warm-Up (5 min)	3→5	15:15–15:45	Easy to Moderate (30 sec)	4–6
5:00–6:00	Moderate (1 min)	5–6	15:45–16:00	Very Fast (15 sec)	8–9
6:00–6:15	Very Fast (15 sec)	8–9	16:00–16:30	Easy to Moderate (30 sec)	4–6
6:15–6:45	Easy to Moderate (30 sec)	4–6	16:30–16:45	Very Fast (15 sec)	8–9
6:45–7:00	Very Fast (15 sec)	8–9	16:45–17:15	Easy to Moderate (30 sec)	4–6
7:00–7:30	Easy to Moderate (30 sec)	4–6	17:15–17:30	Very Fast (15 sec)	8–9
7:30–7:45	Very Fast (15 sec)	8–9	17:30–18:00	Easy to Moderate (30 sec)	4–6
7:45–8:15	Easy to Moderate (30 sec)	4–6	18:00–18:15	Very Fast (15 sec)	8–9
8:15–8:30	Very Fast (15 sec)	8–9	18:15–18:45	Easy to Moderate (30 sec)	4–6
8:30–9:00	Easy to Moderate (30 sec)	4–6	18:45–19:00	Very Fast (15 sec)	8–9
9:00–9:15	Very Fast (15 sec)	8–9	19:00–19:30	Easy to Moderate (30 sec)	4–6
9:15–9:45	Easy to Moderate (30 sec)	4–6	19:30–19:45	Very Fast (15 sec)	8–9
9:45–10:00	Very Fast (15 sec)	8–9	19:45–20:15	Easy to Moderate (30 sec)	4–6
10:00–10:30	Easy to Moderate (30 sec)	4–6	20:15–20:30	Very Fast (15 sec)	8–9
10:30–10:45	Very Fast (15 sec)	8–9	20:30–21:00	Easy to Moderate (30 sec)	4–6
10:45–11:15	Easy to Moderate (30 sec)	4–6	21:00–21:15	Very Fast (15 sec)	8–9
11:15–11:30	Very Fast (15 sec)	8–9	21:15–21:45	Easy to Moderate (30 sec)	4–6
11:30–12:00	Easy to Moderate (30 sec)	4–6	21:45–22:00	Very Fast (15 sec)	8–9
12:00–12:15	Very Fast (15 sec)	8–9	22:00–22:30	Easy to Moderate (30 sec)	4–6
12:15–12:45	Easy to Moderate (30 sec)	4–6	22:30–22:45	Very Fast (15 sec)	8–9
12:45–13:00	Very Fast (15 sec)	8–9	22:45–23:15	Easy to Moderate (30 sec)	4–6
13:00–13:30	Easy to Moderate (30 sec)	4–6	23:15–23:30	Very Fast (15 sec)	8–9
13:30–13:45	Very Fast (15 sec)	8–9	23:30–24:00	Easy to Moderate (30 sec)	4–6
13:45–14:15	Easy to Moderate (30 sec)	4–6	24:00–24:15	Very Fast (15 sec)	8–9
14:15–14:30	Very Fast (15 sec)	8–9	24:15–24:45	Easy to Moderate (30 sec)	4–6
14:30–15:00	Easy to Moderate (30 sec)	4–6	24:45–25:00	Very Fast (15 sec)	8–9
15:00–15:15	Very Fast (15 sec)	8–9	25:00–25:30	Easy to Moderate (30 sec)	4–6
			25:30–30:00	Cool-Down (4.5 min)	5→3

RECOVERY WALK

TIME	ACTIVITY	INTENSITY
0:00–3:00	Warm-Up (3 min)	3→5
3:00–23:00	Moderate Walk (20 min)	5–6
23:00–25:00	Cool-Down (2 min)	5→3

SPEED WALK

ACTIVITY	INTENSITY
Warm-Up (5 min)	3→5
Brisk to Very Fast Walk (times will vary)	6–8
Cool-Down (5 min)	5→3

WOW Winner
Meg Kranzley
GROUP: Exercise and Diet

AGE: 50 HEIGHT: 5'4"
POUNDS LOST: 10½
INCHES LOST: 9½ overall, including 3½ from her waist
MAJOR ACCOMPLISHMENT: Boosted her energy level 43%

More Energy and a Flatter Belly

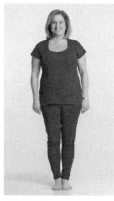

BEFORE

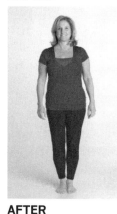

AFTER

MEG KRANZLEY was the one woman on the WOW program who started off with the biggest bang. "Last spring, I bought a linen top with a zipper up the left side. It was a little snug at the waist, but it fit. After the first week [on WOW], I just pulled it over my head and down over my body without even unzipping it!" she exclaimed.

According to the scale, she had lost nearly 5 pounds. "I knew that every week wouldn't be so dramatic, but what a great way to begin," said Meg, who signed on to the WOW team because she wanted to go from "50 and fat" to "50 and fit." She added, "I hit the big 5-0 this year, so I was really determined to make a change."

While Meg was right about the weight loss—some weeks it slowed, others it seemed as if the scale was just plain stuck—her resolve never waivered. "Even on weeks when I didn't lose, my clothes still continued to fit better than they had the previous week, so I knew I was losing inches," she explained.

One of the most valuable lessons Meg learned from the program was not to be so hard on herself. "I've always been an all-or-nothing type of person," she explained. "If I couldn't do it perfectly, then I'd give up. But this program taught me that every little bit counts. So instead of getting discouraged if I couldn't do a longer walk, I'd just sub in a shorter workout, and then do the longer one on an alternate day."

While Meg had always walked for exercise, she'd never done intervals or resistance training before. She credited both for newfound muscles, a firmer butt, slimmer thighs, and a flatter belly. "When you learn to walk heel to toe and squeeze your glutes, it makes all the difference for a speedy walk. It tightens up your tush, too."

Her hard work has paid off in other ways as well. She lost nearly 11 pounds and more than 9 inches through the 8 weeks of WOW. With her fitter, slimmer body, she was able to unpack the entire car at the beach, lugging groceries, suitcases, and beach chairs all by herself. "I didn't feel winded, out of breath, or frazzled by the time I sat down on the beach. It was great to feel so energetic," Meg reported. But her favorite result: "The 3½ inches that are no longer padding my belly!"

P.S. *Three months after the official end of the program, Meg recorded an additional 1¾-pound weight loss and shaved another ½ inch off her figure despite having surgery a few weeks before the follow-up weigh-in, for a grand total of 12¼ pounds and 10 inches lost in 5 months.*

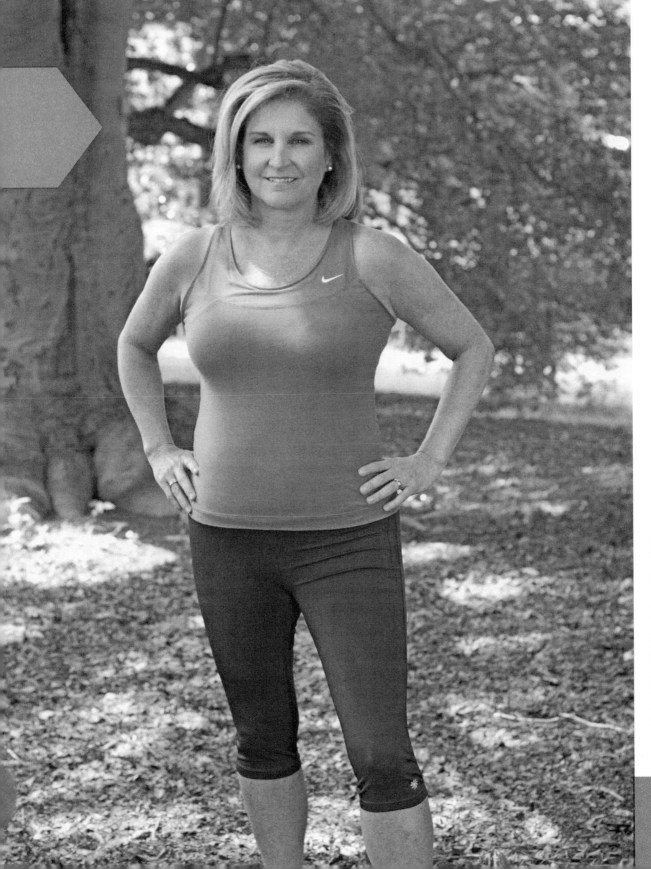

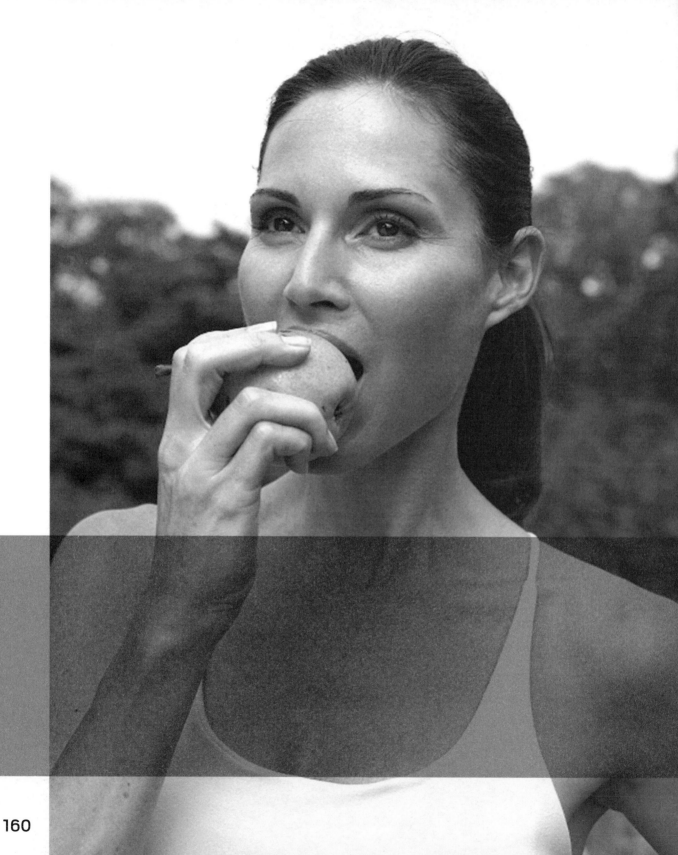

CHAPTER

7

Eating
FOR WEIGHT LOSS
AND EXERCISE

STUDY AFTER STUDY HAS SHOWN THAT YOU CAN LOSE more weight by cutting calories from what you eat than you can by burning them off with exercise. That's why I *had* to include a diet component with the WOW program. I want to give you every advantage to slim down and shape up as quickly as possible—and to keep the pounds and inches off long-term. And to be perfectly honest, most of us will benefit in *many* ways—such as having more energy, boosting our immunity, and protecting ourselves against disease—from making some changes to our diets.

One of the reasons dieting trumps exercise for weight loss is that it's just too easy to eat back the calories you work off. Your body needs fuel to exercise, and the source of that fuel is food. That's why some people report feeling hungrier when they start to work out. It's also why elite athletes require hundreds, even thousands, more calories a day than the average person (you may have heard about Olympian Michael Phelps's 12,000-calorie-a-day diet). If you're trying to lose weight, this could be counterproductive—unless you find the right balance.

To help, registered dietitian and fellow walker Heidi McIndoo, MS, RD, LDN, author of *The Complete Idiot's Guide to Superfoods Cookbook*, has created an eating plan that will energize you for your workouts and help you burn the most fat for the fewest calories—all while making sure you feel satisfied, not deprived.

It worked for our WOW test panel. The women who followed the eating plan in addition to the walking program lost nearly three times more body fat, shed more than twice as much weight, and whittled away 65 percent more inches than the women who followed just the walking program.

FUEL YOUR WALKS WITH PROPER NUTRITION

THE BASIC EATING PLAN IS APPROXIMATELY 1,600 CALORIES, spread out over three meals and one snack. If you're like most women, 1,600 calories is what you need to meet your body's nutritional requirements, fuel your workouts, and promote weight loss. All of our eating plan testers, who ranged in weight from 234 to 144 pounds at the start of the program, followed the 1,600-calorie plan.

But calorie requirements vary from one person to the next, depending on height, gender, activity level, age, current weight, and desired weight. If you find yourself feeling overly hungry—stomach often growling, light-headed—or fatigued, add a 200-calorie snack, which will bring you to 1,800 calories a day. (In the 2-week meal plan beginning on page 177, this is the Optional Snack.)

If you're taller than 5 feet 6 inches and/or you weigh more than 250 pounds, you may do better on 1,800 calories a day. Again, if you're often hungry or fatigued at this calorie level, you may need to add another 200-calorie snack. In this case, you'll be eating three snacks a day and a total of 2,000 calories. At this intake level, you'll still lose weight, though probably a bit more slowly.

Calories are only part of the story when you're trying to walk off weight. Where those calories come from can make or break your workouts.

The typical American diet is filled with refined or simple carbohydrates such as white flours, rices, and pastas, and pastries, sodas, and other sugary foods and drinks. Simple carbohydrates, which lack the fiber found in complex carbs such as whole grains, fruits, and veggies, are metabolized by your body quickly. So while you may feel raring to go after eating them, in no time, that energy boost will be overshadowed by a big energy slump, making it hard to give your all during your workouts.

In addition, if the majority of the foods you eat are metabolized quickly, you'll find yourself feeling hungry more often, which could mean more snacking and a higher calorie intake. Alternatively, a diet based on complex, fiber-rich carbohydrates provides longer-lasting energy and satiety to fuel exercise and prevent overeating.

6 EATING GUIDELINES FOR FASTER WEIGHT LOSS

THE WOW EATING PLAN INCORPORATES THE RIGHT MIX of high-energy foods to rev up your workouts and speed weight loss, all while satisfying your body's nutritional needs. Here are the building blocks used to design the WOW plan.

1. **FIBER** Eat at least 20 grams of fiber per day from whole grains, fruits, and vegetables. Fiber helps keep you feeling full longer—a big benefit when you're trying to lose weight. A 2009 study from Brigham Young University College of Health and Human Performance demonstrated that women who ate more fiber significantly lowered their risk of gaining weight and fat. Each gram of fiber eaten correlated to ½ pound less body weight. The researchers suspect that the higher fiber intake led to a reduction in total calories over time.[1]

2. **CALCIUM AND VITAMIN D** Strive for three servings of calcium-rich and vitamin D–rich foods a day. These nutrients often occur together in foods, especially dairy.

   Recommended Calcium Intake
   Men and women ages 19–50: 1,000 milligrams
   Men and women age 51+: 1,200 milligrams

   Recommended Vitamin D Intake
   Men and women ages 19–50: 200 IU
   Men and women ages 51–70: 400 IU
   Men and women age 71+: 600 IU

Calcium and vitamin D work together in your body, primarily to strengthen your bones. But if the latest research is any indication, both of these nutrients may flex some muscle in your weight loss success. Dairy foods are the prime source of calcium and vitamin D in the diet. In a recent study from Johns Hopkins Bloomberg School of Public Health, college students who came closest to meeting the three-a-day dairy requirement while eating an otherwise healthy diet weighed less, gained less, and actually lost belly fat, compared with students who consumed little or no dairy.[2] Moreover, vitamin D by itself may play a role in weight control. Extra body fat holds on to vitamin D so that the body can't use it. This perceived deficiency interferes with the action of

THE WOW FACTOR

Sit down and savor your meal. When you're stressed, you tend to gulp down your food, eating more than if you were paying attention to every bite. For a study at Brazosport Memorial Hospital in Lake Jackson, Texas, six women were asked to eat slowly, chew thoroughly, and stop when their food no longer tasted as good as when they took their first bite. These women lost 8 pounds, on average, compared to a 3-pound weight *gain* for a control group.[3]

the hormone leptin, whose job is to tell your brain that you're full. And if you can't recognize when you're satiated, you're more likely to overeat.

You may also want to consider a vitamin D supplement. The latest research suggests that this nutrient may be a factor in protecting you from everything from heart disease to memory loss and even chronic pain. Evidence is mounting that we need more than the current recommended intakes, especially as we age, because older skin produces less vitamin D (and sunscreens block the body's ability to use sunlight to produce this vitamin). That's why the leading experts in vitamin D research are now recommending a daily supplement of 1,000 IU of vitamin D_3—the kind most readily used by the body.

3. **GOOD FATS** These include monounsaturated fatty acids and omega-3 fatty acids, found in oils, nuts, avocados, certain fish—and yes, even chocolate! Eat three to four servings daily.

A recent study published in the journal *Appetite* shows how these fats— besides being good for your heart—can help you feel fuller longer after meals. The study participants with a higher intake of omega-3 fatty acids (more than 1,300 milligrams a day either from foods or from supplements) reported feeling less hungry right after their meals, as well as 2 hours later, compared with a lower omega-3 intake (less than 260 milligrams a day).[4] Less hunger means less munching and an easier time keeping calories in check.

More specific research has been done on walnuts, a good source of monounsaturated fats. An Australian study had participants follow a healthy low-fat diet either with walnuts or without. Both groups ate the same number of calories and lost approximately the same amount of weight at 6 months. But during the next 6 months of the year-long study, the walnut-eaters continued to lose weight and body fat while the other group stopped losing—even though they were still following the same diet.[5]

4. **PROTEIN** Aim for three servings of lean protein (such as fish, white meat chicken and turkey, pork loin chops, and lean beef sirloin) per day. In addition to being an essential nutrient, protein helps to keep you feeling full longer, which is a big benefit when you're trying to lose weight. In a small 2009 study, participants who ate a higher-protein breakfast were more satiated afterward (and took in fewer calories at lunch) than those who ate a low-protein breakfast.[6]

5. **WATER** Studies from Stanford Prevention Research Center suggest that water helps promote weight loss in two ways. First, drinking more water—at least 4 cups per day—was linked to a 5-pound weight loss over the course of a year. According to the researchers, this amount of water increases the amount of energy or calories your body burns. Second, substituting water for sugary drinks—sodas, sports drinks, flavored drinks, and sweetened milks, coffees, and teas—resulted in even more weight loss. The exact number of pounds lost

depended on how many sugary drinks were consumed in the first place and how many were replaced with water. Interestingly, switching from sweetened drinks to diet drinks instead of water also resulted in weight loss, but only about 3½ pounds instead of slightly more than 5 with water.[7]

Still don't think you can give up your sodas and mochaccinos? Then consider this: It's been shown that when people consume a certain amount of calories, they're hungrier and more likely to overeat at their next meal when those calories are in liquid rather than in solid form. Translation: If you eat a 200-calorie snack, you'll be more satisfied afterward and eat less later than if you drink a 200-calorie beverage. So frequently drinking calorie-dense beverages could increase both your hunger and your calorie intake throughout the day.

6. **GREEN TEA** Sip at least 3 cups of green tea every day. Catechins, the antioxidants found in high amounts in green tea, have been shown to be helpful in promoting weight loss, specifically belly fat.[8] If caffeine is a concern, decaf tea is an option. Some decaffeination processes, however, can lower the antioxidant content, so you might want to have an extra cup or two.

In a study at the USDA Human Nutrition Research Center on Aging at Tufts University, participants who drank the equivalent of 3 cups of green tea

JAZZ UP YOUR GREEN TEA

HERE IS YOUR GUIDE
to making great green teas! Once you've mastered basic tea brewing, add flavors to prevent beverage boredom. If you prefer iced tea, just chill your tea of choice after brewing.
Basic Brewed Green Tea:
Place 1 green tea bag or a tea ball with 1 teaspoon of loose green tea leaves in your cup. Bring a little more than a cup of cold water to a boil. Remove from the heat and add an ice cube; this will help bring the water to the ideal temperature for brewing tea, which is 180ºF. Pour the water over the tea and let steep

for 3 to 5 minutes.
Blueberry Green Tea:
Brew green tea as previously described, then mix in 2 tablespoons of blueberry juice.
Blueberry Zinger Green Tea:
Brew green tea as previously described in 6 ounces of water and 1 tablespoon of lemon juice. Mix in 2 tablespoons of blueberry juice.
Ginger Green Tea: Steep some green tea together with 1 ginger tea bag or a few slices of fresh ginger as previously described. This is a terrific brew for bouts of digestive distress because ginger can help settle your stomach.

Peppermint Green Tea: Brew green tea together with 1 peppermint tea bag as previously described. The scent of peppermint may help to curb your appetite.
Pomo Power Green Tea:
Brew green tea as previously described. Mix in 2 tablespoons of pomegranate juice.
Raspberry Iced Green Tea:
Brew green tea as previously described. Put in the refrigerator to chill, then pour over ½ cup of frozen raspberries. You can try this with blueberries, strawberries, chopped peaches, or any combination you like.

What a Serving Size Looks Like

3 ounces of cooked meat = *the palm of your hand (excluding your fingers) or a deck of cards*

1 medium piece of fruit = *a tennis ball*

1 ounce of cheese = *1 tube of lipstick*

1 cup = *a closed fist*

$^1\!/_2$ cup = *a computer mouse, half a baseball*

$^1\!/_4$ cup = *half a tennis ball*

1 tablespoon = *half a golf ball, the tip of your thumb (from last knuckle)*

1 teaspoon = *a die*

a day lost twice as much weight as those not drinking tea. The tea-drinking group also lost significantly more belly fat than the non-tea drinkers.

If you like citrus, the news gets better. Replacing some of the tea brewing water with citrus juice, such as lemon, lime, orange, or grapefruit, allows your body to use more of the tea's catechins.[9] You can drink your green tea freshly brewed for a warming hot drink or chill it after brewing for a refreshing cold drink.

WHAT TO EAT

NOW YOU'RE PROBABLY THINKING, "Okay, I'm convinced that I need to add more fiber, calcium, vitamin D, good fats, protein, water, and green tea to my diet. But what do I actually eat?" Don't worry, you won't need to calculate grams of fiber or protein each day. We've done all the math for you. Just follow the simple rules for serving sizes at left, and you'll meet the WOW nutritional guidelines without even thinking about it.

Keep in mind, these lists are examples and are by no means all inclusive. If certain fruits, veggies, or other foods don't appear here, it doesn't mean that you can't eat them. Go ahead and enjoy them. Variety is the spice of life!

WHOLE GRAINS, STARCHY VEGGIES, AND BEANS:
Eat 5–6 servings a day

Bread *(1 serving = 1 slice)*
  Bagel ($^1\!/_2$ mini)
  English muffin ($^1\!/_2$)
  Pita ($^1\!/_2$ small)
  Tortilla (1 small)

Cereal, dry *(1 serving = 1 cup)*

Crackers *(1 serving = 1 ounce)*

Pancake/waffle *(1 serving = 1 medium)*

Popcorn, light **microwave** *(1 serving = 3 cups popped)*

Cooked whole grains *(1 serving = $^1\!/_2$ cup)*
  Couscous
  Hot cereal
  Oatmeal
  Pasta
  Rice

Canned and cooked beans, all kinds *(1 serving = $^1\!/_2$ cup)*

Cooked starchy veggies *(1 serving = $^1\!/_2$ cup)*
  Corn
  Peas
  Potatoes, all kinds

TIP: *When buying foods, check the ingredient list found on the label—the first ingredient should be something such as whole wheat flour, oats, or brown rice—to make sure you are getting whole grains.*

FRUIT: Eat 3 servings a day

Whole fresh fruit
(1 serving = 1 medium piece)

Apple
Banana ½
Grapefruit ½
Kiwifruit
Nectarine
Orange
Peach
Pear
Plum
Tangerine

Canned or cut-up fresh fruit
(1 serving = ½ cup)

Blueberries
Cherries
Grapes
Mango
Melon
Papaya
Pineapple
Pomegranate
Raspberries
Strawberries

Dried fruit
(1 serving = ¼ cup)

Apricots
Craisins
Prunes (dried plums)
Raisins

100% fruit juice, all kinds *(1 serving = ½ cup)*

TIP: *When buying canned or frozen fruit, be sure to avoid sugar- or syrup-packed products.*

VEGETABLES: Eat 4–5 servings a day

Cooked
(fresh, frozen, or canned; 1 serving = ½ cup)

Asparagus (or 3 spears)
Bell pepper
Broccoli
Brussels sprouts
Cabbage
Carrots
Cauliflower
Eggplant
Green beans
Mushrooms
Onion
Spinach
Zucchini

Cut-up raw vegetables
(1 serving = 1 cup)

Baby carrots
Bell pepper
Broccoli
Cauliflower
Cucumber
Greens, all kinds
Lettuce, all kinds
Tomato

100% vegetable juice, all kinds *(1 serving = ½ cup)*

TIP: *When buying frozen vegetables, avoid butter, cheese, or other creamy sauces. When buying vegetable juices, look for reduced-sodium products.*

DAIRY: Eat 3 servings a day

Milk, fat-free or soy *(1 serving = 1 cup)*

Yogurt *(1 serving = 1 cup)*

Shredded or crumbled cheese *(1 serving = ⅓ cup)*

Blue cheese
Cheddar
Feta
Mozzarella

Parmesan
Romano

Sliced or cubed cheese *(1 serving = 1 ounce or 1 slice or 2 domino-sized cubes)*

American
Cheddar
Colby
Monterey Jack
Swiss

Soft cheese *(1 serving = ½ cup)*

Cottage cheese
Ricotta

TIP: *When buying dairy products, choose fat-free or reduced-fat versions whenever possible. If you're lactose intolerant, you can try dividing your dairy into smaller servings throughout the day, making sure to pair them with other foods. Also, look for lactose-reduced foods and beverages, or consider Lactaid or other lactase supplements. You can get some calcium and vitamin D from nondairy foods, such as dark leafy greens and fortified orange juice, or, of course, from supplements.*

HEALTHY FATS: Eat 3-4 servings a day

Monounsaturated fatty acids and omega-3 fatty acids
Avocado (1 serving = 1/3 medium)
Chocolate, dark (1 serving = 1/4 cup chips or a 2-ounce piece)
Fatty fish (1 serving = 3 ounces)
   Herring
   Mackerel
   Salmon
   Sardines
   Trout
Nut butter (1 serving = 1 tablespoon)
   Almond
   Cashew
   Peanut
   Soy

Nuts (1 serving = 1 ounce)
   Almonds (24)
   Cashews (18)
   Peanuts (28)
   Pecan halves (20)
   Pistachios (46)
   Macadamias (12)
   Walnut halves (7)
Oil (1 serving = 2 1/2 teaspoons)
   Canola
   Flaxseed
   Olive
Olives (1 serving = 10 medium)
Pesto (1 serving = 1 tablespoon)

Polyunsaturated and trans fats:
☞ *The following are unhealthy fats and should be eaten sparingly.*
Reduced-fat mayonnaise (1 serving = 2 tablespoons)
Reduced-fat salad dressing (1 serving = 2 1/2 tablespoons)
Regular salad dressing (1 serving = 1 1/2 tablespoons)
Soft/tub/stick margarine, butter, or regular mayonnaise (1 serving = 1 tablespoon)

TIP: *You should limit your total fat consumption to no more than 5 servings per day, so limit unhealthy fats to 1 or 2 servings. Even better, make all 5 servings healthy fats.*

LEAN PROTEIN: Eat 3 servings a day

Meat (1 serving = 3 ounces)
   Beef
   Deli meat (roast beef or ham)
   Ground beef
   Pork, boneless loin
Poultry, white meat preferred (1 serving = 3 ounces)
   Chicken, boneless, skinless
   Chicken or turkey, ground
   Deli meat (chicken or turkey)
   Turkey, boneless, skinless

Seafood, low fat content (1 serving = 3 ounces)
   Shrimp, without shells
   Tuna, canned, water-packed
   Whitefish (such as cod and haddock)
Nonmeat protein (1 serving = 3 ounces)
   Egg, large (1)
   Egg substitute (1/4 cup)
   Tofu or soy foods

TIP: *Choose 2 servings from the meat, poultry, or seafood groups and 1 serving from the nonmeat group per day. If you're a vegetarian, simply choose all 3 servings from the nonmeat group.*

This may look like a lot of food, but keep in mind that you should be dividing it into three meals (breakfast, lunch, and dinner) and one, two, or three snacks a day. Also, you're not limited to only one serving of any given food per meal. For example, it's fine to eat multiple servings of bread or veggies or protein at the same meal. You just want to make sure that you're not eating so many servings at one meal that you're left with little or none for the rest of the day.

The table below gives you an example of how you can spread your food servings over the course of a day. As you'll see, the 2-week suggested menus that we've created for you follow these guidelines, too. So if you don't want to do any math, don't worry—we've done it for you! Remember that you can add water or green tea to any meal or snack.

MEAL	FOOD SERVINGS	EXAMPLE
BREAKFAST	**Grains/Starches:** 2 servings	1 English muffin
	Fruits: 1 serving	$1/2$ grapefruit
	Dairy: 1 serving	1 cup yogurt
	Healthy Fats: 1 serving	1 tablespoon almond butter
	Lean Protein: 1 serving	1 large hard-cooked egg
LUNCH	**Grains/Starches:** 2 servings	1 small pita
	Fruits: 1 serving	1 medium apple
	Vegetables: 2 servings	$1/2$ cup lettuce; $1/2$ cup cucumber; $1/2$ cup raw baby carrots; $1/2$ cup raw bell peppers
	Dairy: 1 serving	$1/3$ cup shredded Cheddar
	Healthy Fats: 1 serving	$1/3$ avocado
	Lean Protein: 1 serving	3 ounces boneless, skinless chicken breast
SNACK	**Fruits:** 1 serving	$1/2$ cup grapes
	Dairy: 1 serving	1 slice American cheese
DINNER	**Grains/Starches:** 1 serving	$1/2$ cup pasta
	Vegetables: 2 servings	$1/2$ cup cooked mushrooms; $1/2$ cup cooked onion
	Healthy Fats: 1 serving	$2^{1}/_{2}$ teaspoons olive oil
	Lean Protein: 1 serving	3 ounces lean ground beef
OPTIONAL SNACK*	**Grains/Starches:** 1 serving	3 cups popped light microwave popcorn
	Vegetables: 1 serving	$1/2$ cup carrot juice
	Healthy Fats: 1 serving	1 tablespoon butter
TOTAL	**Grains/Starches:** 6 servings >> **Fruits:** 3 servings >> **Vegetables:** 5 servings	
	Dairy: 3 servings >> **Healthy Fats:** 4 servings >> **Lean Protein:** 3 servings	

*If you feel hungry on the 1,800-calorie plan, eat two optional snacks for a total of 2,000 calories.

EASY WAYS TO EAT HEALTHY

IN THESE HECTIC TIMES, it can be difficult to do all you need to do in the course of a day. That includes finding time to grocery shop and cook healthfully. Here are some simple strategies that you can use to help make this part of your life a little easier.

Plan Ahead

This is a great time-saver when it comes to creating healthy meals. First, try to make only one big trip to the supermarket each week. It means less time and money spent on multiple grocery runs for one or two items. Before you go, however, plan out your meals for the week. This can be as simple as deciding to make chicken and broccoli one night and fish and carrots another; as detailed as knowing that, on Monday, you'll cook sweet-and-sour chicken with brown rice and steamed broccoli; or something in between. The purpose here is to get an idea of the major ingredients that you should have on hand.

While this may seem like another task you don't have time for, the payoff is worth the investment. First, you'll never again experience that 5:30 p.m. what-are-we-going-to-have-for-dinner panic—which also means no last-minute runs through the drive-thru. Second, you'll have an array of healthy foods from which to create delicious meals all week. Another plus: Shopping once a week allows you to buy and use more fresh produce and rely less on processed foods.

To help you get in the habit of planning ahead, you might want to follow the menus beginning on page 183 for the first couple of weeks. The grocery-shopping lists are included for you, so it couldn't be any easier.

Once you have your groceries home, it's time to make the food easy to use. For example, you can wash and cut up any produce that requires it. Again, it may take a few extra minutes up front, but having everything ready to go means spending less time on meal prep during the week, when time is usually at a premium.

Prepping the food ahead of time also applies to breakfasts and lunches, which you should get ready the day before whenever possible. Like dinnertime, mornings are often busy and rushed. If you can have ingredients measured out, eggs boiled, and so on, sitting down to a healthy breakfast will be that much simpler. Likewise, taking 5 minutes in the evening to pack your lunch for the next day means a calmer morning, as well as less reliance on fast food and convenience store foods.

Be Smart When Dining Out

Learning to cook and eat differently at home as part of your normal everyday routine can be a bit challenging at first. In no time, though, it'll seem like old hat. But what if your day-to-day life has you eating away from home often? Planning ahead is equally important in these situations.

Whenever possible, brown-bag it—whether you're at the office, running errands, or on the road. That way you're not at the mercy of cafeterias, food courts, vending machines, or drive-thrus. Great foods to pack are simple sandwiches, cut-up veggies and fruit, a big salad, even last night's leftovers. As for snacks or even a quick breakfast on those mornings when you're running late, stock your desk or glove compartment with a stash of raisins, instant oatmeal, nuts, and whole grain crackers with a small jar of peanut butter.

In restaurants, between the oversize portions and the seemingly never-ending menu options, selecting your meal will require more thought. First, pay attention to the words used to describe foods. For example, *crispy, breaded,* and *crunchy* all suggest that a food is fried.

Understanding Menu Lingo

Steer clear of . . .	Instead try . . .
Crispy	Grilled
Breaded	Poached
Fried	Sautéed
Cream Sauce	Au Jus
Cheese Sauce	Steamed

Second, don't be afraid to make special requests. Most restaurants are more than happy to accommodate you. So ask to swap the French fries that come with your sandwich for veggies or a baked potato, and order dressings and sauces on the side so you can control how much you use. Also:

- Skip the basket of bread or chips that's meant to tide you over until your meal arrives. It's too tempting to overindulge.
- Keep your meal small and simple—see if half portions are available.
- At fast-food restaurants, stick with a simple burger and salad. It can be a satisfying meal, and it's much better for you than the deluxe burger and extra-large fries.
- Consider taking half of your meal home for lunch the next day. As soon as your meal arrives, ask your server to wrap up half of it to go. This reduces the temptation of overeating.

THE WOW FACTOR

When hunger strikes, take a stand.

New research from the University of Massachusetts shows that sedentary subjects felt 17 percent hungrier than those who moved around throughout the day. Set your watch or computer to alert you to get up and move around every hour.[10]

Fuel Properly for Exercise

There are three nutrients that provide energy, aka calories, to your body, and they're all important for maximizing your workouts. Carbohydrates break down quickly for fast energy, while protein and fats sustain you longer. That's why the WOW meal plans contain a balanced mix of these nutrients. But to ensure that you're properly fueled to give it your all when you exercise, you may need to adjust the timing of your meals and snacks.

Working out on a full stomach can cause cramping because your body is diverting blood to your muscles, not your digestive system. Likewise, exercising on empty can make you feel weak, light-headed, and tired, causing you to slack off or even shorten your workouts and decrease your calorie burn. Ideally, schedule your workouts for 2 to 3 hours after a meal or 1 to 2 hours after a snack. Your body will be done digesting your food and have energy on hand.

If you still feel like you need a little boost before your workout, eat about 150 calories of a quickly digestible low-fat food such as yogurt, a banana, raisins, or a slice of turkey in half of a pita.

What you eat after your workout is also important for refueling and helping your muscles to recover so you're ready for your next workout. If your next meal is more than an hour away, have a 100- to 200-calorie snack that contains both carbohydrates and protein, such as an apple with peanut butter.

To avoid overeating as you fuel and refuel, redistribute your current calories by breaking up meals and snacks and eating them before or after you exercise. And don't forget to make sure that you're drinking enough fluids, as we discussed on page 164. Timing your workouts with your meals and snacks, fueling properly, and staying hydrated will also help to keep your appetite in check.

Curb Your Appetite

It's no shocker that hunger is often one of the big barriers to successful weight loss. Don't get me wrong; hunger can be a *good* thing. It can be a sign that your

CHEW HUNGER AWAY

A RECENT STUDY ASKED participants to chew sugarless gum for 15 minutes of every hour between lunch and a snack. When they did so, they ate 40 fewer calories of their snack than they did on the days when they didn't have gum.[11] Now 40 calories may not seem like a big deal, but it adds up to more than 4 pounds over the course of a year. And that's from just chewing gum! It helped one of our WOW testers, who's surrounded by food all day (she works in a cafeteria), to curb her appetite. She lost 4 to 4½ pounds and more than 5 inches—including 2¾ inches from her belly in just 4 weeks!

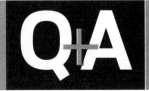

Q: I'm finding it tough to exercise in the morning when I feel so full from breakfast. What can I do?

A: Try dividing your breakfast into two mini-meals or snacks. Have one about an hour before your workout and the other an hour or so afterward. This way, you're not exercising on an empty tank, so to speak, but you're still getting the calories and nutrients you need from a balanced breakfast.

Q: I eat breakfast around 7:00 a.m., and I'm finding myself hungry long before lunch, which I usually eat around 1:00 p.m. Any suggestions?

A: You should avoid going longer than 3 to 4 hours without food. Otherwise, you risk the possibility of overeating at your next meal or—because hunger can lower your willpower—grabbing a quick candy bar or another less-than-healthy temptation. Try splitting your daily snack in two; have half around 10:00 a.m., which should easily get you through to lunch, then save the other half to tide you over between lunch and dinner. If you're still feeling hungry, you may need to eat another snack, increasing to 1,800 calories a day.

Q: Can I use NutriSystem or Jenny Craig food with the WOW eating plan?

A: Preportioned meals and snacks like these, as well as products like Lean Cuisine, Weight Watchers, and Healthy Choice, can easily be worked into a healthy eating plan like WOW. They're often quite low in calories, so pair them with a glass of milk, a salad, and some fruit to form a well-rounded, satisfying meal. If you find yourself turning to these meals several times a week, be aware that some can be high in sodium. Scan the labels to get those lowest in sodium and be sure to choose more whole foods (such as fresh fruits, veggies, grains, lean protein, and low-fat dairy) versus processed foods throughout the day to keep your sodium intake in check. In general, you want to limit yourself to 2,300 milligrams of sodium per day, or about 600 per meal.

Q: Between errands and the kids' activities, I sometimes end up skipping meals or grabbing something quick at a convenience store. What should I do?

A: In the morning, pack a small cooler with bottles of water or green tea, fruit, veggies, cheese sticks, yogurt, and nuts. These make great mini-meals to help you steer clear of the local convenience store, with its colas, jumbo candy bars, and bags of chips.

metabolism is doing its job, using up the calories from your last meal, and your body is ready for more fuel. But feeling hungry within an hour or so after eating or feeling as if you can't satisfy your hunger can be difficult when trying to control your calorie intake.

The first step in dealing with hunger is to determine if what you're feeling is really hunger. We often eat when we're actually thirsty or bored or stressed. So think about what's going on when the urge to eat strikes. Try drinking some water or green tea and see how you feel. If you know you often eat out of boredom, write down a list of projects that can occupy you and post it somewhere easy to see so you can refer to it before heading to the fridge. If you're stressed, call a friend to vent or go for a brisk walk instead of trying to soothe yourself with food.

If you're truly physically hungry—stomach growling, light-headed, and/or fatigued—you may need to increase your calorie intake by having another snack each day.

PUTTING THE PLAN INTO ACTION

KNOWING WHAT AND HOW MUCH YOU EAT is the best way to learn where you need to make changes to produce the weight loss and health benefits you desire. A food log or diary is a great instrument to help you become more aware of what you're putting into your body. Admittedly, it can be time consuming, but it really is an incredible learning tool. "I have always been careful about eating nutritious food, but tracking what I ate made me realize that some foods—like mayonnaise—are just not worth the calories," said WOW test panelist Denise Jennings. "And peanut butter is good for you, but it's easy to load on calories without realizing it."

Researchers at Kaiser Permanente have found that when dieters keep a food log, they lose almost twice as much weight compared with when they're not logging.[12]

The key components of a food diary are the foods and drinks you consume, of course, but also the amounts and the times. In the beginning, you should weigh and measure your food to learn what 3 ounces of chicken or ½ cup of carrots looks like. (You can also use visual cues like those on page 166.) Once you feel comfortable eyeballing your portions, it might be a good idea to do a spot-check on occasion, weighing and measuring a few foods to make sure that you haven't gradually increased (or decreased) the amounts.

Review your diary every 3 to 4 hours to make sure that you're eating at regular intervals throughout the day. This will also allow you to see if you're missing out or going overboard on any food groups.

Once you get in the habit of writing things down, go one step further and try to include calories. Food labels and restaurant and food manufacturer Web sites are the best sources for calorie counts and other nutrient values. For foods without labels or for online tracking, try *Prevention*'s My Health Trackers at prevention.com/healthtracker.

Seeing in print what they eat is often a big "aha" moment for people. Most find that they're eating either too many or far too few calories. That's right: Too few calories can be as bad for weight loss as too many. In particular, your metabolism may slow down, causing you to burn fewer calories as your body protects you from starving. This makes weight loss even more difficult.

Now you may be thinking, "*I know what I eat. I don't need to write it down.*" But after counseling people about healthy eating for more than 15 years, Heidi (our WOW dietitian) has found that perception doesn't always match the reality. Give journaling a try and see what it reveals about your eating habits. If nothing else, it may help you to eat better. Putting things in writing often makes them seem more real and honest. So just knowing that you have to document what goes into your mouth may be enough to help you steer clear of the doughnuts in the break room or stave off a late-night ice cream binge.

BREAKFAST BONUS

THE OLD SAYING ABOUT breakfast being the most important meal of the day really has some merit. As the first meal after a long period of not eating, breakfast wakes up your metabolism for the day. Also, the foods that make up a healthy breakfast, such as whole grains, fruits, and fat-free milk, pack a nutritional punch—a great opportunity to get a head start on your daily requirements for fiber, calcium, and an assortment of other nutrients.

Breakfast plays a role in weight loss, too. Countless studies have shown that people who regularly eat breakfast are less likely to be overweight than those who skip this morning meal. The explanation for this may have been revealed, at least in part, by recent research in which breakfast-eaters ended up taking in fewer calories throughout the entire day than non-breakfast-eaters. The a.m. eaters also had a lower body mass index (BMI), a measure-

ment commonly used to assess how healthy a person is based on her height and weight.[13]

Another study, in the *Journal of Nutrition*, found women who ate a high-fiber, low-sugar breakfast burned more fat when exercising.[14]

Fat burning was higher immediately after eating the higher-fiber breakfast as well as 3 hours later when the women took a 60-minute walk. In addition, lunch was more satiating after the higher-fiber breakfast.

"I took baby steps and lost big"

Laura Chiles experienced typical results, losing about ½ pound a week, as one of our 8-week exercise-only test panelists. After the official program, she added the WOW eating plan, and over an additional 8 weeks she lost more than six times as much weight (20 pounds versus 3¼) and more than twice as many

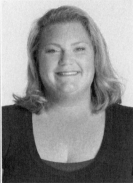

inches (8¾ versus 4¼) as she had during the 8 weeks in which she was doing only the WOW workouts.

Combining healthy eating with exercise definitely can improve weight loss, but I doubt that alone was responsible for Laura's fantastic turnaround. "Since I'm seeing good results, I notice that I'm really pushing harder when exercising and even doing more than required," she reported.

At first Laura was disappointed to be assigned to the exercise-only group, but now she credits her success in part to starting slowly. "Making many changes all at once never worked in the past because I got so overwhelmed," said the mother of three.

During those first 8 weeks, she kept herself from getting discouraged by her modest results by focusing on other good things that exercise was doing for her body. After just 1 week, for example, she could bend over more easily to pick up her kids' toys. After 3 weeks, she could carry on a conversation with her friends as they walked, rather than huffing and puffing.

Even playing kickball and dodgeball with her kids felt good to Laura after 8 weeks of regular exercise. Once she added the eating plan, it felt even better!

2 WEEKS OF WOW MENUS

HERE'S A 2-WEEK MENU PLAN to get you started and to show you how the WOW eating guidelines work in real life. It's by no means a strict diet that must be followed to a T. Feel free to use it for inspiration or to pick and choose what looks good—whatever works for you.

We all have different likes and dislikes. If a meal calls for a particular fruit or vegetable that you don't care for, swap it out for one you do like, referring to the lists beginning on page 166 for an appropriate serving size. Several meals include a tossed salad; this is simply any combination of your favorite salad-type veggies, such as lettuce, tomatoes, cucumbers, shredded carrots, and radishes.

You will come across some name brands in the menus. These are merely examples and not required; use the brand you prefer. Generally, the menus call for soft/tub/stick margarine because of its healthier nutrition profile, though you will see a few recipes with butter, which has a better flavor. You can certainly use margarine for cooking as well.

The meals and snacks that are higher in sodium (more than 650 milligrams) are marked with an asterisk. There are certain foods that, while healthy in other ways, are high in sodium, such as ham, lean deli meat, canned seafood, and so on. For most of us, there's no problem in enjoying these foods once in a while as long as you balance out the rest of the day with lower-sodium choices. Limit yourself to no more than 2,300 milligrams of sodium per day.

All meals and snacks make one serving unless otherwise noted.

For some quick, time-saving strategies, read through the menus in their entirety before you jump in. You'll see several foods that can be made ahead, which is a huge advantage when you're pressed for time.

You'll notice, too, that some meals include beverages while others do not. The meals without beverages are perfect opportunities to make progress toward your water and green tea quotas. Remember, you're striving for 3 cups of green tea and four 8-ounce glasses of water each day. If you can't start the day without your morning java, go ahead and wake up with 1 to 2 cups of coffee. Just remember, the milk and sugar in your coffee also add calories!

Speaking of calories, the meals in these menus loosely follow certain caloric guidelines. The goal for breakfast is 375 calories, lunch is 475, dinner is 550, and snacks are 200. Keep in mind, though, these are rough guidelines. There are days when breakfast may be closer to 300 or 400 or dinner may be barely 500 or a little over 600. The idea is, as in life, it all balances out in the end.

HERE YOU'LL FIND ALL of the foods that you'll need to follow the WOW 2-week meal plan. The pantry items that you may already have on hand appear first, followed by the shopping lists for Weeks 1 and 2. After each item, we've included the amount that you'll use in 1 or both weeks, so you can buy an appropriate quantity or see if you already have enough at home.

PANTRY ITEMS FOR BOTH WEEKS

Baking Needs
All-purpose flour (about $3\frac{1}{2}$ cups)
Almond extract ($\frac{1}{2}$ teaspoon)
Apple cider vinegar ($\frac{1}{2}$ tablespoon)
Baking powder (about 2 teaspoons)
Baking soda (about 1 teaspoon)
Black pepper (about $1\frac{3}{4}$ teaspoons)
Brown sugar (about 9 tablespoons)
Canola oil (about 4 teaspoons)
Cornstarch (about 3 teaspoons)
Granulated sugar (about $1\frac{1}{2}$ cups)
Olive oil (about 8 tablespoons)
Salt (about 3 teaspoons)
Semisweet chocolate chips (2 tablespoons)
Vanilla extract ($2\frac{1}{4}$ teaspoons)
White wine vinegar (about $\frac{1}{4}$ cup)

Condiments
All-fruit spread (2 teaspoons)
Chocolate syrup (2 tablespoons)
Garlic chili sauce or hot sauce (optional)
Honey (about 7 tablespoons)
Honey mustard (1 tablespoon)
Ketchup (1 teaspoon)
Maple syrup (3 tablespoons)
Mustard ($\frac{1}{2}$ tablespoon)
Peach preserves ($2\frac{1}{2}$ tablespoons)
Peanut butter ($\frac{1}{2}$ cup)
Pizza sauce (2 tablespoons)
Raspberry jelly (1 tablespoon)
Reduced-fat mayonnaise (7 tablespoons)
Reduced-fat salad dressing (about $1\frac{1}{4}$ cups)
   (such as Kraft Light Done Right!)

Reduced-sodium soy sauce (3 tablespoons)
Taco sauce ($\frac{1}{2}$ cup)
Worcestershire sauce ($\frac{1}{2}$ teaspoon)

Dairy
Butter (optional) (2 teaspoons)
Reduced-fat cream cheese (about 5 ounces)
Reduced-fat sour cream ($\frac{1}{2}$ cup)
Soft/tub/stick margarine (about
   8 tablespoons)

Grains
Plain bread crumbs (about 7 tablespoons)
Saltines (4)
Seasoned bread crumbs (2 tablespoons)
Whole-grain bread (12 slices)
Whole-grain crackers (about 13)

Herbs & Spices
Chili powder (about $1\frac{1}{2}$ tablespoons)
Dried onion flakes (use to taste)
Garlic powder (about $\frac{1}{2}$ teaspoon)
Ground cinnamon (about 3 teaspoons)
Ground cumin ($1\frac{1}{2}$ teaspoons)
Ground ginger (a dash)
Ground nutmeg (a dash)
Ground red pepper ($\frac{1}{8}$ teaspoon)
Onion powder (about 1 teaspoon)
Paprika ($\frac{1}{2}$ teaspoon; use more as garnish)
Red-pepper flakes (a dash)
Salt-free Italian seasoning
   (about $\frac{1}{8}$ teaspoon)

GROCERIES FOR WEEK 1

Baking Needs
Almonds, slivered ($^1/_4$ cup)
Cherries, dried (2 tablespoons)
Cranberries, dried (3 tablespoons)
Nonfat dry milk ($^3/_4$ cup + 1 tablespoon)
Raisins ($^3/_4$ cup)
Walnuts, chopped ($1^1/_2$ cups)

Cans/Bottles/Jars
100% cranapple or your favorite flavor juice ($^1/_2$ cup)
Beans, black (1 can, 15.5 ounces)
Beans, red (1 can, 15.5 ounces)
Corn (1 can, 8.75 ounces)
Mandarin oranges, juice-packed (1 small can)
Pineapple, crushed, juice-packed (2 cans, 8 ounces each)
Salmon, canned (1 can, 4 ounces)
Salsa, chunky (1 small jar)
Chicken stock (2 cups)
Tomatoes, diced (1 can, 15 ounces)
Tomato juice (1 small can)
Tomato paste (2 tablespoons)
Tomato sauce (2 cans, 8 ounces each)
Tuna, water-packed (1 can, 3 ounces)

Condiments
Capers (2 tablespoons)
Hummus ($^1/_3$ cup) (such as Tribe brand)
Olives (8 large)

Dairy
Cheddar cheese, reduced-fat (1 ounce)
Cheddar cheese, reduced-fat, shredded (8 ounces)
Cottage cheese, 1 carton ($^3/_4$ cup)
Eggs (13 large)
Feta cheese, crumbled (1 tablespoon)
Liquid egg substitute (4 tablespoons)
Milk, fat-free (1 gallon)
Parmesan cheese, grated ($3^1/_2$ tablespoons)
Pudding cup, fat-free, chocolate (1)
Romano cheese, grated (2 tablespoons)
Yogurt, fat-free, plain (4 cups)
Yogurt, low-fat, blueberry (1 container, 6 ounces)

Frozen Foods
Blueberries ($^3/_4$ cup)
Edamame ($^1/_2$ cup)
Raspberries ($^1/_2$ cup)
Snow peas (1 cup)
Veggie burgers (1)

Grains & Rice
Brown rice ($^1/_2$ cup)
Ciabatta roll (1 small)
Couscous, plain ($^1/_3$ cup)
Orzo ($^3/_4$ cup)
Quick oats ($3^1/_3$ cups)
Whole-grain elbow macaroni ($1^1/_2$ cups)
Whole-grain English muffins (1)
Whole-wheat bagel (1 mini)
Whole-wheat flour (1 cup)
Whole-wheat hamburger bun (1)
Whole-wheat tortilla (one 7-inch or 1.5 ounce)

Herbs & Spices
Garlic (4 cloves)

(continued)

GROCERIES FOR WEEK 1 *(continued)*

Meat/Poultry/Fish

Bacon, center-cut (2 strips)
Chicken breasts, boneless and skinless
    (4, about 4 ounces each)
Cod ($\frac{1}{2}$ pound)
Deli turkey, thinly sliced (2 ounces)
Ground beef, 93–95% lean ($\frac{1}{2}$ pound)
Pork loin chops, boneless
    (2, 4 ounces each)
Salmon fillet, cooked (3 ounces)
Shrimp, raw ($\frac{1}{2}$ pound medium/large)

Produce

Apples (1 Granny Smith, 1 your favorite)
Asparagus ($\frac{3}{4}$ cup)
Avocado (1 small)
Baby carrots* (1 cup)
Baby spinach (8 ounces)
Bananas (4)
Bell peppers, red (4 small)
Blueberries ($\frac{1}{4}$ cup)
Broccoli coleslaw (such as Mann's; 1 cup)
Carrots* (3 medium)

If you prefer, you can buy 1 to 2 pounds whole carrots to shred and cut sticks yourself, skipping the baby carrots and shredded carrots.

Carrots, shredded* (2 cups)
Cauliflower ($\frac{3}{4}$ cup)
Cucumbers (2 medium)
Grapes (about $\frac{1}{4}$ pound)
Green beans ($\frac{1}{2}$ cup)
Lemons (2)
Melon ($\frac{3}{4}$ cup)
Nectarines (2)
Onion, red (1 small)
Onion, white (2)
Orange (1 medium)
Peaches (2)
Plum (1)
Salad greens ($\frac{3}{4}$ cup)
Strawberries (2 quarts)
Tomatoes (2 medium)
Zucchini (1 small)

Snacks

Graham crackers (2)
Microwave popcorn, light (3 cups)
Tortilla chips, baked (1 ounce)

GROCERIES FOR WEEK 2

Baking Needs
Almonds, slivered (1$\frac{1}{2}$ tablespoons)
Cranberries, dried (2 tablespoons)
Raisins (2 tablespoons)
Sesame seeds ($\frac{1}{2}$ teaspoon)
Walnuts, chopped ($\frac{3}{4}$ cup)

Cans/Bottles/Cartons
Chicken stock ($\frac{1}{2}$ cup)
Cranberry sauce, jellied (2 tablespoons)
100% cranapple or your favorite flavor
    juice ($\frac{3}{4}$ cup)
100% orange juice ($\frac{1}{2}$ cup)
100% pineapple juice ($\frac{1}{2}$ cup)
Pesto (1 tablespoon)
Pineapple, crushed, juice-packed
    (8 ounces)
Pineapple chunks, canned, juice-packed
    (8 ounces), or fresh ($\frac{1}{2}$ cup)
Salmon, canned (2 ounces)
White wine (2 tablespoons)

Dairy
American cheese (1 slice)
Cheddar cheese, reduced-fat (5 ounces)
Cheddar cheese, reduced-fat, shredded
    (2 tablespoons)
Cottage cheese, 1% ($\frac{3}{4}$ cup)
Eggs (3 large)
Milk, fat-free (1 gallon plus 1 pint)
Mozzarella, reduced-fat, shredded
    (1 tablespoon)
String cheese, reduced-fat (2 sticks)
Yogurt, fat-free, plain (2 containers,
    1 cup each)
Yogurt, low-fat, vanilla (2 containers,
    6 ounces each) (such as Yoplait)
Yogurt, low-fat, your choice of flavors
    (1 container, 6 ounces)

Frozen Foods
Cheese pizza (one 12-inch) (such as
    Amy's 4 cheese)
Peas ($\frac{1}{2}$ cup)
Whole-grain waffles (2)

Grains & Rice
Bagel (one 3-inch)
Cheerios (1 cup)
Graham crackers (3$\frac{1}{4}$)
Jasmine rice ($\frac{1}{2}$ cup)
Long-grain rice ($\frac{1}{4}$ cup)
Whole-grain elbow macaroni ($\frac{1}{2}$ cup)
Whole-grain English muffins (2)
Whole-grain flake cereal ($\frac{3}{4}$ cup)
Whole-wheat spaghetti (4 ounces)
Whole-wheat tortillas (two 7-inch or
    1.5 ounces each)

Herbs & Spices
Chives (1 teaspoon)
Cilantro (1 teaspoon)
Garlic (3 cloves)
Ginger, fresh (1 teaspoon)

Meat/Poultry/Fish
Chicken breasts, boneless and skinless
    (4; about 4 ounces each)
Deli roast beef, low-sodium, thinly sliced
    (2 ounces)
Haddock or other white fish fillet
    ($\frac{1}{2}$ pound)
Ham steak (3 ounces)
Pork loin chop, boneless (4 ounces)
Salmon fillet (4 ounces)

(continued)

GROCERIES FOR WEEK 2 *(continued)*

Produce

Apples (1 Granny Smith, 1 your favorite)
Asparagus ($\frac{1}{2}$ cup)
Avocado (1 small)
Baby carrots* (1 cup)
Baking potatoes (2 small)
Bananas (3 medium)
Bell peppers, red (1 medium, 1 small)
Blueberries (1 cup)
Broccoli coleslaw (such as Mann's; $\frac{1}{2}$ cup)
Broccoli florets (3 cups)
Carrots, shredded* ($\frac{1}{2}$ cup)
Cucumber (1 medium)

If you prefer, you can buy 1 pound whole carrots to shred and cut sticks yourself, skipping the baby carrots and shredded carrots.

Grapes (1 cup or about $\frac{1}{2}$ pound)
Kiwifruit (1)
Lemon (1)
Melon ($1\frac{1}{2}$ cups)
Salad greens (5 cups)
Scallions (2)
Strawberries (1 cup)
Sweet potatoes (3 small, 1 large)
Tomatoes (2 or 3 small to medium)

Snacks

Cashews, unsalted or lightly salted (2 ounces)
Fun-size candy bars (3) (such as Milky Way)

BREAKFAST

Banana-Maple-Walnut Oatmeal (page 184)

¹/₂ cup cranapple juice

> PER SERVING: *423 calories, 7 g fat, 0 g saturated fat, 15 g protein, 79 g carbohydrates, 5 g fiber, 385 mg calcium, 212 mg sodium*

LUNCH

Ciabatta Turkey Sandwich: 1 small ciabatta roll cut in half, spread with 1 tablespoon raspberry jelly and layered with 2 ounces thinly sliced turkey breast, a medium-size lettuce leaf, and 1 slice red onion

¹/₂ cucumber, sliced, with ¹/₂ tablespoon reduced-fat dressing

1 medium fresh peach or ¹/₂ cup thawed frozen peaches

1 cup fat-free milk

> PER SERVING: *519 calories, 7 g fat, 1 g saturated fat, 32 g protein, 83 g carbohydrates, 5 g fiber, 388 mg calcium, 937 mg sodium**

SNACK

1 slice of Bananaberry Bread (page 185) topped with ¹/₂ tablespoon of peanut butter (or other nut butter)

> PER SERVING: *197 calories, 8 g fat, 1.5 g saturated fat, 5 g protein, 29 g carbohydrates, 2 g fiber, 22 mg calcium, 278 mg sodium*

DINNER

1 serving Cod Piccata (page 186)

¹/₂ cup cooked brown rice

1 cup baby carrots, steamed

1 cup fat-free milk

1 green apple

> PER SERVING: *550 calories, 11 g fat, 3 g saturated fat, 34 g protein, 83 g carbohydrates, 11 g fiber, 336 mg calcium, 650 mg sodium**

OPTIONAL SNACK

¹/₂ toasted whole-grain or whole-wheat mini bagel (2¹/₂-inch) with 2 teaspoons all-fruit spread

¹/₄ cup blueberries

1 cup fat-free milk

> PER SERVING: *190 calories, 1 g fat, 0 g saturated fat, 11 g protein, 36 g carbohydrates, 3 g fiber, 313 mg calcium, 192 mg sodium*

* Higher in sodium; remember to limit yourself to no more than 2,300 mg of sodium per day.

CHAPTER 7 EATING FOR WEIGHT LOSS AND EXERCISE

Banana-Maple-Walnut Oatmeal

TOTAL TIME: 5 MINUTES

½ cup Oatmeal Mix (see recipe below)
½ small banana, chopped
1 tablespoon maple syrup
1 tablespoon chopped walnuts
1 cup fat-free milk, divided

1. Combine the Oatmeal Mix, banana, syrup, walnuts, and ½ cup of the milk in a medium microwaveable bowl.

2. Microwave on high for 1 minute. Stir and continue to microwave at 30–second intervals until it reaches the desired consistency. Serve with the remaining ½ cup milk.

Makes 1 serving

MAKE-AHEAD

Oatmeal Mix

3 cups quick-cooking oats
¼ cup + 1 tablespoon nonfat dry milk
2 tablespoons brown sugar
1 teaspoon ground cinnamon
¼ teaspoon salt

Combine the oats, dry milk, brown sugar, cinnamon, and salt in a large bowl. Store in an airtight container.

Makes 4 cups

MAKE-AHEAD

Bananaberry Bread

TOTAL TIME: 1 HOUR

3 medium ripe bananas
½ teaspoon baking soda
3 tablespoons tub margarine
¼ cup mashed ripe avocado
¾ cup sugar
3 large eggs
½ cup whole-wheat flour
1½ cups all-purpose flour
1 teaspoon salt
1 teaspoon baking powder
3 tablespoons cold water
1 teaspoon vanilla extract
¾ cup frozen blueberries

1. Preheat the oven to 350ºF.

2. Mash the bananas and baking soda together in a small bowl and set aside.

3. Cream the margarine, avocado, and sugar together in a medium bowl. Add the eggs one at a time, mixing after each. Add the flours, salt, and baking powder and combine until just mixed. Stir in the water and vanilla. Add the banana mixture and mix until well combined. Fold in the blueberries.

4. Pour the batter evenly into two 8-inch loaf pans. Bake for 40 to 50 minutes, until a cake tester inserted in the center of the bread comes out clean. Let cool before turning out.

Makes 16 1"-thick slices

NOTE: *After cooling completely, store half a loaf in the refrigerator; it should keep about 1 week. Wrap and freeze the remainder for future use.*

Cod Piccata

TOTAL TIME: 15 MINUTES

2 tablespoons all-purpose flour
$\frac{1}{8}$ teaspoon black pepper
$\frac{1}{2}$ pound cod fillet
2 teaspoons canola oil
$\frac{1}{2}$ cup low-sodium chicken stock
$\frac{1}{2}$ teaspoon cornstarch
$1\frac{1}{2}$ teaspoons water
1 tablespoon freshly squeezed lemon juice
$1\frac{1}{2}$ teaspoons butter or tub margarine
2 tablespoons drained capers

1. Mix the flour and pepper in a pie plate. Dredge the fish in the flour mixture to coat.

2. Heat the oil in a large nonstick skillet over medium–high heat. Add the fish and cook until brown, about 2 minutes. Turn the fish and cook the other side for 1 to 2 minutes longer. Remove the fish to a plate and keep warm.

3. Increase the heat to high. Add the stock to the skillet and bring to a boil. Cook for about 3 minutes, or until reduced by half.

4. In a cup, dissolve the cornstarch in the water and whisk into the stock. Cook for 1 minute, then stir in the lemon juice and butter.

5. Put the fish back into the skillet along with the capers to warm up and let the sauce thicken for a minute or two.

Makes 2 servings

BREAKFAST

1 poached egg

1 toasted whole-grain English muffin with 1 teaspoon tub margarine

³/₄ cup cubed melon

1 cup fat-free milk

> eZg hZgk^c\ 0 369 calories, 10 g fat, 2 g saturated fat, 21 g protein, 51 g carbohydrates,
> 4 g fiber, 385 mg calcium, 471 mg sodium

LUNCH

Spinach Salad (page 188)

1 cup fat-free plain yogurt mixed with ¹/₂ cup drained mandarin oranges

> eZg hZgk^c\ 0 449 calories, 22 g fat, 5 g saturated fat, 23 g protein, 49 g carbohydrates,
> 8 g fiber, 427 mg calcium, 752 mg sodium*

SNACK

1 ounce baked tortilla chips with 3 tablespoons chunky salsa and
2 tablespoons mashed avocado

> eZg hZgk^c\ 0 180 calories, 7 g fat, 1 g saturated fat, 3 g protein, 27 g carbohydrates,
> 5 g fiber, 4 mg calcium, 497 mg sodium

DINNER

1 serving Chicken Cutlets Pomodoro (page 189)

¹/₂ cup cooked orzo

¹/₂ cup steamed green beans seasoned with ¹/₈ teaspoon salt-free Italian seasoning

> eZg hZgk^c\ 0 660 calories, 24 g fat, 6 g saturated fat, 41 g protein, 71 g carbohydrates,
> 5 g fiber, 184 mg calcium, 549 mg sodium

OPTIONAL SNACK

2 graham crackers (2¹/₂" squares)

1 medium nectarine

¹/₂ cup fat-free milk

> eZg hZgk^c\ 0 167 calories, 2 g fat, 0 g saturated fat, 7 g protein, 32 g carbohydrates,
> 3 g fiber, 137 mg calcium, 150 mg sodium

* Higher in sodium; remember to limit yourself to no more than 2,300 mg of sodium per day.

Spinach Salad

TOTAL TIME: 10 MINUTES

Dressing

> 1 tablespoon olive oil
> 1 teaspoon sugar
> 1 teaspoon ketchup
> ½ teaspoon white wine vinegar
> ½ teaspoon Worcestershire sauce
> Pinch of salt

Salad

> 4 ounces baby spinach (roughly chopped, if desired)
> 1 slice center-cut bacon, cooked and diced
> ½ small tomato, chopped
> 1 large hard-cooked egg, sliced

1. For the dressing: Combine the oil, sugar, ketchup, vinegar, Worcestershire sauce, and salt in a cup and mix well.

2. For the salad: Toss together the spinach, bacon, and tomato in a serving bowl. Top with the egg and drizzle the dressing on top.

MAKE-AHEAD

Chicken Cutlets Pomodoro

TOTAL TIME: 20 MINUTES

½ cup all-purpose flour
1 egg, beaten
¼ cup + 2 tablespoons plain dry bread crumbs
3 tablespoons Parmesan cheese
3 boneless, skinless chicken breasts (4 ounces each),
    pounded to ¼" thickness
2 tablespoons olive oil
2 tablespoons grated or minced onion
2 tablespoons sugar
2 cloves garlic, grated or minced
1 cup chicken stock
2 tablespoons tomato paste
Dash of salt
Dash of black pepper

1. Preheat the oven to 400°F.

2. Place ¼ cup + 2 tablespoons of the flour in one shallow bowl and the egg in another. Mix the bread crumbs and Parmesan in a third shallow bowl. Dredge the chicken in the flour and dip in the egg, then in the bread crumb mixture. In a large nonstick skillet, sauté the chicken in 1 tablespoon of the oil over medium-low heat for 2 minutes on each side, until browned. Place the chicken on a baking sheet and bake for 10 minutes.

3. Meanwhile, wipe out the skillet, then add the remaining 1 tablespoon oil and heat over medium heat. Add the onion and 1 tablespoon of the sugar. Cook until the onion is softened and slightly brown. Add the garlic and cook for a few seconds, then add the remaining 2 tablespoons flour and cook for 1 minute longer. Whisk in the stock, tomato paste, salt, pepper, and the remaining 1 tablespoon sugar. Cook on medium heat until thickened, about 5 minutes.

4. Remove the chicken from the oven. Set one cutlet aside to cool, and then refrigerate to use on Day 4. Pour the sauce over the remaining 2 cutlets and serve.

Makes 3 servings

BREAKFAST

1 cup fat-free plain yogurt mixed with $\frac{1}{2}$ cup diced strawberries and $\frac{1}{4}$ cup chopped walnuts

> **PER SERVING:** *318 calories, 19 g fat, 2 g saturated fat, 15 g protein, 29 g carbohydrates, 4 g fiber, 342 mg calcium, 136 mg sodium*

LUNCH

Salmon Melt (page 191)

$\frac{1}{2}$ cucumber, sliced, with 1 tablespoon reduced-fat dressing for dipping

1 medium plum

1 cup fat-free milk

> **PER SERVING:** *567 calories, 21 g fat, 5 g saturated fat, 40 g protein, 54 g carbohydrates, 6 g fiber, 466 mg calcium, 675 mg sodium**

SNACK

1 medium red bell pepper cut into sticks, with $\frac{1}{3}$ cup flavored hummus

> **PER SERVING:** *169 calories, 8 g fat, 0 g saturated fat, 4 g protein, 20 g carbohydrates, 5 g fiber, 8 mg calcium, 427 mg sodium*

DINNER

1 serving Stovetop Mac 'n' Cheese (page 192)

1 cup steamed snow peas

> **PER SERVING:** *567 calories, 53 g fat, 11 g saturated fat, 28 g protein, 57 g carbohydrates, 6 g fiber, 577 mg calcium, 733 mg sodium**

OPTIONAL SNACK

$\frac{1}{2}$ cup edamame

1 ounce reduced-fat Cheddar cheese

> **PER SERVING:** *191 calories, 10 g fat, 5 g saturated fat, 15 g protein, 9 g carbohydrates, 4 g fiber, 253 mg calcium, 442 mg sodium*

* Higher in sodium; remember to limit yourself to no more than 2,300 mg of sodium per day.

Salmon Melt

TOTAL TIME: 10 MINUTES

> 3 ounces cooked salmon fillet, flaked
> 2 teaspoons reduced-fat mayonnaise
> 1 whole-wheat English muffin, toasted
> 2 slices tomato
> 1 tablespoon reduced-fat shredded Cheddar cheese

1. Preheat the oven or toaster oven broiler.

2. Combine the salmon and mayonnaise in a small bowl. Spread evenly on the muffin halves. Top each half with a tomato slice and sprinkle the cheese evenly over the tops.

3. Place on a baking sheet and broil until the cheese melts.

NOTE: *Salmon is used in this recipe to provide omega–3 fatty acids, but you may substitute tuna. If you're short on time, you may use canned/pouched salmon, but the sodium content is much higher.*

Stovetop Mac 'n' Cheese

TOTAL TIME: 20 MINUTES

> 1 cup whole-grain elbow macaroni
> 1½ tablespoons olive oil
> 2 tablespoons all-purpose flour
> Dash of salt
> Dash of black pepper
> ½ cup fat-free milk
> ½ can (8 ounces) diced tomatoes, drained
> 1 cup reduced-fat shredded Cheddar cheese

1. Cook the macaroni according to package directions.

2. Meanwhile, in a medium saucepan, heat the oil over medium heat. Add the flour, salt, and pepper and whisk until bubbly, about a minute.

3. Gradually add the milk and stir until thickened. Add the tomatoes and stir. Add the cheese and stir until melted.

4. Add the drained pasta to the sauce pan and stir until it is evenly coated with sauce.

Makes 2 servings

BREAKFAST

Touch-of-Honey Berry Smoothie (page 194)

1 slice toasted whole-grain bread with $\frac{1}{2}$ teaspoon tub margarine

> PER SERVING: *335 calories, 5 g fat, 2 g saturated fat, 11 g protein, 63 g carbohydrates, 4 g fiber, 298 mg calcium, 238 mg sodium*

LUNCH

Chicken Garden Salad: 2 cups greens, $\frac{1}{2}$ medium tomato, chopped, and $\frac{1}{2}$ cucumber, sliced, topped with a chicken breast (left over from Day 2), sliced, and 2 tablespoons reduced-fat dressing

3 whole-grain crackers

1 medium nectarine

1 cup fat-free milk

> PER SERVING: *543 calories, 15 g fat, 3 g saturated fat, 42 g protein, 63 g carbohydrates, 10 g fiber, 370 mg calcium, 661 mg sodium**

SNACK

10 medium strawberries dipped into 1 fat-free chocolate pudding cup

> PER SERVING: *163 calories, 0 g fat, 0 g saturated fat, 3 g protein, 37 g carbohydrates, 4 g fiber, 85 mg calcium, 200 mg sodium*

DINNER

1 serving Bean-Lover's Chili (page 195)

4 saltine crackers

1 cup tossed salad with $1\frac{1}{2}$ tablespoons reduced-fat dressing

1 cup fat-free milk

> PER SERVING: *590 calories, 13 g fat, 4 g saturated fat, 28 g protein, 93 g carbohydrates, 17 g fiber, 459 mg calcium, 858 mg sodium**

OPTIONAL SNACK

10 unsalted walnut halves mixed with 3 tablespoons dried cranberries

> PER SERVING: *205 calories, 13 g fat, 1 g saturated fat, 3 g protein, 21 g carbohydrates, 2 g fiber, 20 mg calcium, 0 mg sodium*

* Higher in sodium; remember to limit yourself to no more than 2,300 mg of sodium per day.

Touch-of-Honey Berry Smoothie

TOTAL TIME: 5 MINUTES

1 container (6 ounces) reduced-fat blueberry yogurt
½ cup frozen raspberries
¼ cup fat-free milk
1½ teaspoons honey

Combine the yogurt, raspberries, milk, and honey in a blender. Blend until smooth. Pour into a glass.

Bean-Lover's Chili

TOTAL TIME: 40 MINUTES

2 teaspoons olive oil
2 tablespoons chopped onion
¼ cup chopped red bell pepper
½ can (7.75 ounces) black beans, rinsed and drained
½ can (7.75 ounces) red beans, rinsed and drained
1 cup frozen corn
½ can (7.25 ounces) unsalted, diced tomatoes, not drained
½ can (4 ounces) unsalted tomato sauce
1½ teaspoons chili powder
¼ cup reduced-fat shredded Cheddar cheese

1. Heat the oil in a medium saucepan over medium heat. Add the onion and pepper and cook, stirring often, until tender, about 5 to 10 minutes. Add the black beans, red beans, corn, tomatoes (in sauce), tomato sauce, and chili powder. Mix well. Reduce the heat to low, cover, and simmer for 30 minutes, stirring occasionally.

2. Sprinkle 1 tablespoon of the cheese evenly in the bottom of each bowl. Add the chili, then sprinkle with the remaining cheese.

Makes 2 servings

BREAKFAST

Florentine Omelet (page 197)

2 slices toasted whole-grain bread with 1 teaspoon tub margarine

1 medium orange

> **PER SERVING:** *367 calories, 13 g fat, 4 g saturated fat, 23 g protein, 41 g carbohydrates, 7 g fiber, 188 mg calcium, 541 mg sodium*

LUNCH

Tuna Sandwich: 2 slices toasted whole-grain bread topped with 3 ounces canned water-packed tuna, drained and mixed with $1/2$ tablespoon reduced-fat mayonnaise

1 serving Carrot-Broccoli Salad (page 198)

> **PER SERVING:** *441 calories, 12 g fat, 3 g saturated fat, 30 g protein, 53 g carbohydrates, 8 g fiber, 134 mg calcium, 915 mg sodium**

SNACK

1 Cream Cheese–Filled Carrot Cake Gem (page 199)

$1/2$ cup fat-free milk

> **PER SERVING:** *209 calories, 6 g fat, 2 g saturated fat, 9 g protein, 32 g carbohydrates, 1 g fiber, 164 mg calcium, 226 mg sodium*

DINNER

1 serving Honey Baked Shrimp (page 200)

$3/4$ cup steamed asparagus with $1/2$ teaspoon tub margarine

Lemon-Scented Couscous: $1/3$ cup plain couscous cooked according to the package directions, but replace $1/2$ cup of the water with chicken stock and add 1 teaspoon olive oil and the zest of half a lemon

$1/2$ cup fat-free milk

> **PER SERVING:** *684 calories, 14 g fat, 2 g saturated fat, 42 g protein, 100 g carbohydrates, 6 g fiber, 237 mg calcium, 716 mg sodium**

OPTIONAL SNACK

$1/2$ cup light churned ice cream or frozen yogurt topped with $3/4$ cup sliced strawberries and 1 tablespoon chopped walnuts

> **PER SERVING:** *198 calories, 7 g fat, 1 g saturated fat, 5 g protein, 30 g carbohydrates, 4 g fiber, 127 mg calcium, 46 mg sodium*

* Higher in sodium; remember to limit yourself to no more than 2,300 mg of sodium per day.

Florentine Omelet

TOTAL TIME: 8 MINUTES

> 1 large egg
> 2 large egg whites
> 2 teaspoons water
> 2 tablespoons finely chopped fresh baby spinach
> ¼ small tomato, diced
> 1 tablespoon feta cheese, crumbled

1. Heat a small nonstick skillet over medium heat. Scramble the egg, egg whites, and water together in a small bowl. Pour into the hot skillet, tilting and turning the skillet to coat the entire bottom. With a spatula or spoon, while tilting the pan slightly, scrape the edges of the cooked egg toward the center of the pan and allow the uncooked egg to flow out onto the pan. Continue doing this until the egg is almost set.

2. Spread the spinach, tomato, and feta evenly over half of the egg mixture. Fold the other half of the egg over the spinach. Continue to cook until the spinach is heated through and the egg is cooked.

CHAPTER 7 EATING FOR WEIGHT LOSS AND EXERCISE

MAKE-AHEAD

Carrot-Broccoli Salad

TOTAL TIME: 5 MINUTES

    2 tablespoons reduced-fat sour cream
    2 tablespoons reduced-fat mayonnaise
    1 teaspoon freshly squeezed lemon juice
    Dash of salt
    1 teaspoon brown sugar
    1 cup shredded carrots
    1 cup packaged broccoli coleslaw (such as Mann's)
    ¼ cup raisins
    2 tablespoons drained crushed pineapple

1. Combine the sour cream, mayonnaise, lemon juice, salt, and sugar in a large bowl and mix well.

2. Stir in the carrots, coleslaw, raisins, and pineapple until well coated. Chill and reserve 1 serving to use on Day 7.

Makes 2 servings

MAKE-AHEAD

Cream Cheese–Filled Carrot Cake Gems

TOTAL TIME: 45 MINUTES

Filling

> 4 ounces reduced-fat cream cheese, softened
> ¼ cup sugar
> 2 tablespoons liquid egg substitute

Muffins

> 1¼ cups all-purpose flour
> ½ cup whole-wheat flour
> ¼ teaspoon salt
> ¼ teaspoon baking soda
> ¾ teaspoon baking powder
> 1 teaspoon ground cinnamon
> 2 tablespoons canola oil

> ¼ cup low-fat sour cream
> 2½ tablespoons brown sugar
> 2½ tablespoons sugar
> 1 egg
> 1 teaspoon vanilla
> 1 cup freshly grated carrots
> ½ cup drained crushed pineapple

1. Preheat the oven to 375°F. Coat a 12-cup muffin tin with nonstick spray.

2. For the filling: Beat together the cream cheese, sugar, and egg substitute in a small bowl.

3. For the muffins: In a large bowl, combine the flours, salt, baking soda, baking powder, and cinnamon. Set aside.

4. In a medium bowl, cream together the oil, sour cream, and sugars until well blended. Beat in the egg and vanilla. Stir in the carrots and pineapple.

5. Make a well in the center of the dry ingredients and add the wet ingredients all at once. Stir just until combined. The batter will be thick, so don't overmix.

6. Fill the muffin cups about one-quarter of the way with the batter. Add 1 tablespoon of the filling, then top with more batter (it may not cover completely).

7. Bake for 20 to 25 minutes, until a cake tester or toothpick inserted in the center of a muffin comes out clean. Let cool for 10 minutes before removing from the pan.

Makes 12 muffins

NOTE: *Freeze 10 of the muffins to keep them fresh longer. Reserve 1 muffin for Day 8.*

CHAPTER 7 EATING FOR WEIGHT LOSS AND EXERCISE

Honey Baked Shrimp

TOTAL TIME: 40 MINUTES

¼ cup reduced-fat Italian dressing
1 clove garlic, grated or minced
¼ cup honey
½ pound peeled and deveined medium or large raw shrimp

1. Combine the dressing, garlic, and honey in a medium bowl. Add the shrimp and toss to coat. Cover and refrigerate for 30 minutes.

2. Preheat the oven to 400ºF. Place the shrimp in an even layer on a baking sheet and drizzle with any remaining marinade. Bake for 5 to 6 minutes, or until the shrimp turn pink all over.

Makes 2 servings

BREAKFAST
Cherry-Almond Oatmeal (page 202)

½ cup orange juice

> **PER SERVING:** *410 calories, 8 g fat, 0 g saturated fat, 19 g protein, 67 g carbohydrates, 7 g fiber, 361 mg calcium, 221 mg sodium*

LUNCH
Veggie burger on a whole-grain bun

1 serving Waldorf Salad (page 202)

> **PER SERVING:** *444 calories, 13 g fat, 2 g saturated fat, 18 g protein, 67 g carbohydrates, 10 g fiber, 118 mg calcium, 664 mg sodium**

SNACK
1 cup fat-free plain yogurt mixed with ½ cup sliced strawberries and 2 tablespoons slivered almonds

> **PER SERVING:** *204 calories, 7 g fat, 1 g saturated fat, 13 g protein, 28 g carbohydrates, 3 g fiber, 349 mg calcium, 136 mg sodium*

DINNER
1 serving Skillet Meatloaf in Pepper Rings (page 203)

¼ cup cooked orzo mixed with ½ tablespoon Parmesan cheese and ⅛ teaspoon black pepper

½ cup sliced, steamed zucchini

> **PER SERVING:** *515 calories, 12 g fat, 5 g saturated fat, 39 g protein, 59 g carbohydrates, 6 g fiber, 202 mg calcium, 381 mg sodium*

OPTIONAL SNACK
1 cup baby carrots with ¼ cup flavored hummus

> **PER SERVING:** *153 calories, 6 g fat, 0 g saturated fat, 3 g protein, 22 g carbohydrates, 5 g fiber, 27 mg calcium, 380 mg sodium*

* Higher in sodium; remember to limit yourself to no more than 2,300 mg of sodium per day.

Cherry-Almond Oatmeal

TOTAL TIME: 5 MINUTES

$\frac{1}{2}$ cup Oatmeal Mix (page 184)
2 tablespoons dried cherries
1$\frac{1}{2}$ tablespoons slivered almonds
1 cup fat-free milk

1. Combine the Oatmeal Mix, cherries, almonds, and $\frac{1}{2}$ cup of the milk in a microwaveable bowl.

2. Microwave on high for 1 minute. Stir and continue to microwave at 30–second intervals until it reaches the desired consistency. Serve with the remaining $\frac{1}{2}$ cup milk.

MAKE-AHEAD

Waldorf Salad

TOTAL TIME: 5 MINUTES

1 tablespoon reduced-fat mayonnaise
1 tablespoon fat-free plain yogurt
1$\frac{1}{2}$ teaspoons sugar
$\frac{1}{2}$ teaspoon freshly squeezed lemon juice
Pinch of salt
1 large apple, cored and diced
2 tablespoons chopped walnuts
$\frac{1}{4}$ cup raisins

In a medium bowl, combine the mayonnaise, yogurt, sugar, lemon juice, and salt. Add the apple, walnuts, and raisins and stir well. Chill and reserve 1 serving to use on Day 8.
Makes 2 servings

Skillet Meatloaf in Pepper Rings

TOTAL TIME: 45 MINUTES

½ pound lean ground beef (93–95% lean)
¼ cup + 2 tablespoons oats
½ teaspoon onion powder
2 tablespoons liquid egg substitute
½ can (2.25 ounces) low-sodium tomato juice
2 tablespoons grated Romano cheese
Dash of salt
Dash of black pepper
1 tablespoon olive oil
2 small red bell peppers or 1 large
1 can (8 ounces) unsalted tomato sauce
2 tablespoons maple syrup
1 clove garlic, minced or grated

1. Preheat the oven to 375ºF.

2. In a medium bowl, combine the beef, oats, onion powder, egg substitute, tomato juice, Romano, salt, and pepper. Set aside.

3. In an ovenproof skillet, heat the oil over medium-high heat. Seed and core the peppers and slice into four 1" rings. Press the meatloaf mixture evenly into the pepper rings. Sauté the meat-filled rings for about 5 minutes per side, until golden brown.

4. In a small bowl, combine the tomato sauce, syrup, and garlic. Pour evenly over the meat and peppers. Place the skillet in the oven and bake for about 20 minutes, or until cooked through.

Makes 2 servings

BREAKFAST

2 slices whole-grain bread, toasted and topped with 1 teaspoon tub margarine and $\frac{1}{4}$ teaspoon cinnamon

1 medium peach

Amaretto Steamer (page 205)

PER SERVING: *361 calories, 5 g fat, 1 g saturated fat, 15 g protein, 69 g carbohydrates, 12 g fiber, 457 mg calcium, 334 mg sodium*

LUNCH

Lean Green Wrap (page 205)

$\frac{1}{2}$ cup grapes

1 serving Carrot-Broccoli Salad (left over from Day 5)

$\frac{1}{2}$ cup fat-free milk

PER SERVING: *606 calories, 15 g fat, 5 g saturated fat, 34 g protein, 77 g carbohydrates, 7 g fiber, 331 mg calcium, 717 mg sodium**

SNACK

$\frac{1}{2}$ cup 1% cottage cheese mixed with 4 ounces crushed pineapple, drained

PER SERVING: *149 calories, 1 g fat, 1 g saturated fat, 15 g protein, 21 g carbohydrates, 1 g fiber, 87 mg calcium, 460 mg sodium*

DINNER

1 serving Peachy Pork Olé (page 206)

$\frac{1}{2}$ cup cooked brown rice

$\frac{3}{4}$ cup steamed cauliflower topped with $\frac{1}{2}$ teaspoon melted butter mixed with $1\frac{1}{2}$ teaspoons plain dry bread crumbs

$\frac{1}{2}$ cup fat-free milk

PER SERVING: *495 calories, 16 g fat, 5 g saturated fat, 27 g protein, 55 g carbohydrates, 4 g fiber, 165 mg calcium, 542 mg sodium*

OPTIONAL SNACK

3 cups popped light microwave popcorn mixed with 2 tablespoons raisins and 1 tablespoon peanut butter (or other nut butter)

PER SERVING: *262 calories, 10 g fat, 2 g saturated fat, 8 g protein, 36 g carbohydrates, 5 g fiber, 13 mg calcium, 292 mg sodium*

* Higher in sodium; remember to limit yourself to no more than 2,300 mg of sodium per day.

Amaretto Steamer

TOTAL TIME: 3 MINUTES

1 cup fat-free milk
1 tablespoon chocolate syrup
½ teaspoon almond extract

Heat the milk, syrup, and almond extract together in a small saucepan or microwaveable cup.

Lean Green Wrap

1 tablespoon honey mustard
1 medium (7" or 1.5 ounce) whole-wheat tortilla
2 ounces chopped cooked boneless, skinless chicken breast
½ cup raw baby spinach
2 tablespoons reduced-fat shredded Cheddar cheese

Spread the mustard on the tortilla. Fill with the chicken, spinach, and cheese and roll up.

Peachy Pork Olé

TOTAL TIME: 30 MINUTES

> 2 boneless pork loin chops (4 ounces each), trimmed of excess fat and cut into bite-size pieces
> 1½ teaspoons taco seasoning (see recipe below)
> 1 teaspoon canola oil
> ½ cup taco sauce
> 2½ tablespoons peach preserves

1. Coat the pork with the taco seasoning.

2. Heat the oil in a large nonstick skillet over medium–high heat. Add the pork and cook about 6 to 8 minutes or until lightly browned, stirring occasionally.

3. Add the taco sauce and preserves. Lower the heat, cover, and simmer for 15 to 20 minutes, or until the sauce is slightly thickened and the pork is firm but not hard.

Makes 2 servings

MAKE-AHEAD

Taco Seasoning

> 1 tablespoon chili powder
> ¼ teaspoon garlic powder
> ¼ teaspoon onion powder
> ⅛ teaspoon ground red pepper
> ½ teaspoon paprika
> 1½ teaspoons ground cumin
> ½ teaspoon salt
> 1 teaspoon black pepper

Combine the chili powder, garlic powder, onion powder, red pepper, paprika, cumin, salt, and black pepper in a cup and mix well. Store in an airtight container.

Makes 2⅓ tablespoons

BREAKFAST

¾ cup whole-grain flake cereal with 2 tablespoons chopped walnuts and ½ medium banana, sliced

1 cup fat-free milk

PER SERVING: *369 calories, 11 g fat, 1 g saturated fat, 16 g protein, 59 g carbohydrates, 7 g fiber, 279 mg calcium, 245 mg sodium*

LUNCH

Ham-and-Sweet-Potato Bake (page 208)

1 serving Waldorf Salad (left over from Day 6)

½ cup fat-free milk

PER SERVING: *561 calories, 15 g fat, 3 g saturated fat, 24 g protein, 87 g carbohydrates, 8 g fiber, 205 mg calcium, 1,281 mg sodium**

SNACK

1 Cream Cheese–Filled Carrot Cake Gem (left over from Day 5), cut in half and heated in a nonstick skillet or toaster oven

½ cup low-fat vanilla yogurt

PER SERVING: *164 calories, 6 g fat, 2 g saturated fat, 4 g protein, 25 g carbohydrates, 1 g fiber, 39 mg calcium, 161 mg sodium*

DINNER

1 boneless, skinless chicken breast (4 ounces) sprinkled with salt-free seasoning and grilled

1 serving Stuffed Baked Potatoes (page 209)

½ cup steamed broccoli with ½ teaspoon tub margarine and sprinkled with dried minced onion

1 cup tossed salad with 1½ tablespoons reduced-fat dressing and 2 tablespoons chopped walnuts

½ cup fat-free milk

1 cup cut-up watermelon (or other melon)

PER SERVING: *592 calories, 22 g fat, 5 g saturated fat, 40 g protein, 68 g carbohydrates, 10 g fiber, 310 mg calcium, 486 mg sodium*

OPTIONAL SNACK

1 slice toasted whole-grain bread topped with 1 tablespoon peanut butter (or other nut butter)

PER SERVING: *164 calories, 9 g fat, 2 g saturated fat, 7 g protein, 15 g carbohydrates, 3 g fiber, 27 mg calcium, 185 mg sodium*

* Higher in sodium; remember to limit yourself to no more than 2,300 mg of sodium per day.

Ham-and-Sweet-Potato Bake

TOTAL TIME: 35 MINUTES

3 ounces ham steak
1 tablespoon brown sugar
½ can (4 ounces total) crushed pineapple, drained
1 small baked sweet potato, peeled and sliced

1. Heat the oven to 350ºF.

2. Place the ham slice on a large piece of foil. Sprinkle with the brown sugar, then with the pineapple. Arrange the potato slices on top. Seal the foil packet and place on a baking sheet. Bake for 30 minutes. Carefully open the packet to serve.

MAKE-AHEAD

Stuffed Baked Potatoes

TOTAL TIME: 60 MINUTES

> 2 small baking potatoes
> 1 tablespoon fat-free milk
> 1 teaspoon tub margarine
> 2 tablespoons reduced-fat sour cream
> 2 tablespoons reduced-fat shredded Cheddar cheese
> $\frac{1}{8}$ teaspoon black pepper
> Ground paprika

1. Preheat the oven to 400°F.

2. Scrub the potatoes and poke a few times with a fork. Bake for about 45 minutes, or until soft.

3. Remove the potatoes from the oven and reduce the oven temperature to 350°F. Let the potatoes cool slightly. Cut in half lengthwise. Scoop out the potato flesh, leaving about a $\frac{1}{8}$"-thick skin. Set aside.

4. Combine the potato flesh with the milk, margarine, sour cream, cheese, and pepper. Beat with an electric mixer until well combined. Divide the mixture evenly among the potato skins. Sprinkle with the paprika. Return to the oven for 15 to 20 minutes, or until heated through.

NOTE: *The potatoes can be prepared earlier in the day. After sprinkling with the paprika, refrigerate until ready to eat. Then heat in the oven for 30 minutes.*

Makes 2 servings

BREAKFAST

Egg & Avocado Breakfast Sandwich (page 211)

¹/₂ cup raspberries

³/₄ cup fat-free milk

> PER SERVING: *399 calories, 8 g fat, 2 g saturated fat, 23 g protein, 60 g carbohydrates, 3 g fiber, 301 mg calcium, 569 mg sodium*

LUNCH

Simple Salmon Macaroni Salad (page 211)

¹/₂ cup pineapple chunks, fresh or canned and drained

³/₄ cup fat-free milk

> PER SERVING: *510 calories, 13 g fat, 3 g saturated fat, 29 g protein, 73 g carbohydrates, 8 g fiber, 315 mg calcium, 526 mg sodium*

SNACK

1 ounce reduced-fat Cheddar cheese melted over 5 whole-grain crackers

> PER SERVING: *191 calories, 11 g fat, 5 g saturated fat, 10 g protein, 17 g carbohydrates, 3 g fiber, 203 mg calcium, 332 mg sodium*

DINNER

¹/₂ Frozen Pizza Deluxe: Cook a frozen cheese pizza according to package directions. Halfway into the cooking time, top with 1 medium tomato, diced, and 1 medium red bell pepper, seeded and diced.

1 cup tossed salad with 1¹/₂ tablespoons reduced-fat dressing

1 cup fat-free milk

> PER SERVING: *347 calories, 12 g fat, 2 g saturated fat, 16 g protein, 45 g carbohydrates, 4 g fiber, 325 mg calcium, 643 mg sodium**

OPTIONAL SNACK

¹/₂ toasted whole-wheat English muffin, topped with 1 tablespoon peanut butter (or other nut butter) and ¹/₂ medium banana, sliced

> PER SERVING: *210 calories, 9 g fat, 2 g saturated fat, 7 g protein, 30 g carbohydrates, 4 g fiber, 53 mg calcium, 183 mg sodium*

* Higher in sodium; remember to limit yourself to no more than 2,300 mg of sodium per day.

Egg & Avocado Breakfast Sandwich

TOTAL TIME: 8 MINUTES

1 large egg, lightly beaten
1 tablespoon mashed avocado
1 bagel (3"), halved and toasted

1. Coat a small nonstick skillet with cooking spray and place over medium heat.

2. Add the egg and cook until set.

3. Spread the avocado on half of the bagel. Top with the egg and the remaining half of the bagel.

Simple Salmon Macaroni Salad

TOTAL TIME: 20 MINUTES

½ cup whole-grain elbow macaroni
2 ounces boneless canned salmon, drained
1½ tablespoons reduced-fat mayonnaise
½ cup baby peas, frozen
⅛ teaspoon garlic powder
⅛ teaspoon onion powder

1. Cook the macaroni according to the package directions.

2. In a small bowl, combine the salmon, mayonnaise, peas, garlic powder, and onion powder. Add the drained pasta and mix well.

NOTE: *Salmon is used in this recipe to provide omega-3 fatty acids, but you may also substitute tuna.*

BREAKFAST

1 slice Bananaberry Bread (left over from Day 1), toasted and topped with 1 tablespoon reduced-fat cream cheese

1 large hard-cooked egg spread with $\frac{1}{2}$ teaspoon tub margarine

$\frac{1}{2}$ cup raspberries

PER SERVING: *285 calories, 13 g fat, 4 g saturated fat, 11 g protein, 35 g carbohydrates, 2 g fiber, 71 mg calcium, 398 mg sodium*

LUNCH

Turkey Cranberry Wrap: Spread a medium (7") whole-wheat tortilla with 2 tablespoons jellied cranberry sauce, then top with 2 ounces thinly sliced turkey breast, $1\frac{1}{2}$ ounces reduced-fat Cheddar cheese, and $\frac{1}{4}$ green apple, thinly sliced

$\frac{3}{4}$ green apple

PER SERVING: *468 calories, 14 g fat, 7 g saturated fat, 27 g protein, 58 g carbohydrates, 7g fiber, 315 mg calcium, 777 mg sodium**

SNACK

1 small banana dipped into 2 tablespoons melted semisweet chocolate chips

PER SERVING: *230 calories, 8 g fat, 5 g saturated fat, 3 g protein, 41 g carbohydrates, 5 g fiber, 5 mg calcium, 1 mg sodium*

DINNER

4 ounces broiled salmon

$\frac{1}{2}$ cup steamed asparagus with 1 teaspoon tub margarine

$\frac{1}{2}$ cup cooked brown rice

1 cup tossed salad with $1\frac{1}{2}$ tablespoons reduced-fat dressing

1 cup fat-free milk

PER SERVING: *531 calories, 20 g fat, 4 g saturated fat, 40 g protein, 47 g carbohydrates, 6 g fiber, 327 mg calcium, 456 mg sodium*

OPTIONAL SNACK

1 cup fat-free plain yogurt mixed with 10 cut-up grapes and 2 tablespoons unsalted cashews

PER SERVING: *232 calories, 8 g fat, 2 g saturated fat, 13 g protein, 33 g carbohydrates, 1 g fiber, 313 mg calcium, 139 mg sodium*

* Higher in sodium; remember to limit yourself to no more than 2,300 mg of sodium per day.

BREAKFAST
Banana Smoothie (page 214)

½ toasted whole-wheat English muffin with ½ teaspoon tub margarine

> PER SERVING: *386 calories, 6 g fat, 3 g saturated fat, 15 g protein, 67 g carbohydrates, 3 g fiber, 479 mg calcium, 310 mg sodium*

LUNCH
English Muffin Pizza (page 214)

1 cup baby carrots

½ cup grapes

1 container (6 ounces) any flavor low-fat yogurt

> PER SERVING: *477 calories, 6 g fat, 3 g saturated fat, 18 g protein, 89 g carbohydrates, 7 g fiber, 647 mg calcium, 637 mg sodium**

SNACK
1 medium apple, cut up, with 1½ tablespoons peanut butter (or other nut butter)

> PER SERVING: *237 calories, 12 g fat, 2 g saturated fat, 6 g protein, 30 g carbohydrates, 6 g fiber, 11 mg calcium, 114 mg sodium*

DINNER
1 serving Garlic Butter Baked Haddock (page 215)

1 serving Rice Amandine (page 215) or cooked plain brown rice (if you're short on time)

1 medium baked or microwaved sweet potato with 1 teaspoon tub margarine

½ cup fat-free milk

> PER SERVING: *529 calories, 17 g fat, 7 g saturated fat, 33 g protein, 58 g carbohydrates, 5 g fiber, 241 mg calcium, 610 mg sodium*

OPTIONAL SNACK
3 fun-size candy bars

> PER SERVING: *231 calories, 8 g fat, 6 g saturated fat, 2 g protein, 36 g carbohydrates, 1 g fiber, 59 mg calcium, 85 mg sodium*

* Higher in sodium; remember to limit yourself to no more than 2,300 mg of sodium per day.

CHAPTER 7 EATING FOR WEIGHT LOSS AND EXERCISE

Banana Smoothie

TOTAL TIME: 5 MINUTES

1 container (6 ounces) low-fat vanilla yogurt
½ ripe banana, roughly chopped
½ cup fat-free milk
¼ teaspoon vanilla extract
¼ graham cracker, crushed

1. Combine the yogurt, banana, milk, and vanilla in a blender. Blend until smooth.

2. Pour into a glass. Sprinkle with graham cracker.

English Muffin Pizza

TOTAL TIME: 15 MINUTES

2 tablespoons pizza sauce
1 whole-wheat English muffin, halved
3 tablespoons reduced-fat shredded mozzarella cheese
1 tablespoon drained crushed pineapple

1. Preheat the oven to 375ºF.

2. Spread the sauce evenly over the muffin halves. Top with the mozzarella and pineapple. Bake for 10 minutes, until the cheese is melted.

Garlic Butter Baked Haddock

TOTAL TIME: 35 MINUTES

½ pound haddock or other whitefish fillet
2 tablespoons white wine
1 tablespoon butter or tub margarine, melted
1 clove garlic, minced or grated
⅛ cup seasoned dried bread crumbs

1. Preheat the oven to 350ºF. Place the fish on the nonshiny side of a large piece of foil.

2. Combine the wine, butter, garlic, and bread crumbs in a small bowl and sprinkle over the fish.

3. Seal the foil packet, then bake for 30 minutes, or until the fish flakes easily with a fork.

Makes 2 servings

Rice Amandine

TOTAL TIME: 30 MINUTES

1½ teaspoons butter
1 tablespoon diced onion
¼ cup long-grain rice
½ cup heated chicken stock
Pinch of salt
1½ tablespoons slivered almonds

1. Melt the butter over medium heat in a medium saucepan. Add the onion and rice and cook for a couple of minutes, until light brown.

2. Add the stock and salt. Reduce the heat to low, then cover and simmer for about 20 minutes, or until most of the liquid is absorbed.

3. Add the almonds and let sit, covered, until the rest of the liquid is absorbed, about 5 minutes.

Makes 2 servings

BREAKFAST
Cranberry-Walnut Oatmeal (page 217)

¹/₂ cup orange juice

> PER SERVING: *385 calories, 7 g fat, 1 g saturated fat, 16 g protein, 65 g carbohydrates, 5 g fiber, 331 mg calcium, 219 mg sodium*

LUNCH
Chicken Salad Sandwich (page 217)

1 kiwifruit

1 cup fat-free milk

> PER SERVING: *517 calories, 15 g fat, 2 g saturated fat, 40 g protein, 55 g carbohydrates, 11 g fiber, 595 mg calcium, 626 mg sodium**

SNACK
1 ounce (about 18 whole) unsalted or lightly salted cashews mixed with 2 tablespoons raisins

> PER SERVING: *228 calories, 13 g fat, 3 g saturated fat, 5 g protein, 25 g carbohydrates, 2 g fiber, 23 mg calcium, 10 mg sodium*

DINNER
1 serving General's Chicken (page 218)

¹/₂ cup cooked jasmine rice

1 cup tossed salad with 1 tablespoon reduced-fat dressing

1 cup fat-free milk

> PER SERVING: *501 calories, 11 g fat, 2 g saturated fat, 37 g protein, 63 g carbohydrates, 4 g fiber, 322 mg calcium, 547 mg sodium*

OPTIONAL SNACK
³/₄ cup 1% cottage cheese mixed with ¹/₂ cup blueberries

> PER SERVING: *164 calories, 2 g fat, 1 g saturated fat, 22 g protein, 15 g carbohydrates, 2 g fiber, 108 mg calcium, 689 mg sodium**

* Higher in sodium; remember to limit yourself to no more than 2,300 mg of sodium per day.

Cranberry-Walnut Oatmeal

TOTAL TIME: 5 MINUTES

½ cup Oatmeal Mix (page 184)
2 tablespoons dried cranberries
1 tablespoon chopped walnuts
1 cup fat-free milk

1. Combine the Oatmeal Mix, cranberries, walnuts, and ½ cup of the milk in a microwaveable bowl.

2. Microwave on high for 1 minute. Stir and continue to microwave at 30–second intervals until it reaches the desired consistency. Serve with the remaining ½ cup milk.

Chicken Salad Sandwich

TOTAL TIME: 10 MINUTES

4 teaspoons reduced-fat mayonnaise
½ teaspoon canola oil
½ cup diced cooked skinless chicken breast
1 teaspoon chopped cilantro
1 teaspoon chopped chives
½ scallion, chopped
¼ cup sliced cucumber, with skin
½ cup mixed salad greens
½ teaspoon sesame seeds
2 slices 100% whole-grain bread

1. Mix together the mayonnaise and oil in a medium bowl. Add the chicken and mix well. Add the cilantro, chives, and scallion and combine well.

2. Layer the chicken salad, cucumber, mixed greens, and sesame seeds on 1 slice of the bread, topping with the remaining slice.

General's Chicken

TOTAL TIME: 15 MINUTES

1 tablespoon olive oil
½ pound boneless, skinless chicken breast or tenders, cut into bite-size pieces
2 tablespoons sugar
1 tablespoon low-sodium soy sauce
½ cup pineapple juice
2 tablespoons white wine vinegar
2 cloves garlic, minced or grated
Pinch of crushed red-pepper flakes
1 teaspoon grated fresh ginger
Pinch of ground red pepper
2¼ teaspoons cornstarch
1½ tablespoons cold water
1½ cups steamed broccoli
1 scallion, sliced (optional)

1. Heat the oil in a medium skillet over medium heat. Add the chicken and sauté until golden brown, about 6 to 8 minutes.

2. In a small saucepan, combine the sugar, soy sauce, pineapple juice, vinegar, garlic, pepper flakes, ginger, and red pepper and heat gently.

3. Meanwhile, in a cup, dissolve the cornstarch in the water. Add it to the saucepan, stirring until thickened. Pour the sauce over the chicken, add the broccoli, and stir to coat. Sprinkle the scallion over top, if using.

Makes 2 servings

BREAKFAST

2 whole-grain frozen waffles topped with 1 tablespoon peanut butter (or your favorite nut butter) and $1/2$ cup sliced strawberries

1 cup fat-free milk

PER SERVING: *392 calories, 14 g fat, 3 g saturated fat, 19 g protein, 51 g carbohydrates, 6 g fiber, 363 mg calcium, 626 mg sodium*

LUNCH

Pesto Grilled Cheese (page 220)

$1/2$ cup sliced strawberries

1 cup fat-free milk

PER SERVING: *464 calories, 22 g fat, 6 g saturated fat, 23 g protein, 45 g carbohydrates, 6 g fiber, 630 mg calcium, 784 mg sodium**

SNACK

3 graham crackers ($2^1/2$" squares)

$3/4$ cup fat-free milk mixed with 1 tablespoon chocolate syrup

PER SERVING: *206 calories, 2 g fat, 0 g saturated fat, 9 g protein, 38 g carbohydrates, 1 g fiber, 193 mg calcium, 237 mg sodium*

DINNER

1 lean boneless pork chop (4 ounces) seasoned with salt-free seasonings and pan-fried in 1 teaspoon olive oil

1 serving Twice-Baked Sweet Potato (page 221)

$3/4$ cup steamed broccoli florets drizzled with lemon juice, to taste, and $1/2$ teaspoon olive oil

1 cup tossed salad with $1^1/2$ tablespoons reduced-fat dressing

1 cup fat-free milk

PER SERVING: *572 calories, 22 g fat, 5 g saturated fat, 34 g protein, 62 g carbohydrates, 9 g fiber, 388 mg calcium, 511 mg sodium*

OPTIONAL SNACK

2 sticks reduced-fat string cheese

5 whole-grain crackers

PER SERVING: *200 calories, 9 g fat, 3 g saturated fat, 15 g protein, 18 g carbohydrates, 3 g fiber, 300 mg calcium, 510 mg sodium*

* Higher in sodium; remember to limit yourself to no more than 2,300 mg of sodium per day.

CHAPTER 7 EATING FOR WEIGHT LOSS AND EXERCISE

Pesto Grilled Cheese

TOTAL TIME: 8 MINUTES

> 2 slices whole-grain bread
> 1 tablespoon store-bought pesto
> 1 slice tomato
> 1 slice American cheese
> 2 teaspoons tub margarine

1. Heat a small skillet over medium heat.

2. Spread 1 slice of the bread with the pesto, then top with the tomato and cheese. Add the second slice of bread.

3. Spread the margarine on the outside of both sides of the sandwich and place in the hot skillet. Grill the sandwich to desired doneness, flipping it occasionally, until both sides are golden.

MAKE-AHEAD

Twice-Baked Sweet Potato

TOTAL TIME: 80 MINUTES

1 large sweet potato
1 tablespoon fat-free milk
1 teaspoon tub margarine
2 tablespoons brown sugar
$\frac{1}{8}$ teaspoon ground cinnamon
Dash of ground nutmeg
Dash of ground ginger

1. Preheat the oven to 400°F.

2. Scrub the potato and poke a few times with a fork. Bake for 60 to 75 minutes, or until soft.

3. Remove the potato from the oven and reduce the oven temperature to 350°F. Let the potato cool slightly. Cut in half lengthwise. Scoop out the potato flesh, leaving about a $\frac{1}{8}$"-thick skin. Set aside.

4. Combine the potato with the milk, margarine, brown sugar, cinnamon, nutmeg, and ginger. Beat with an electric mixer until well combined. Divide the mixture evenly among the potato skins. Return to the oven for 15 to 20 minutes, or until heated through.

Makes 2 servings

NOTE: *The sweet potato can be prepared earlier in the day. Once the mixture is added to the potato skins, refrigerate until ready to eat. Then heat in the oven for 30 minutes.*

BREAKFAST

1 cup Cheerios

$^1/_2$ medium banana, sliced

1 tablespoon chopped walnuts

1 cup fat-free milk

$^3/_4$ cup cranapple juice

> PER SERVING: *376 calories, 7 g fat, 1 g saturated fat, 14 g protein, 69 g carbohydrates, 5 g fiber, 374 mg calcium, 341 mg sodium*

LUNCH

Roast Beef Wrap: Spread a medium (7") whole-wheat tortilla with $^1/_2$ tablespoon mustard, then top with 2 ounces thinly sliced, low-sodium, lean deli roast beef (such as Boar's Head), and 1$^1/_2$ ounces reduced-fat Cheddar cheese

1 cup cubed honeydew melon (or other melon)

1 cup fat-free milk

> PER SERVING: *496 calories, 16 g fat, 8 g saturated fat, 39 g protein, 489 g carbohydrates, 3 g fiber, 564 mg calcium, 663 mg sodium**

SNACK

1 large hard-cooked egg

1 ounce reduced-fat Cheddar cheese

5 whole-grain crackers

> PER SERVING: *269 calories, 16 g fat, 7 g saturated fat, 16 g protein, 16 g carbohydrates, 3 g fiber, 228 mg calcium, 394 mg sodium*

DINNER

1 serving Thai Pepper Pasta (page 223)

1 cup tossed salad with 1$^1/_2$ tablespoons reduced-fat dressing

1 cup fat-free milk

> PER SERVING: *538 calories, 16 g fat, 3 g saturated fat, 26 g protein, 78 g carbohydrates, 13 g fiber, 317 mg calcium, 672 mg sodium**

OPTIONAL SNACK

8 ounces fat-free plain yogurt mixed with $^1/_4$ cup blueberries

> PER SERVING: *121 calories, 0 g fat, 0 g saturated fat, 10 g protein, 24 g carbohydrates, 1 g fiber, 302 mg calcium, 135 mg sodium*

* Higher in sodium; remember to limit yourself to no more than 2,300 mg of sodium per day.

Thai Pepper Pasta

TOTAL TIME: 15 MINUTES

4 ounces whole-wheat spaghetti
1 teaspoon canola oil
1 small red bell pepper, cut into short, thick strips
2 tablespoons water
2½ tablespoons peanut butter
1 tablespoon reduced-sodium soy sauce
½ tablespoon apple cider vinegar
Dash of ground red pepper
1 teaspoon honey
½ cup shredded carrots
½ cup packaged broccoli coleslaw (such as Mann's)
Garlic chili sauce or hot sauce (optional)

1. Cook the pasta according to the package directions.

2. In a small skillet, heat the oil over medium heat and sauté the red bell pepper until tender, about 8 to 10 minutes. Set aside.

3. In a small saucepan over medium heat, combine the water, peanut butter, soy sauce, vinegar, ground red pepper, and honey. Stirring occasionally until smooth and warmed through, about 5 minutes.

4. Place the drained pasta in a large bowl. Stir in the bell peppers, peanut butter sauce, carrots, coleslaw, and chili sauce, if using. Mix well and serve.

Makes 2 servings

A Flatter Belly in 2 Weeks

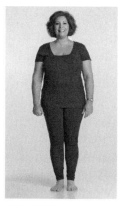

BEFORE

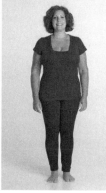

AFTER

GERI KREMPA knew she needed a wake-up call—and in 2009, she got one. "At my annual checkup, my doctor told me I'd put on 30 pounds since 2001—and I'd piled on a dozen of them in just the last year!" So when the WOW program came her way, she was already brimming with motivation.

When she heard that the majority of the exercise was walking, she didn't think it was going to be that tough. "I'd always thought I was a pretty hearty walker," said Geri. "My girlfriends and I would look for the best hills and then go for an hour-long walk a few times a week. So I was surprised that just 30 minutes could kick my butt. I got a better workout in less time"—a big plus for this busy mother of three very active kids.

The workouts also helped Geri shape up her eating habits. Once she figured out which meals she liked best, she got into a groove: oatmeal for breakfast at 8:00 a.m.; a healthy (packed) lunch, usually a turkey wrap, by 1:00 p.m.; and dinner at 6:00 p.m. Then she'd walk at night, have a healthy snack such as a slice of Bananaberry Bread

(page 185) with peanut butter, and go to bed early—no more mindless snacking. "I was exhausted by 10:00, and I slept like a baby," said Geri, adding that she used to regularly wake up in the middle of the night.

"I felt like a new person by day 14," exclaimed Geri, whose husband commented that her face looked less puffy. "This is a man who doesn't notice haircuts!" she added. "It was really noticeable, and not just in my face. My belly bloat was gone, too. And I had tons more energy during the day."

After 8 weeks, she not only had lost pounds and inches, she also had lowered her cholesterol by 10 points, her blood sugar by 11 points, and her resting heart rate—an indicator of fitness—by 8 beats per minute.

"I've lost weight on other diets, but I feel like the walking, especially the intervals, and the strength exercises have changed my metabolism," said Geri. "The weight came off more easily this time, and I've been able to maintain it without being superstrict about my diet."

P.S. *Three months after the official end of the program, Geri recorded an additional 4½-pound weight loss and shaved another 3¾ inches off her figure, for a grand total of 16 pounds and 13¼ inches lost in 5 months. Six weeks later, she walked the Philadelphia half-marathon, completing the 13.1-mile course in 3 hours 19 minutes.*

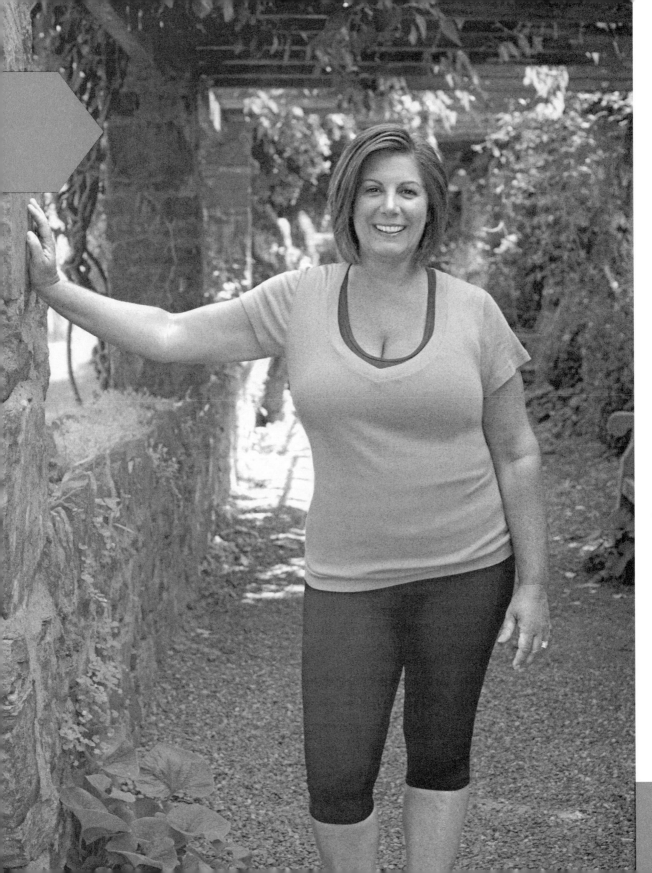

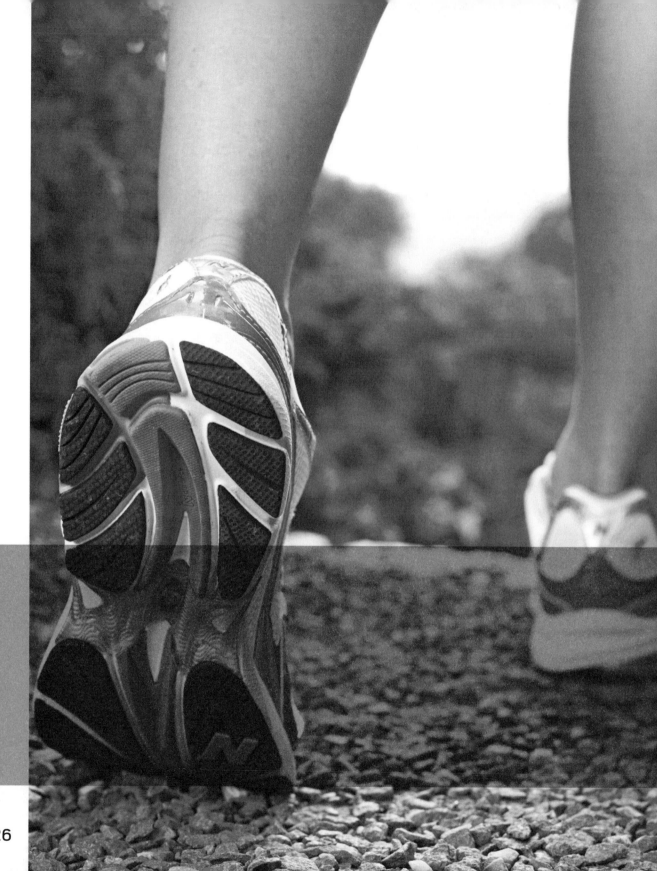

Overcoming
OBSTACLES

BARRIERS TO EXERCISE come in many shapes and sizes, from bunions and blisters to long workdays and bad weather. Excuses and obstacles know no limits, and they can eat away at your resolve to stick with any exercise program.

In this chapter, I'm going to give you the tools you need to overcome these and many other physical, mental, and environmental obstacles. My goal is to help you stay on track with your workouts, make exercise a lifelong habit, and finally get the body you want.

PHYSICAL OBSTACLES

Shin Pain

Shin pain was the most common complaint among our test panelists. The good news: Within a week or two of starting the WOW program, nearly everyone's shin pain disappeared or diminished significantly—and no one had to stop walking because of it.

Unlike some of the other physical obstacles in this chapter, shin pain, in most cases, is not an injury. Instead, it's the result of challenging this particular group of muscles, which includes the anterior tibialis. They're responsible for pulling your toes up when you plant your heel, so your foot rolls instead of flopping on the ground. The faster you go, the more steps you take, and the harder your shins have to work—which is why unconditioned shins can start to hurt. It's similar to the burning feeling you'd get from doing endless leg lifts or crunches. Once your muscles become conditioned, though, the pain eases up. "Just stick with it," recommended WOW participant Kristina Donatelli, whose shin pain eased after the first week. "It goes away as you get stronger."

Many people refer to shin pain as shin splints, but not all shin pain is due to shin splints. Runners are more susceptible to this injury than walkers are because they experience more impact. Shin splints are the result of tears in the tissue that attaches the shin muscles to the bones in the lower leg. If your shin pain occurs when you start to walk faster and subsides when you slow down, it's probably not the result of shin splints but rather of deconditioned shin muscles. Ease up a little and build your speed more slowly. Also, try the following measures, keeping in mind that the pain should disappear within a week or two. If it doesn't, or if it occurs even apart from your workouts, check with your doctor.

SHOES Wearing sneakers that are worn out or that don't provide enough stability can make you more susceptible to shin pain and shin splints. For advice on when to replace your shoes and how to find the right pair for your feet, turn to page 32.

SQUEEZE This is a great shin-protecting trick I learned from my good friend Lee Scott, a walking coach based in Toronto. Focus on squeezing your butt every time your heels land on the ground. This activates your glutes, which shortens your stride and helps your shins not work so hard. Plus, squeezing your butt with every step takes concentration, so you'll be distracted from any discomfort in your shins.

STRETCH Tight shin and calf muscles can contribute to the problem, so make sure you're doing the WOW stretching routine (page 56) after every workout.

Also, add this shin-targeted move to the series: After you do the Lunge & Reach stretch (page 56), stay in the lunge position (feet 2 to 3 feet apart, with your front knee bent, your back leg straight, and your toes pointing forward). Hold onto something for balance, then flip your back foot so that the tops of your toes are on the ground. Bend that knee a little and press the tops of your toes, foot, and ankle toward the ground until you feel a stretch in your shin. Hold for 10 seconds, then release. (If you don't feel a stretch, try it barefoot.) You may want to point and flex or circle your foot a few times before repeating the stretch on the opposite foot. Do three times on both sides. Several of our WOW testers reported that stopping for a few seconds to stretch during their walks when their shins started to burn helped alleviate the ache. Balancing on one leg, point and flex your foot and then circle it in both directions, 5 to 10 times with each foot or until the pain eases. If a particular motion works better for you, stick with that one.

STRENGTHEN To tone your shin muscles more quickly, tag this move onto

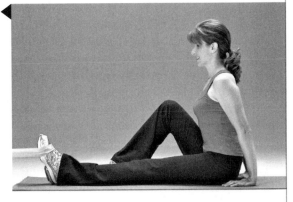

your Lower-Body Strength Workout (page 81): Tie a resistance band around a sturdy sofa leg or a railing at floor height so that it forms a loop. Sit on the floor with your right leg bent and your right foot flat on the floor; extend your left leg with the band looped around the top of your left foot. You may need to move back a little so that the band is taut. Keeping a slight bend in your left leg, flex your foot, pulling your toes toward you and against the band. Then release as if you were going to point your toes, but don't; otherwise, the band may slip off your foot. Do 10 to 20 reps with each foot, two or three times a week.

You can also strengthen your shins anytime with these moves. Just don't do all of these strengthening moves on the same day.

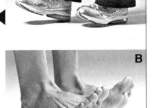

1. Walk on your heels with your toes lifted beginning with 15 to 30 seconds and working up to 2 minutes, two or three times a week. Don't do this during an actual walking workout.

2. Do double toe taps while you're sitting: With bare feet, first lift your toes, keeping the rest of your feet on the floor (A), then lift the balls of your feet, keeping only your heels on the floor (B). Lower in the opposite order.

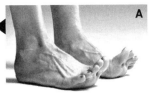

A

B

Foot Pain

Your feet have 26 bones, 33 joints, and more than 100 tendons, ligaments, and muscles that support the rest of your body. So it's not surprising that pain can hit in a variety of areas for a variety of reasons, and it's one of the fastest routes back to the couch. Your best offense: a good pair of walking shoes that are right for your feet (see pages 32 to 36). Your best defense: Pay attention at the first signs of trouble and take action immediately.

Unlike shin pain, foot pain is not something to just push through. To help, here's a look at some of the most common problems you may encounter and first-line strategies to resolve them. If you don't notice any improvement within a week, or if things get worse, see a podiatrist. (See Resources on page 320 for where to find a podiatrist.)

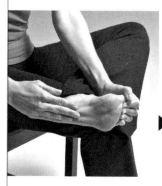

PROBLEM: Pain in the heel and/or arch

Is the pain most severe in the morning or after sitting for a long time, and does it decrease with activity? It may be plantar fasciitis, an inflammation of the fascia (a band of fibrous connective tissue) on the bottom of the foot.

FIX: Try this stretch.

▶ While seated, cross your legs so that the ankle of your injured foot is resting on the thigh of the other leg. Pull your toes toward your shin with your hand until you feel a stretch in the arch. Run the opposite hand along the sole of your foot; you should feel a taut band of tissue. Repeat 10 times, holding for 10 seconds each time. Research from the University of Rochester found this stretch to be more effective than others at relieving heel and arch pain.[1]

Also, get in the habit of stretching your calves frequently and putting on supportive shoes before you get out of bed. Wear them all day for a week or two, until the pain subsides—no walking barefoot or wearing unsupportive shoes. (I know it's not very fashionable, but it works.) During this time, reduce the amount of walking you're doing, especially the high-intensity workouts. You might need to stop walking altogether. It's a last resort, but you don't want plantar fasciitis to develop into a chronic condition. I know people who've battled this problem for months, even years. Take the time now to let it heal properly so it doesn't sideline you long-term. To relieve acute pain, roll your foot over a frozen bottle of water.

PROBLEM: Pain slightly above the heel, with or without a bump.

It may be Achilles tendonitis, an inflammation of the tendon that runs up the calf of the leg.

FIX: Rest and stretch.

Take a break from walking and ice the area a few times a day. For
acute pain, use an anti-inflammatory medication, like ibuprofen.
Wearing a heel lift in both shoes or wearing a shoe with a little bit of
a heel can be helpful as you recover.

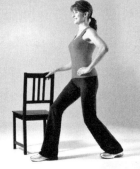

Also, try some gentle stretching. To target the area, add this twist to
the Lunge & Reach stretch (page 56): While you're in the lunge position (feet 2 to 3 feet apart, with your front knee bent, your back leg
straight, and your toes pointing forward), grasp onto something for
balance. Shift your weight back slightly and bend your back knee a little, keeping that heel on the floor. You should feel a stretch lower in
your calf, closer to your heel. Hold for 10 seconds, then repeat two more times.
Switch legs and repeat.

PROBLEM: Pain on the bottom of your foot

If it feels as though you're walking on a pebble, and the painful spots look similar
to calluses but with one or more tiny black pinpoints, they may be plantar warts.

FIX: Apply an over-the-counter wart treatment.

This product should contain salicylic acid. For stubborn, painful warts, see a
podiatrist to confirm the diagnosis and discuss treatments, which can include
surgery, laser or chemical removal, or freezing.

PROBLEM: Painful corns and calluses

These thick, hardened layers of skin develop when your skin tries to protect
itself from friction and pressure.

FIX: Pad them with moleskin.

Avoid medicated corn pads, especially if you have diabetes or vascular disease.
These contain acid, which can cause chemical burns.

Since friction and pressure from poorly fitting shoes or rubbing against a
seam are often the culprits, you may want to try out some new shoes. Another
common cause is a bony deformity of the foot; your doctor or podiatrist may
be able to recommend a permanent fix for this problem.

Never cut corns or calluses with any instrument. Your doctor or a podiatrist can trim large ones, which may help.

PROBLEM: Itchy toes or feet

If you have dry, scaly skin, itching, inflammation, and small blisters usually
on the bottom of your foot and between your toes, it may be athlete's foot.

FIX: Use an over-the-counter antifungal cream.

If you don't get relief within 2 weeks, ask your doctor about a prescription antifungal. Powders and liquid sprays work best between toes; creams work better on exposed skin. You can also try tea tree oil (found in health food stores). Stop using if irritation occurs.

PROBLEM: Painful bunion

Genetics are the usual cause of this bony bump that forms at the base of your big toe. Wearing narrow or pointed shoes can aggravate the problem and cause more pain.

FIX: Try the Bunion Aid.

You can wear this flexible splint 24-7 and inside shoes (unlike standard rigid splints, which can be worn only at night) to ease foot pain and possibly delay the need for surgery indefinitely. In a German study of patients with bunions, the splint reduced the misalignment of the big toe by 18 degrees, on average, while a night splint resulted in only an 11 degree improvement.[2] (See Resources on page 320 for more information on where to buy the Bunion

9 STEPS TO HAPPY FEET
(Even When You're Not Walking)

HOW YOU TREAT your feet when you're not exercising can have a big impact on your workouts. Here's how to keep them in tip-top walking shape.

Go barefoot only in safe areas like your home. It's the most important thing you can do to protect your feet from injury and infection.

Wear appropriate shoes. Your shoes should fit the activity you are performing: well-cushioned shoes for long periods of standing and activity-specific ones for exercise.

Don't wear the same pair every day. When you put your feet in moist, dark confines all day, they love to breed bacteria.

By giving shoes a day off, you thwart germ procreation.

Stick with heels no higher than ¾ inch. Heels contribute to knee and back problems, falls, and an awkward, unnatural gait. Over time, you may start to walk incorrectly when you're *not* wearing heels, which can cause more trouble.

Measure your feet every time you buy shoes. Try on both shoes, and walk in them. Make sure that there are no uncomfortable pressure points, that your toes aren't squeezed, and that your heels don't slip.

Choose socks that wick sweat away from your feet. Also, avoid tight socks or

nylons. They can squeeze your toes or bunch under your feet, both of which can lead to foot pain and ingrown toenails.

Really dry your feet, including between your toes. Podiatrists swear by this extra step after showering as a key to preventing fungal infections.

Protect yourself from germs. Always wear shower shoes in public facilities. At home, clean and disinfect your shower at least once a week with ¼ cup chlorine bleach mixed in a bucket of water.

Cut toenails straight across. Curved toenails are more likely to grow into your skin (aka ingrown toenails).

Aid.) Also, make sure that all of your shoes have wide toe boxes and good support to avoid putting extra pressure on the bunion. Sometimes custom orthotics can slow the progression of a bunion by controlling abnormal motion of the foot. Apply ice and take anti-inflammatories for temporary relief of acute pain. If the pain is interfering with your daily activities, see a doctor for an x-ray to determine if orthotics or surgery is necessary.

PROBLEM: Foot slapping

If you hear a slapping sound as you walk, it means that the front of your foot is dropping flat to the ground as it lands instead of rolling.

FIX: Strengthen your shins.

This will help you to land on your heel and roll through your foot and onto your toes to step quietly. To build stronger shins, practice toe taps and heel walking. (See page 63 for instructions and more suggestions.) If you don't notice any improvement after about a week of these exercises, see your doctor. You should schedule an appointment right away if you feel any numbness in your leg or foot or if you can't flex your foot toward your shin.

WOW WINNER Theresa Bahnick 53, lost 5½ pounds and 3 inches overall after 4 weeks

"Don't make the same mistake I did"

Theresa Bahnick has this advice to offer: "Buy a good pair of walking shoes before you start [the WOW program]." That was her plan, too, but we all know how other things can get in the way of our best intentions. Unfortunately this time, the consequence was particularly disappointing.

In Theresa's first week of keeping a journal, she noted that the muscles in her right foot were bothering her. "Nothing I can't overcome, though!" she wrote. She suspected that she might be experiencing a flare-up of plantar fasciitis, which she'd had in the past. She made a point of stretching more but kept walking.

Four weeks into the program, a favorite black dress that Theresa couldn't have worn a month earlier "zipped up beautifully," and "a good friend who I haven't seen in a month told me that my arms look amazing." But her foot still hurt, and she was still wearing her old sneakers.

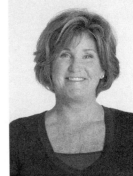

When Theresa picked up her pace for the Supercharged Interval Walks the following week, she really noticed the lack of support in her sneakers. So she laced them really tightly, took off "almost bouncing in my walk to push harder," and ended up with sharp, shooting pain in her other foot. The diagnosis: a minor stress fracture, an injury that develops over time. Her doctor suspects that her tight calf muscles may have contributed, and she's awaiting tests to determine if low bone density may have been a factor.

Either way, Theresa is convinced—and I concur—that new sneakers would have helped prevent the plantar fasciitis and maybe the stress fracture, too. The good news: She is back to walking, and she's lost more weight. Her new walking shoes feel great, too.

ACHES FROM HEAD TO TOE

THE ADVICE BELOW IS FOR GENERAL ACHES AND PAINS, not specific injuries. In many cases, you should get some relief almost instantly. If you don't notice any improvement within a week or if things get worse, see a doctor. (For a list of the types of doctors and other health care professionals that can help and how to find one in your area, see Resources on page 320.)

PROBLEM: Neck or upper back pain
FIX: Keep your shoulders down.

Often, when you start bending your arms and swinging them faster, you tense your upper body, which pulls your shoulders up toward your ears. Make sure you're not clenching your fists, either.

PROBLEM: Achy arms
FIX: Unclench your fists.

Holding your hands tight can lead to tension and even pain in your arms and up into your shoulders and neck. And tense muscles can cause you to fatigue faster. Let your fingertips just touch each other; imagine that you're holding something fragile, like an egg, and if you squeeze too hard, you'll break it.

PROBLEM: Bouncing breasts
FIX: Buy a supportive sports bra.

For the most comfort, make sure you get one that fits properly and is designed for your cup size. Also check your walking technique; proper posture and a smoother stride—that is, rolling from heel to toe—can help.

PROBLEM: Swollen hands
FIX: Check your arm swing.

You may be bending your wrists or extending your elbows. Swelling often occurs if you're walking for long periods of time with your arms down at your sides. The swinging action forces blood down your arms, causing it to pool in your hands. Keeping your arms bent and your wrists in line with your forearms reduces the pooling and swelling. If you notice your fingers getting puffy (often on a longer walk), raise your arms overhead as you walk, and clench and release your fists a few times. Repeat as often as needed.

PROBLEM: Side stitch
FIX: Slow down and breathe deeply.

A side stitch is believed to be a cramp or spasm in your diaphragm. There are several theories as to why it occurs. Easing your pace and taking deep belly breaths often provide relief. If not, massage or press on the area where you feel pain while bending forward slightly. Some experts say that you'll have fewer side stitches as you become more fit, while others claim that strengthening your abs helps (so keep doing the Core Strength Workout on page 97).

PROBLEM: Stomach cramps
FIX: Wait at least 1 hour after eating to walk.

Also, try to avoid caffeine and limit dairy foods prior to walking. These types of foods often cause problems for many people. And check your form; too much bouncing can upset your stomach, too.

PROBLEM: Lower back pain
FIX: Stand up straight.

If you're bending at the waist, your lower back muscles have to support the weight of your entire upper body—which, not surprisingly, can lead to soreness. You should be leaning slightly forward as you walk, but it should be coming from your ankles, not your waist. To become aware of the difference, stand with your back against a wall. Now lean forward slightly from your heels so that your entire body comes off the wall. That's what you want to do while you're walking. Now for what you don't want to do: Get back against the wall and lean forward, only this time bend at your waist so that your butt stays against the wall. Unfortunately, this is often common walking posture, especially when you try to speed up. So be aware.

PROBLEM: Frequent urination or leakage
FIX: See your doctor.

There are so many treatment options today that you shouldn't let urinary incontinence get in the way of an active lifestyle. Until you see a doctor, you might want to try wearing a tampon. In one study, 86 percent of women with exercise-induced incontinence had no leakage when they wore a tamponlike sponge while working out.[3] When inserted normally, a tampon pushes on the vaginal wall, which compresses the urethra. For comfort, you may want to apply K-Y Jelly to the tampon. Only wear tampons for a short period of time (no more than an hour) when you aren't menstruating. Also, practice Kegel exercises daily (tightening the vaginal and pelvic muscles as if to stop urinating) to develop better urinary control.

PROBLEM: Front-of-hip pain
FIX: Practice your push-off.

Using your back foot more to propel you and swing your leg forward means that your hip muscles won't have to work so hard. Also, check your posture to make sure that you're not leaning back or collapsing into your hips. Bring your weight to the front of your feet. To strengthen your hip flexors as you walk, spend a few minutes during your warm-up raising your knees as if you're marching.

PROBLEM: Chafing
FIX: Lubricate with petroleum jelly.

This, or other lubricants such as Body Glide, will prevent irritation in areas that may rub together as you walk, such as your thighs and underarms. Switch to wicking fabrics such as CoolMax, or try different styles of clothes to avoid edges or seams that rub against your skin.

PROBLEM: Back-of-knee pain
FIX: Don't lock your knee.

Keep your weight forward and soften your knee when your foot lands—but not too much. You don't want to bounce as you walk.

MENTAL OBSTACLES

SOMETIMES THESE TYPES OF BARRIERS can be harder to overcome than the physical ones, but with a little perseverance, they're surmountable, too.

PROBLEM: Can't get started or get back on track
FIX: Write down what motivates you.

If your get-up-and-go got up and went (it happens to all of us at some point), you may need to remember what inspires you. Maybe you want to be able to run around after your grandkids, or you're determined to look good for your 20-year high school reunion. Whatever it is, pinpointing why you really want to make a change can help you stick with it—especially if you write it down.

In fact, do it now, while you're feeling really motivated. Get out a piece of paper and draw a line down the middle. On one side, write all the pros for exercising and eating healthy; on the other side, write the cons. Then save the list. That way, if you hit a snag down the road, you'll have your list to remind you of why you started this program in the first place. That's why I also encouraged you to sign a contract (page 76), which you might want to review for additional inspiration.

PROBLEM: A tough day at work
FIX: Exercise in the morning.

I don't normally recommend a specific time of day to exercise, because I believe that the best time to work out is a personal preference. And you'll get the best results by doing it when you're most likely to stick with it. For instance, if you're not a morning person, an a.m. workout isn't likely to happen on a consistent basis.

In this case, however, I'm making an exception because of new research findings. As it turns out, it's not just your imagination that exercise feels harder after you've had a rough day. Only it's your mind, not your muscles, that's fatigued.

When people were asked to complete a mentally challenging task before a workout, they reported that exercise felt harder, and they ended their workout sessions 15 percent sooner than those who didn't receive the task.[5] While the mental fatigue doesn't physically tire your muscles, lungs, and heart, it does affect how you perceive exercise intensity, say researchers.

Whenever you know you have a stressful day ahead of you, exercise in the morning to ensure that you don't skip or cut short your workout later in the day. That sweat session may even help you to better handle the day's challenges. And if an earlier workout is out of the question, just knowing that exercise feels tough because of stress (not muscles) might be enough for you to push through a workout.

PROBLEM: Too self-conscious
FIX: Find a buddy.

That's what some of our test panelists did, especially if they felt uncomfortable doing the Toning Walks with a resistance band or pumping their arms like a racewalker. University of Southern California researchers found that working out with a friend is the best predictor of exercise satisfaction[6]—and other research shows that partnering can improve your odds of sticking with your workout program.[7] If that's not possible, walk in a busy park or at a track where everyone will be focused on their own workouts and you'll blend into the crowd.

It's also important to treat yourself to new exercise clothes that will make you look and feel more comfortable. If you're still walking around in sweats you've had for 10 years, it's no wonder you don't feel like being seen in public. And the best news is that today's workout clothing comes in lots of styles for all sizes.

PROBLEM: Lack of motivation
FIX: Work out for a cause.

Most women are great at doing things for others but not so good at taking care of themselves (myself included). Now here's a way you can help others and reap some healthy benefits yourself. Every time you take a walk, you can raise cash to help better the environment or fund cancer research—without it costing you anything more than your burned calories (and who doesn't want to give calories away?).

Plus3network.com, a new social networking Web site, pairs worthy causes (such as the Environmental Defense Fund or the Breast Cancer Research Foundation) with corporate sponsors willing to donate money (ranging from a fraction of a penny to 5 cents) for each mile that you exercise. Proof that those pennies add up: The site raised $9,000 in its first 6 months.

Or sign up for a charity walk that's beyond your current abilities, such as a 10-K, a half marathon, or a full marathon, to give yourself incentive to train. When you're collecting pledges from friends, family, and co-workers, bailing out is not an option.

PROBLEM: Other things getting in the way
FIX: Have a plan B and C and D and E . . .

Let's face it: Real life happens. But it shouldn't sideline your workouts, if you can help it. Having backup plans at the ready—whether they're in your mind, in your diary, or on index cards—will keep you prepared if you run into a snag.

With a little brainstorming, you'll find multiple ways to sneak in your walks, even on the most hectic days. The key is to have lots of options, including a variety of walking routes at work, at home, and around the kids' schools or sports practice areas. One of our WOW walkers, Gail Rarick, would have her husband drop her off a mile or two from a party or their kids' games, and she'd walk the rest of the way. You can also split up your workouts. On the WOW program, for instance, you could do the walk in the morning and the toning exercises at night, after you get home (or vice versa). If you're really crunched, you can do half your walk in the morning and half at lunch—or whatever suits your schedule. Remember doing something (even if it's not the entire workout) is better than doing nothing.

PROBLEM: No energy
FIX: Follow the 10-minute rule.

We all have those days when it feels impossible to exercise. It happens to the best of us. Maybe you're overstressed or fatigued, or you just plain don't feel like getting off your keister. When this happens to me, I follow the 10-minute rule. I tell myself, "All I have to do is walk for 10 minutes, and then I can stop." It's a great trick because 10 minutes is the amount of time needed for those feel-good brain chemicals to kick in. So, usually, once you get to 10 minutes, you'll feel like doing more. And even if you don't, you'll probably feel so much better after 10 minutes that you'll be more likely to get out for another jaunt later in the day. If not, at least you did something!

PROBLEM: Boredom
FIX: Try some tunes.

Music takes your mind off your work. Researchers at Brunel University in London discovered that runners who listened to motivational rock or pop music (think Queen or Madonna) exercised up to 15% longer—and felt better doing it.[8] Walking to the beat also encourages you to speed up.

Both of these changes may help explain why, in another study from Fairleigh Dickinson University in Teaneck, New Jersey, overweight walkers who listened to tunes of their choice lost twice as much weight as a group walking without music.[9] Remember to watch the volume or to wear just one earbud so you can hear oncoming traffic, dogs, and more in your surroundings and stay safe.

PROBLEM: An all-or-nothing mind-set ("If I can't do it all, I won't do it")
FIX: Set flexible goals.

Instead of saying that you're going to do every workout, which on the WOW program translates to exercising 6 days a week, give yourself a range of, say, 4 to 6 days a week. That way, even if you miss one (or two) workouts, you've still succeeded. That will help inspire you for future workouts.

Now, of course, I would love for you to do all the workouts, but that's not always realistic. If you miss a workout, don't make a big deal out of it. All-or-nothing thinking is a surefire way to fail—if you don't do anything, you'll never achieve the results you aspire to. I can't say it enough: Some exercise is better than none.

PROBLEM: Guilt
FIX: Multitask (and get your kids involved some of the time).

Many women (think I'm at the top of the list for this one!) feel guilty about taking time to exercise because it takes them away from their families. It doesn't have to be that way—and, in fact, it's really important that it isn't.

Health is a family affair, and getting the kids—and hubby—involved is a great way to spend quality time together. WOW walker Deb Baer made a habit of loading up her daughter's bike so that her daughter could ride while she walked at a local park. Another participant, Laura Chiles, found a track that had a grassy middle where she could walk around and keep an eye on her children, who played with soccer balls and toys while she exercised.

Remember, too, that you'll be a better mom and wife—not just by becoming a fantastic role model but by taking such good care of yourself, you'll reduce stress, sleep better, have more energy, and improve your mood so you'll enjoy your family and your life more.

PROBLEM: Not enough willpower
FIX: Use skillpower.

Skillpower is the ability to solve problems and strategize when things get tough and willpower fades. Studies show that determination and resolve are stronger at the beginning of each day because that's when you're most rested. And just like physical energy, mental energy—which is what willpower is—wears out each time you face a challenging situation, whether it's a project deadline or a German chocolate cake!

The key to staying strong in the long run is being able to keep your head when life throws you curveballs. For example, you could agree to meet a friend for coffee and end up facing down a cinnamon roll (using up that precious willpower), or you could get your coffee to go and then chat while taking a brisk, cinnamon-roll-free walk together. That's the smarter skillpower strategy. Or, if you find yourself raiding the office candy bowl, compartmentalize this one slipup and redouble your efforts by making a healthy dinner. That's skillpower, too. According to a Brown University study of 142 people, if you get back on the diet-and-exercise track right after a binge, your weight loss efforts won't suffer.[10]

PROBLEM: Feeling overwhelmed by your weight-loss goal
FIX: Set smaller, more doable goals—and celebrate small victories.

While it's always great to have a goal to improve your health, be careful not to focus on too big a chunk all at one time. Yes, you might need to lose 50 pounds—but you didn't put it on all at once, and you shouldn't expect to take it off overnight. Instead, set a goal that feels doable.

For instance, if 8 weeks seems like a long time to be on a program, then just focus on this week, or even on this day. If you went for a walk today, then you succeeded. Don't forget to celebrate by at least taking notice! And as you complete each week, plan a little reward for yourself—a new watch to time your intervals, a sports top, or a new hydration pack. Linking the rewards for your weekly achievements back to your healthy goals continues a positive spiral toward a healthier you.

PROBLEM: Negative self-talk ("I don't think that I can do it")
FIX: Ditch the pessimistic thinking.

Don't buy into negative "I can't" messages; they can be crippling. Fight pessimistic thoughts with positive statements such as "*I am walking!*" or "*Look how well I did yesterday.*" And any time you notice toxic thoughts creeping in, think—or say—a loud "*No!*"

If even that seems too hard, then just smile. And no, you don't have to be sincere about it. Studies show that faking a smile or a chuckle can boost your mood. Researchers suspect that smiling or laughing, whether faux or factual, triggers those good-mood brain chemicals.[11]

PROBLEM: Forgotten good intentions
FIX: Motivate with a note.

A visual nudge can help you stick to your goals—but only if you notice it, says Paddy Ekkekakis, PhD, an exercise psychologist at Iowa State University in Ames. In one study, a sign urging people to use the stairs rather than the nearby escalator increased the number of people who climbed on foot by nearly 200 percent.[12]

Put your prompt near a decision point—such as a sticky note on your alarm clock, your steering wheel, or your office door—to remind you of your workouts. And remember: The boost you get from a reminder usually fades after a few days, so change the color (and the content) of the motivating messages often.

ENVIRONMENTAL OBSTACLES

PROBLEM: Allergies
FIX: Wash up immediately.

If you're able to continue exercising outdoors, shower and change your clothes as soon as you finish, to reduce any further exposure to allergens.

Depending on the severity of your allergies, your best bet may be to move your workout indoors. One no-cost option is to walk in a mall. Many open early just for walkers, so you can stroll without crowds. The air is filtered, the temperature is comfortable, and it's dry. Other options: a treadmill (see page 49) or a short-term health club membership. Some of our test panelists walked in place or around their homes in a pinch.

PROBLEM: Rain
FIX: Buy an extra pair of walking sneakers.

Then get out there and walk in the rain. It's only water! With the right gear (see page 41) and a dry pair of shoes to wear the next day, it can be a fun, empowering experience. Approach it as though you're an athlete in training: They wouldn't let a little thing like rain stop them—and neither should you.

The first time I worked out in the rain as an adult was when I was preparing for a 3-day, 60-mile breast cancer walk. It gives you a whole new sense of accomplishment and usually a great story to tell. When I put this challenge out to our test panelists, several took me up on it, including Denise Jennings, who said, "Even though it was dark, the rain was actually refreshing, not depressing." Go ahead—give it a try!

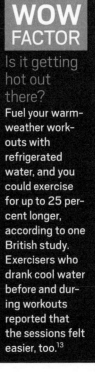

THE WOW FACTOR

Is it getting hot out there?
Fuel your warm-weather workouts with refrigerated water, and you could exercise for up to 25 percent longer, according to one British study. Exercisers who drank cool water before and during workouts reported that the sessions felt easier, too.[13]

WALKING IN ALL WEATHER

DON'T LET summer heat or winter cold sidetrack your walking workout! With a little extra preparation, you can stay comfortable outdoors, no matter what the temperature.

Hot Weather Walking

Be an early bird or a night owl. Plan to walk in the early morning or late evening to avoid the steamiest part of the day—usually between 10:00 a.m. and 2:00 p.m.

Seek out shade. Direct sun can make the temperature feel up to 15 degrees hotter! Check your area to see if there are parks with shaded trails.

Expose your skin. Sweat can evaporate more easily from bare arms and legs. (Wear plenty of sunscreen, though, even under your shirt.)

Just add water. Wet your shirt or a bandana to tie around your neck, and you'll have on-the-spot air-conditioning!

Cover your head. Wear a breathable hat (not a visor—it will protect only your face, not your head), and wet that, too.

Reduce friction. Heat and sweat can contribute to chafing. To help prevent it, apply a small amount of petroleum jelly to areas where skin rubs against skin—between your toes and thighs and under your arms. Or use Meuller Lube Stick for Runners, a nonstaining cream made from lanolin, zinc oxide, and benzocaine. It can be found in many sporting goods stores.

Walk in water. It provides about 15 times more resistance than exercising on land—and it cools you off, too.

Listen to your body. Your body will tell you when you can push yourself and when it's time to coast. If you develop a headache or become dizzy or weak, stop exercising and head for a cool place. Drink plenty of cool fluids and rest. If symptoms don't improve, call your doctor.

Cold Weather Walking

Warm up indoors. Start by walking around your house or marching in place and circling your arms. This will help get blood to the muscles you'll need for your walk before you expose your body to the cold air. That way, your heart doesn't have to work so hard, and exercise will feel easier.

Wear dark colors. They'll absorb the sunlight to keep you warmer.

Double up on gloves. Slip a thin pair under your heavy ones. That way, if your hands heat up (mine always do), you can take off one pair without exposing your fingers.

Leave jewelry at home. Take off earrings, bracelets, watches, and necklaces. It's more than just a safety issue; metal gets cold, which can make you chillier.

Muff your ears. If your hat doesn't cover your ears, invest in a new one with soft fleece flaps. Ears can get painfully cold very quickly. I cover mine with a headband even on mildly cool days to avoid cutting my workouts short. Other good choices: earmuffs or earbags (these fit directly over your ears). See Resources on page 320 for where to find earbags.

Check for gaps. Icy wind can sneak in if you don't check your wrists, waist, ankles, and neck areas. You may need to add a scarf, knee-high socks, longer gloves, or tuck in a shirt to avoid bone-chilling leaks.

Wear sunscreen and sunglasses. Sun reflecting off snow can give you a nasty sunburn, and the glare isn't good for your eyes either. Choose an SPF of at least 30 and cover any exposed skin, including your lips.

Breathe easier. When it's really cold or windy, cover your mouth and nose with a scarf or a face mask to warm the air when you inhale.

Know the warning signs. If you suspect frostbite—watch for paleness, numbness, and loss of feeling or a stinging sensation—get out of the cold immediately and slowly warm the affected area without rubbing. If numbness continues, seek emergency care.

PROBLEM: High wind
FIX: Walk into it to start.

You'll have more energy to face into the wind as you head out. Then when you're tired, turn around, and the wind will be at your back to help you along. If it's chilly, wear a lightweight nylon jacket or a windproof jacket made of tightly woven fabric to block the wind. Add a fleece jacket underneath if it's really cold, and a hat, earmuffs, or headband to protect your ears. Then charge ahead, knowing that you're burning more calories because of the wind resistance. Now, if you're talking hurricane-force winds or other dangerous conditions, choose an indoor option (see page 48).

PROBLEM: Shorter days
FIX: Light up your appendages.

It's especially important to have reflective material on your wrists and ankles (reflective bands, socks, and shoes can all work), because moving parts do a better job of catching the attention of motorists. (For more tips about reflective gear, see page 44.)

HEAT AND YOUR HEART

WHEN THE TEMPERATURE begins to approach 90°F, your heart has to work up to twice as hard, pumping blood both to the muscles you're using and to your skin to help keep you cool. Anybody at risk for heart disease shouldn't be exercising outdoors in those conditions, advises Bryant Stamford, PhD, professor and chair of the department of exercise science at Hanover College in Indiana. Hot, humid weather causes your heart rate and breathing to speed up, so your body is working harder even if you walk a bit slower.

The good news is, if this weather is typical of your area, your body will naturally adjust to the climate in a week or two. Then you should be able to walk normally. Just take it easy until then, and always listen to your body. If you start feeling clammy, dizzy, or nauseated, stop walking and head indoors. If symptoms persist, call your doctor.

WOW Winner
Deb Baer
GROUP: Exercise Only

AGE: 41 HEIGHT: 5'6"
POUNDS LOST: $9^3/_4$
INCHES LOST: $7^1/_2$ overall, including 2 from her waist
MAJOR ACCOMPLISHMENT: Boosted her energy level by 30 percent. Lowered her blood glucose level by 22 points.

Turning 40 Was Her Turning Point

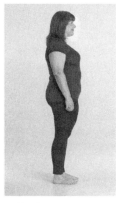

BEFORE

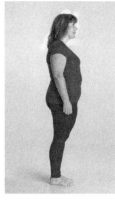

AFTER

DEB BAER turned 40 in 2009, and those milestone birthdays can provide a hefty dose of motivation to get in shape. "Life is short, and I want to live however many years I have to the fullest," she said, citing things like going for bike rides and hikes with her husband and two children, ages 4 and 8.

Like many people, Deb didn't think of walking as *real* exercise, much less a way to lose weight. That's not surprising, since it hadn't been helping her up to now. Then again, she hadn't done walking like the WOW program before. "I'd run intervals years ago, when I was much more active, but I'd never even thought about interval walking," admitted Deb.

The technique advice like "head up, arms up" was particularly helpful. "Now I notice if I'm hunched over, I immediately correct it," said Deb. "As soon as I do, I can feel the energy flowing powerfully through my body, and I move faster." By the end of the program, she was able to walk a mile 2 minutes and 23 seconds quicker than at the start. And the improvements didn't stop there.

"I saw that if I put in the effort,

I got the returns," said Deb, adding that sometimes she had to be patient, though. "I was getting frustrated because I was working my tail off, and the scale didn't show a thing the first few weeks. But I'm so glad I didn't give up, because when the weight did come off, it came off big!"

The program—and the resulting weight loss—also helped with her chronic back pain. "I had a herniated disk when my son was born and had back trouble for many years," explained Deb. "Every morning I'd wake up achy, crabby, and in no mood to move a muscle."

When the alarm rings now, things are much different. "The pain is gone, I'm full of energy. I can practically leap out of bed in the morning! I don't snap at my kids as much either. My whole being feels better," exclaimed Deb.

Even Deb's husband noticed the pounds melting away. "One day, I was bending over to look for something, and he said, 'Hmm, I think that program is working,'" recalled Deb. "I get a haircut and he doesn't notice! So I was happy to hear anything positive about my weight."

P.S. *Three months after the official end of the program, Deb recorded an additional $1^1/_2$-pound weight loss and shaved another $2^1/_4$ inches off her figure, despite being sick for several weeks. That adds up to a grand total of $11^1/_4$ pounds and $9^3/_4$ inches lost in 5 months.*

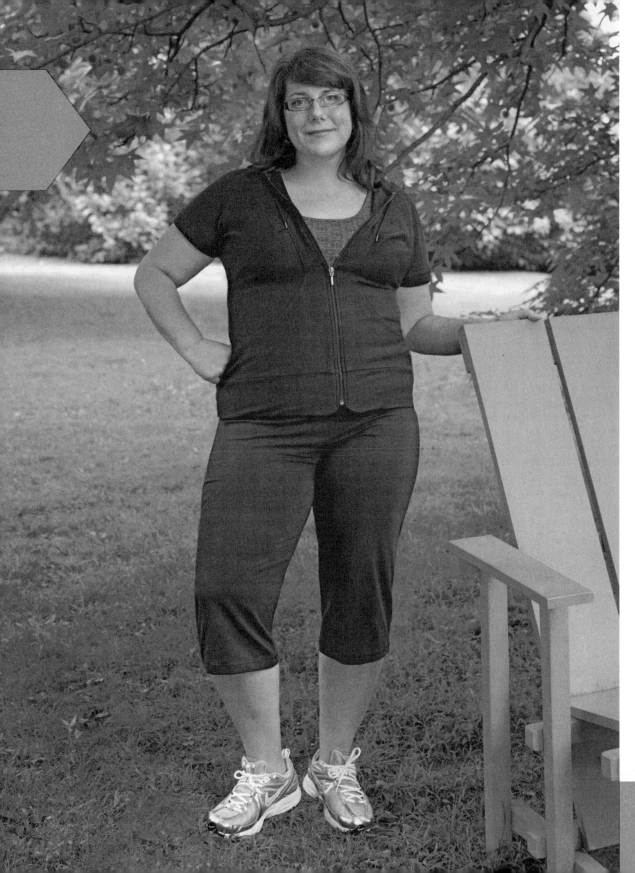

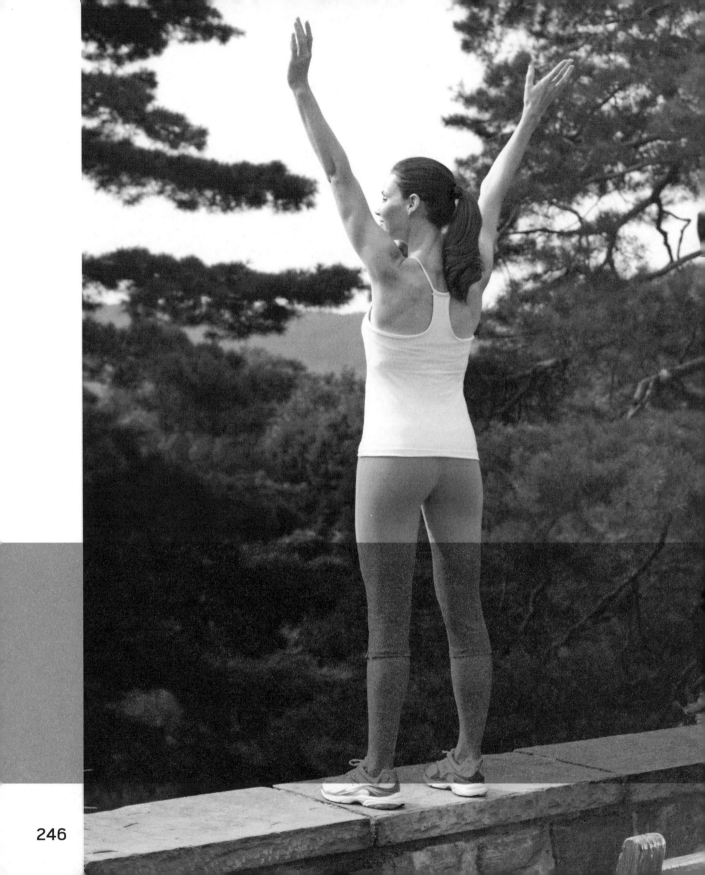

BEYOND
8 WEEKS

DON'T STOP NOW! Whether you're looking to lose a few more pounds, get firmer, or just maintain the results you've already achieved, here's how to continue the WOW program to meet your goals. And remember that no matter what type of workouts you're doing or what your goals are, the WOW menu plan and eating guidelines will keep you satisfied and provide all the nutrients you need.

TO LOSE MORE WEIGHT

DO THE BASIC LOSE MORE PLAN (below; it's the same as Week 4) for 4 to 6 weeks. Then do the Supercharged Lose More Plan (at right; it's the same as Week 8) for the next 4 to 6 weeks. Or alternate these plans weekly for 10 to 12 weeks.

Continue with one or both of these cycles until you reach your goal weight, then switch to the WOW maintenance plan (pages 252–253). While following the Lose More plans, try some of the Make It Harder options for the toning workouts from weeks 1 to 8 or the new variations of these routines (Lower-Body Strength Workout II, Core Strength Workout II, and Upper-Body Strength Workout on pages 258–293) and new interval workouts (pages 254–255) for variety and faster results. Remember, challenging your body in new ways will keep the scale moving and help you avoid a plateau.

BASIC Lose More Plan
YOUR WORKOUT AT A GLANCE

DAY	ACTIVITY//WORKOUT	TOTAL
1	Basic Interval Walk II (45 min) // Lower-Body Strength Workout (15 min)	60 min
2	Toning Walk II (25 min)	25 min
3	Basic Interval Walk II (45 min) // Core Strength Workout (15 min)	60 min
4	Toning Walk II (25 min)	25 min
5	Basic Interval Walk II (45 min) // Lower-Body Strength Workout (15 min)	60 min
6	Long Walk (1–2 hours) // Core Strength Workout (15 min)	75–135 min
7	Rest	

WHAT YOU'LL DO THIS WEEK

**2 x Basic Interval Walk II ○ 2 x Lower-Body Strength Workout
2 x Toning Walk II ○ 2 x Core Strength Workout ○ 1 x Long Walk**

SUPERCHARGED Lose More Plan

YOUR WORKOUT AT A GLANCE

DAY	ACTIVITY//WORKOUT	TOTAL
1	Supercharged Interval Walk II (30 min)	30 min
2	Recovery Walk (20 min) // Total-Body Strength Workout (20 min)	40 min
3	Supercharged Interval Walk II (30 min)	30 min
4	Recovery Walk (20 min) // Total-Body Strength Workout (20 min)	40 min
5	Supercharged Interval Walk II (30 min)	30 min
6	Speed Walk // Total-Body Strength Workout (20 min, optional)	<50 min
7	Rest	

WHAT YOU'LL DO THIS WEEK

**3 x Supercharged Interval Walk ○ 2 x or 3 x Total-Body Strength Workout
2 x Recovery Walks ○ 1 x Speed Walk**

PICK THE RIGHT WEIGHT

THE NEW STRENGTH WORKOUTS in this chapter include dumbbells for a fresh way to challenge your muscles. You want to choose a weight that fatigues your muscles by 8 to 12 repetitions. If you can't do at least 8 reps, you'll need a lighter dumbbell. When you can easily do an exercise 12 times and feel as if you could do more, it's time to increase the weight. Since

some muscles are bigger and stronger than others, you'll need to adjust the amount of weight you're lifting for different exercises. You'll be able to use heavier dumbbells (8 to 15 pounds) for moves that target lower-body muscles such as your quads and glutes and upper-body muscles such as your chest, upper back, and biceps. Smaller muscle groups such as your shoulders

and triceps will require lighter weights (3 to 10 pounds). Most of us tend to underestimate our abilities, so don't be afraid to challenge yourself. And don't worry, you won't get big and bulky from lifting weights—because muscles are firm and more compact than fat, strength training helps you shrink inches. See Resources on page 320 for where to find weights.

TO GET FIRMER

THIS PLAN IS SIMILAR to the Lose More Weight option on the previous pages with the key difference being that you'll increase the challenge of your toning workouts.

Follow the Basic Get Firmer Plan (below) for 4 to 6 weeks, doing the Make It Harder variations for the toning workouts or trying the new routines beginning on page 259 (you can reduce the number of reps to work up to these harder moves).

Then switch to the Supercharged Get Firmer Plan (at right) for the next 4 to 6 weeks. Again, you can do either the Make It Harder variations for the toning workouts or the Lower-Body Strength Workout II and Core Strength Workout II. There's also a new upper-body routine—Upper-Body Strength Workout (page 276)—that doesn't involve walking. Continue this cycle until you are as toned as you want to be. During that time, try some of the new interval workouts (pages 254–255) for variety and faster results. Remember, challenging your body with new exercises and more resistance will sculpt shapelier muscles faster. Then move on to the WOW maintenance plan (pages 252–253).

BASIC Get Firmer Plan
YOUR WORKOUT AT A GLANCE

DAY	ACTIVITY//WORKOUT	TOTAL
1	Basic Interval Walk II (45 min) // Lower-Body Strength Workout: Make It Harder variations or new routine (15 min)	60 min
2	Toning Walk II (25 min) or Upper-Body Strength Workout (15 min) plus Recovery Walk (25 min)	25 or 40 min
3	Basic Interval Walk II (45 min) // Core Strength Workout: Make It Harder variations or new routine (15 min)	60 min
4	Toning Walk II (25 min) or Upper-Body Strength Workout (15 min) plus Recovery Walk (25 min)	25 or 40 min
5	Basic Interval Walk II (45 min) // Lower-Body Strength Workout: Make It Harder variations or new routine (15 min)	60 min
6	Long Walk (1–2 hours) // Core Strength Workout: Make It Harder variations or new routine (15 min)	75–135 min
7	Rest	

WHAT YOU'LL **DO THIS WEEK**

3 x Basic Interval Walk II ○ **2 x Lower-Body Strength Workout: Make It Harder variations or new routine** ○ **2 x Toning Walk or Upper-Body Strength Workout + Recovery Walk** ○ **2 x Core Strength Workout: Make It Harder variations or new routine** ○ **1 x Long Walk**

SUPERCHARGED Get Firmer Plan
YOUR WORKOUT AT A GLANCE

DAY	ACTIVITY//WORKOUT	TOTAL
1	Supercharged Interval Walk II (30 min)	30 min
2	Recovery Walk (20 min) // Total-Body Strength Workout: Make It Harder variations or new routine (20 min)	40 min
3	Supercharged Interval II (30 min)	30 min
4	Recovery Walk (20 min) // Total-Body Strength Workout: Make It Harder variations or new routine (20 min)	40 min
5	Supercharged Interval Walk II (30 min)	30 min
6	Speed Walk II // Total-Body Strength Workout: Make It Harder variations or new routine (20 min, optional)	<50 min
7	Rest	

|||||||||||||||||||||||||||||||||||||||||||||||||||||||||||||||||||||||||||||||||||||||

WHAT YOU'LL DO THIS WEEK

3 x Supercharged Interval Walk II ○ **2 x or 3 x Total-Body Strength Workout: Make It Harder variations or new routine** ○ **2 x Recovery Walk** ○ **1 x Speed Walk II**

|||||||||||||||||||||||||||||||||||||||||||||||||||||||||||||||||||||||||||||||||||||||

TO MAINTAIN

DO THE BASIC MAINTENANCE PLAN (below) for 4 to 6 weeks, then switch to the Supercharged Maintenance Plan (at right) for the next 4 to 6 weeks. Or alternate the plans weekly for 10 to 12 weeks.

Continue with one or both of these cycles, mixing in some of the alternate toning and interval workouts (on pages 254–293) for variety.

BASIC Maintenance Plan
SAMPLE WEEKLY WORKOUT SCHEDULE

DAY	ACTIVITY//WORKOUT	TOTAL
1	Basic Interval Walk II (45 min) // Lower-Body Strength Workout (15 min)	60 min
2	Toning Walk II (25 min)	25 min
3	Basic Interval Walk IV (45 min) // Core Strength Workout (15 min)	60 min
4	Rest	
5	Lower-Body Strength Workout II (15 min)	15 min
6	Long Walk (1 hour)	60 min
7	Rest	

WHAT YOU'LL DO THIS WEEK

2 x 45-minute or 3 x 30-minute Basic Interval Walk ○ 4 x toning workout (be sure to hit each body part—lower, core, upper—once each week; one part will get worked twice each week, so alternate that part from one week to the next) ○ 1 x Long Walk

SUPERCHARGED Maintenance Plan
SAMPLE WEEKLY WORKOUT SCHEDULE

DAY	ACTIVITY//WORKOUT	TOTAL
1	Supercharged Interval Walk I (20 min)	20 min
2	Recovery Walk (25 min) // Total-Body Strength Workout II (20 min)	45 min
3	Supercharged Interval Walk III (20 min)	20 min
4	Total-Body Strength Workout II (20 min)	20 min
5	Supercharged Interval Walk I (20 min)	20 min
6	Speed Walk	<20 min
7	Rest	

IIIIIIIIIIIIIIIIIIIIIIIIIIIIIIIIIIIIIIIIIIIIIIIIIIIIIIIIIIIIIIIIIIIIIIIIIIIIIIIIIIIIIIIIIIIIIIIIIIIIIIIIIIIIIIIIIIIIIIIII

WHAT YOU'LL DO THIS WEEK

2 x 30-minute or 3 x 20-minute Supercharged Interval Walk
○ **1 x Recovery Walk** ○ **2 x toning workout** ○ **1 x Speed Walk II**

IIIIIIIIIIIIIIIIIIIIIIIIIIIIIIIIIIIIIIIIIIIIIIIIIIIIIIIIIIIIIIIIIIIIIIIIIIIIIIIIIIIIIIIIIIIIIIIIIIIIIIIIIIIIIIIIIIIIIIIII

MORE INTERVAL ROUTINES

BASIC INTERVAL WALK III

TIME	ACTIVITY	INTENSITY
0:00–4:00	Warm-Up (4 min)	3→5
4:00–5:00	Moderate (1 min)	5–6
5:00–6:00	Fast (1 min)	7–8
6:00–8:00	Moderate (2 min)	5–6
8:00–9:00	Fast (1 min)	7–8
9:00–11:00	Moderate (2 min)	5–6
11:00–12:00	Fast (1 min)	7–8
12:00–14:00	Moderate (2 min)	5–6
14:00–15:00	Fast (1 min)	7–8
15:00–17:00	Moderate (2 min)	5–6
17:00–18:00	Fast (1 min)	7–8
18:00–20:00	Moderate (2 min)	5–6
20:00–21:00	Fast (1 min)	7–8
21:00–23:00	Moderate (2 min)	5–6
23:00–24:00	Fast (1 min)	7–8
24:00–26:00	Moderate (2 min)	5–6
26:00–30:00	Cool-Down (4 min)	5→3

BASIC INTERVAL WALK IV

TIME	ACTIVITY	INTENSITY
0:00–4:00	Warm-Up (4 min)	3→5
4:00–5:00	Moderate (1 min)	5–6
5:00–5:30	Fast (30 sec)	7–8
5:30–7:30	Moderate (2 min)	5–6
7:30–8:30	Fast (1 min)	7–8
8:30–10:30	Moderate (2 min)	5–6
10:30–12:30	Fast (2 min)	7–8
12:30–14:30	Moderate (2 min)	5–6
14:30–15:00	Fast (30 sec)	7–8
15:00–17:00	Moderate (2 min)	5–6
17:00–18:00	Fast (1 min)	7–8
18:00–20:00	Moderate (2 min)	5–6
20:00–22:00	Fast (2 min)	7–8
22:00–24:00	Moderate (2 min)	5–6
24:00–24:30	Fast (30 sec)	7–8
24:30–26:30	Moderate (2 min)	5–6
26:30–27:30	Fast (1 min)	7–8
27:30–29:30	Moderate (2 min)	5–6
29:30–31:30	Fast (2 min)	7–8
31:30–33:30	Moderate (2 min)	5–6
33:30–34:00	Fast (30 sec)	7–8
34:00–36:00	Moderate (2 min)	5–6
36:00–37:00	Fast (1 min)	7–8
37:00–39:00	Moderate (2 min)	5–6
39:00–41:00	Fast (2 min)	7–8
41:00–42:00	Moderate (1 min)	5–6
42:00–45:00	Cool-Down (3 min)	5→3

SUPERCHARGED INTERVAL WALK III

TIME	ACTIVITY	INTENSITY
0:00–4:00	Warm-Up (4 min)	3→5
4:00–5:00	Moderate (1 min)	5–6
5:00–5:15	Very Fast (15 sec)	8–9
5:15–6:15	Easy to Moderate (1 min)	4–6
6:15–6:45	Very Fast (30 sec)	8–9
6:45–7:45	Easy to Moderate (1 min)	4–6
7:45–8:30	Very Fast (45 sec)	8–9
8:30–9:30	Easy to Moderate (1 min)	4–6
9:30–10:30	Very Fast (1 min)	8–9
10:30–11:30	Easy to Moderate (1 min)	4–6
11:30–12:15	Very Fast (45 sec)	8–9
12:15–13:15	Easy to Moderate (1 min)	4–6
13:15–13:45	Very Fast (30 sec)	8–9
13:45–14:45	Easy to Moderate (1 min)	4–6
14:45–15:00	Very Fast (15 sec)	8–9
15:00–16:00	Easy to Moderate (1 min)	4–6
16:00–20:00	Cool-Down (4 min)	5→3

SUPERCHARGED INTERVAL WALK IV

TIME	ACTIVITY	INTENSITY
0:00–4:00	Warm-Up (4 min)	3→5
4:00–5:00	Moderate (1 min)	5–6
5:00–5:30	Very Fast (30 sec)	8–9
5:30–7:30	Easy to Moderate (2 min)	4–6
7:30–8:00	Very Fast (30 sec)	8–9
8:00–10:00	Easy to Moderate (2 min)	4–6
10:00–10:30	Very Fast (30 sec)	8–9
10:30–12:30	Easy to Moderate (2 min)	4–6
12:30–13:00	Very Fast (30 sec)	8–9
13:00–15:00	Easy to Moderate (2 min)	4–6
15:00–15:30	Very Fast (30 sec)	8–9
15:30–17:30	Easy to Moderate (2 min)	4–6
17:30–18:00	Very Fast (30 sec)	8–9
18:00–20:00	Easy to Moderate (2 min)	4–6
20:00–20:30	Very Fast (30 sec)	8–9
20:30–22:30	Easy to Moderate (2 min)	4–6
22:30–23:00	Very Fast (30 sec)	8–9
23:00–25:00	Easy to Moderate (2 min)	4–6
25:00–25:30	Very Fast (30 sec)	8–9
25:30–27:30	Easy to Moderate (2 min)	4–6
27:30–30:00	Cool-Down (2.5 min)	5→3

LOWER-BODY STRENGTH WORKOUT II

ALL OF THESE MOVES are based on research showing that they're supereffective at strengthening and firming your legs and butt. In fact, they activate muscles up to 30% more than traditional moves.[1] Do 1 or 2 sets of 10 to 12 reps of each move on both sides when appropriate.

Side Lunge
(targets glutes, hips, quads, inner and outer thighs, and lower back)

MAIN MOVE

Holding a dumbbell in each hand, stand with your feet together and your arms down at your sides. Take a big step to the right, bending your right knee and hips, keeping your feet facing forward. Sit back into a deep side lunge, keeping your left leg straight. Lower the dumbbells toward the floor. Push off with your right foot to stand back up. Repeat to the left side.

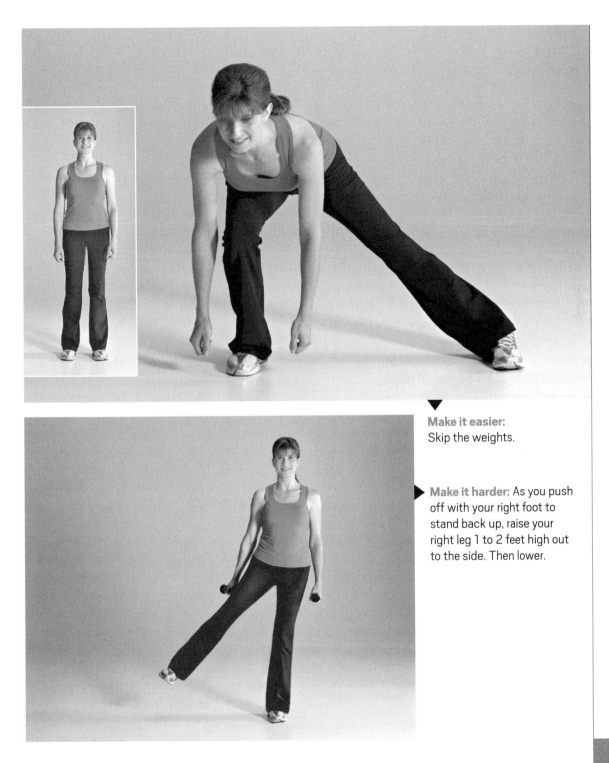

Make it easier:
Skip the weights.

Make it harder: As you push off with your right foot to stand back up, raise your right leg 1 to 2 feet high out to the side. Then lower.

Side Leg Lift
(targets hips and outer thighs)

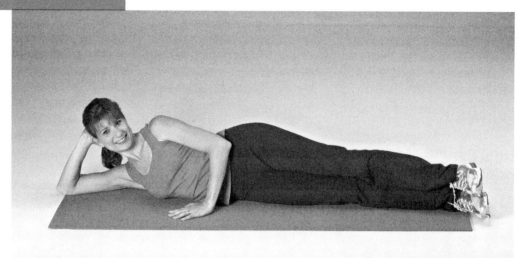

MAIN MOVE

Lie on your right side with your legs stacked. Bend your right arm and support your head on your right hand. Rest your left hand on the floor in front of your chest for balance. Raise your left leg about 2 feet, keeping your foot flexed and squeezing your butt. Pause, then slowly lower. Complete all reps, then switch sides.

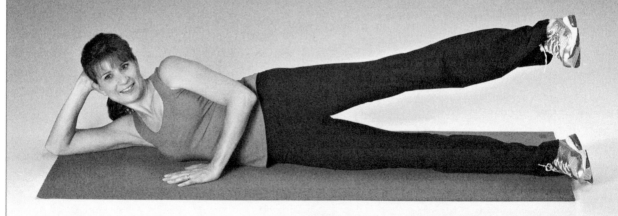

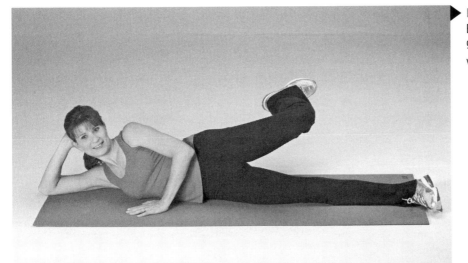

Make it easier: Bend your top leg 90 degrees, and lift with your leg bent.

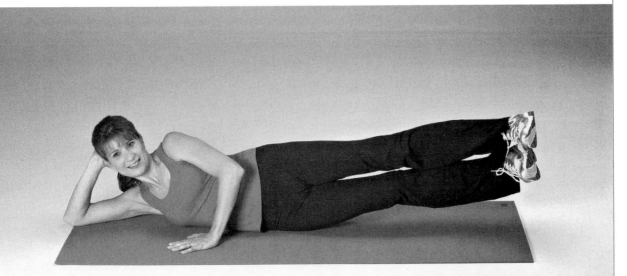

Make it harder: Double up: Once you've raised your top leg, raise your bottom leg to meet your top leg, pause, and then lower one leg at a time.

Kneeling Leg Lift
(targets glutes and hamstrings)

MAIN MOVE
Kneel on the floor on all fours with your hands directly beneath your shoulders and your knees beneath your hips. Place a dumbbell behind your right knee and grasp it with your leg. Contract your right glutes, keep your foot flexed, and lift your right leg, keeping your knee bent, until your thigh is parallel to the floor. Keep your abs tight. Press your heel toward the ceiling and squeeze your glutes at the top of the lift, then slowly lower almost to the floor. Complete one set, then switch legs.

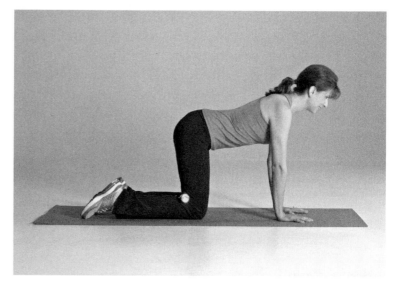

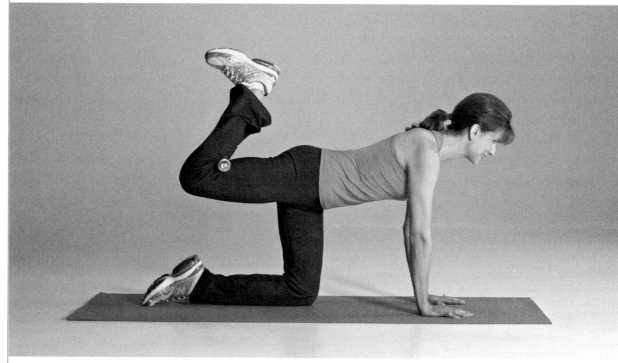

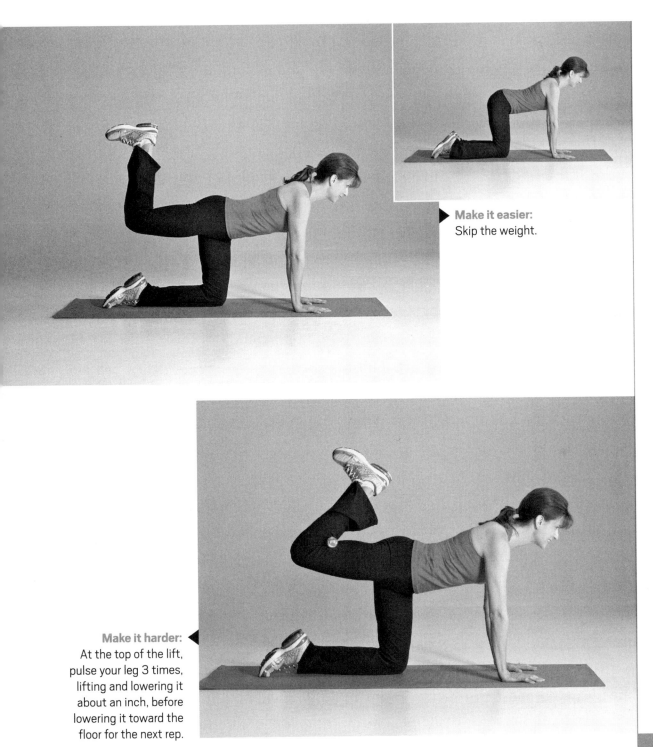

Make it easier:
Skip the weight.

Make it harder:
At the top of the lift, pulse your leg 3 times, lifting and lowering it about an inch, before lowering it toward the floor for the next rep.

Wall Squat with Ball
(targets quads, glutes, hamstrings, and inner thighs)

MAIN MOVE
Holding a soft ball or pillow, stand with your back against a wall, with your feet about 6 inches apart, 18 inches from the wall, and your toes pointed forward. Slide down the wall until your thighs are about parallel to the floor. Place the ball or pillow between your knees and adjust your feet so that your knees are directly over your ankles. Rest your hands on your hips and squeeze the ball with your knees for a count of 4, then relax for 4, while still holding the ball with knees and maintaining the squat position. Repeat, working up to 60 seconds.

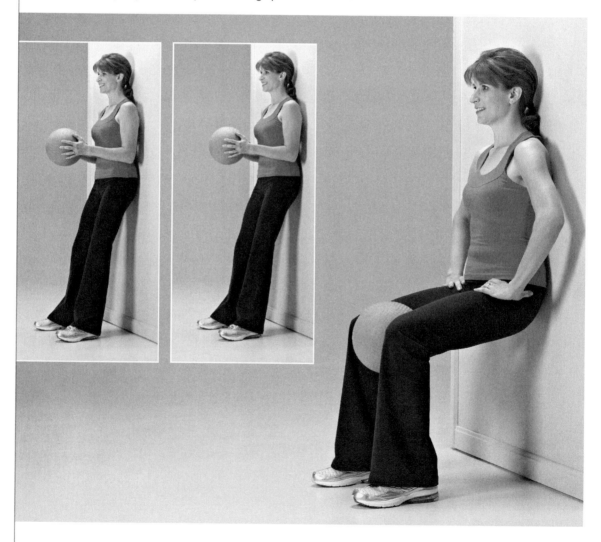

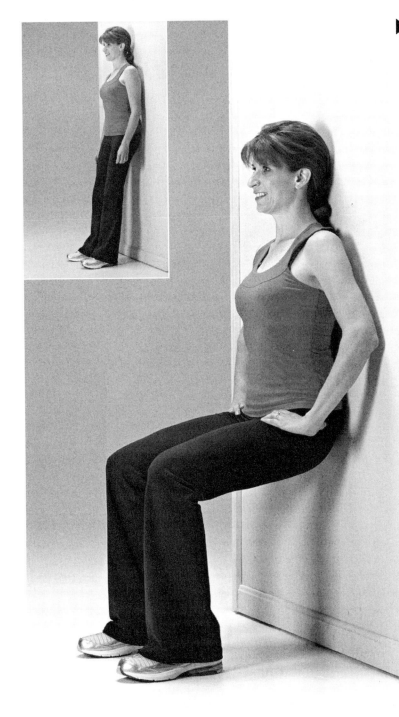

▶ **Make it easier:** Do the squat without a ball, simply holding the position.

Make it harder: While holding the squat position, squeeze the ball and release to a count of 1.

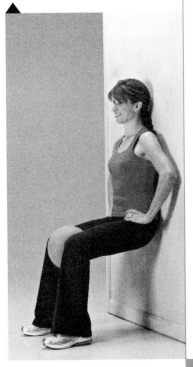

CORE STRENGTH WORKOUT II

THIS WORKOUT IS BASED ON RESEARCH showing that using a stability ball (see Resources on page 320 for where to find stability balls) can tone twice as many muscle fibers[2] and that Pilates moves are superior to traditional crunches for firming up your midsection.[3] The result: a firmer core and flatter abs in less time. Work up to doing 15 repetitions of each exercise on both sides when appropriate, unless otherwise indicated.

Elevated Plank

(targets abs, back, glutes, chest, shoulders, and triceps)

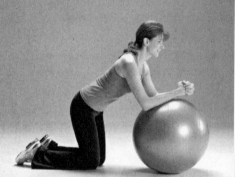

MAIN MOVE

Kneel on the floor and place your forearms on a large stability ball, fingers interlaced. Extend your legs straight behind you, supporting yourself on your toes. Exhale, pulling your belly button in toward your spine. Hold for 30 to 60 seconds, keeping your back flat and your body in a straight line. Rest for 30 seconds, then repeat. Do 3 times.

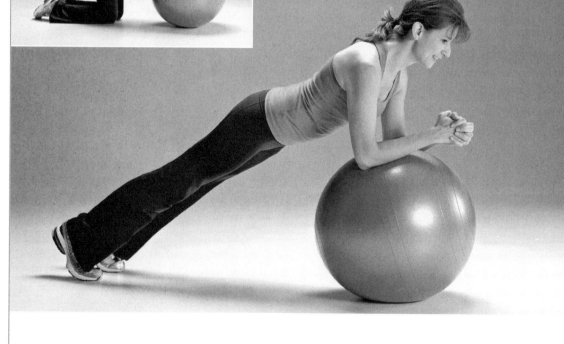

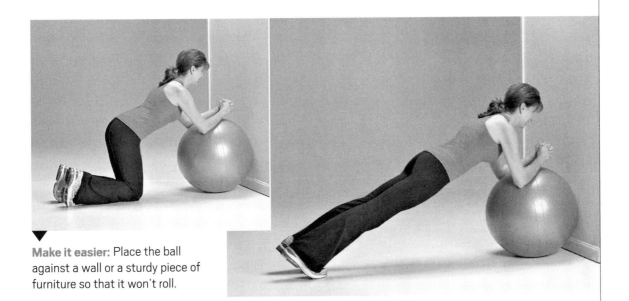

Make it easier: Place the ball against a wall or a sturdy piece of furniture so that it won't roll.

Make it harder: From the plank position on the ball, bring one knee at a time toward your chest.

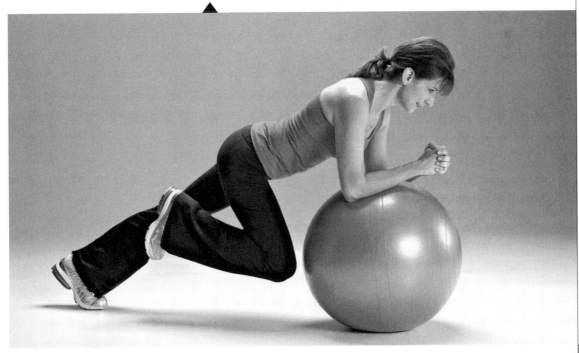

Ball Balance
(targets back, abs, and glutes)

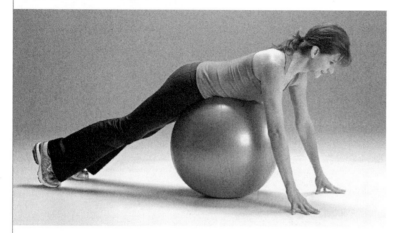

MAIN MOVE

Lie on the ball with your fingers and toes on the floor. Exhale, pulling your abs in to stabilize. Then raise your left arm forward and your right leg back. Breathe and hold for 10 seconds, using your ab and back muscles to keep the ball steady and your body in a straight line. Lower, then repeat with the opposite arm and leg. Do 5 times on each side.

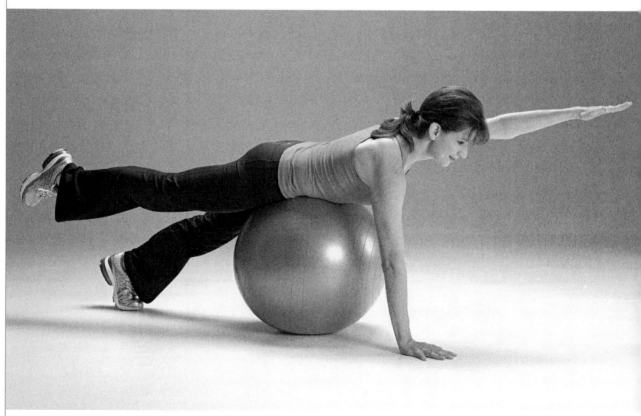

Make it easier: Lift just your left arm for 5 reps, then lift just your right leg for 5 reps. Switch sides and repeat.

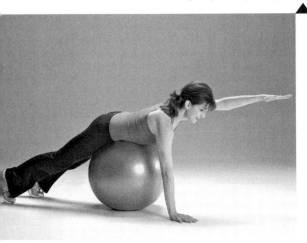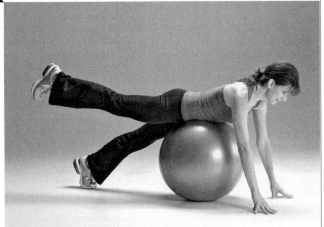

Make it harder: Hold the raised position as you draw 5 small circles with the extended arm and then with your leg. Switch sides and repeat.

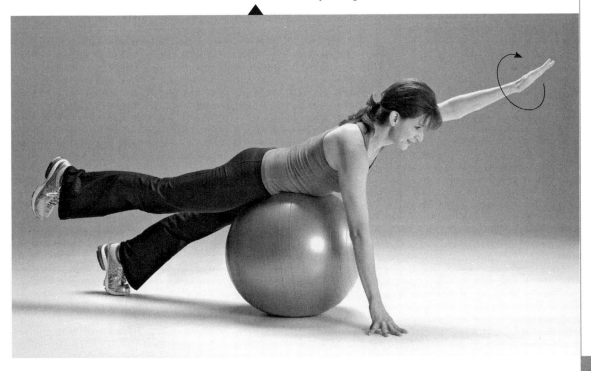

Twisting Crunch on a Ball
(targets abs, back, glutes, and thighs)

MAIN MOVE

Sit on a ball. Walk your feet forward and roll your torso down until your hips are just off the ball and your middle and upper back are on the ball. Your feet should be hip-width apart. Place your fingertips behind your head with your elbows out. Exhale, contracting your abs. Curl up and twist to the right, as if you're trying to bring your left shoulder toward your right hip. Keep your chin tucked slightly, as if you were holding an orange under it. Hold for a second. Inhale and lower. Repeat, twisting to the opposite side.

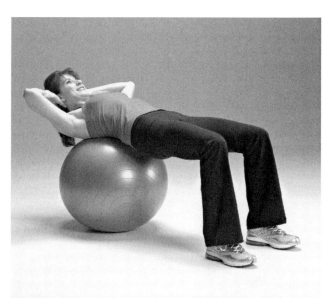

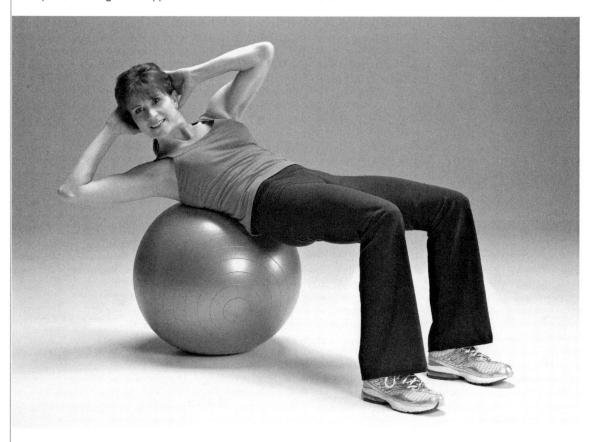

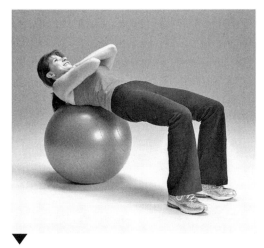

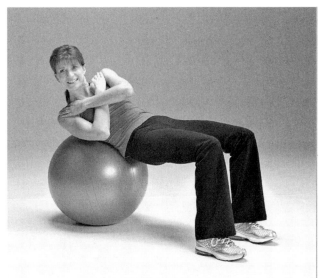

Make it easier: Place your feet more than hip-width apart for greater stability, and cross your arms over your chest.

▶ **Make it harder:** Bring your feet together, so you're less stable.

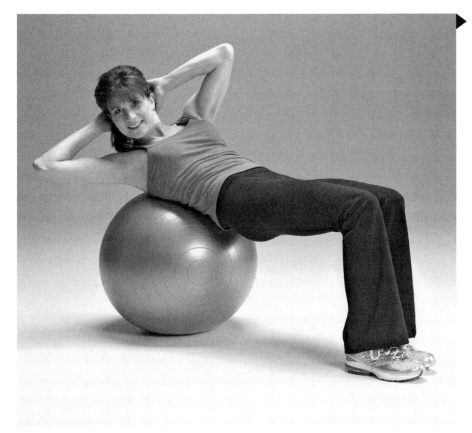

Roll-Up
(targets abs, back, and hips)

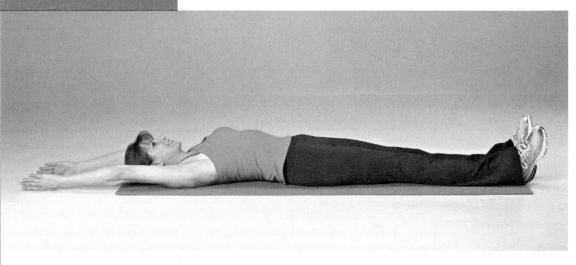

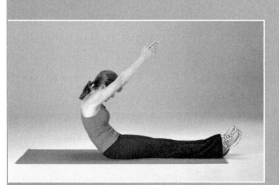

MAIN MOVE

Lie on your back with your legs fully extended and your arms stretched overhead. Inhale and raise your arms toward the ceiling. Exhale slightly, tuck your chin to your chest, pull your belly button in toward your spine, and curl forward to touch your toes (or as far as comfortable). Inhale and roll down one vertebra at a time.

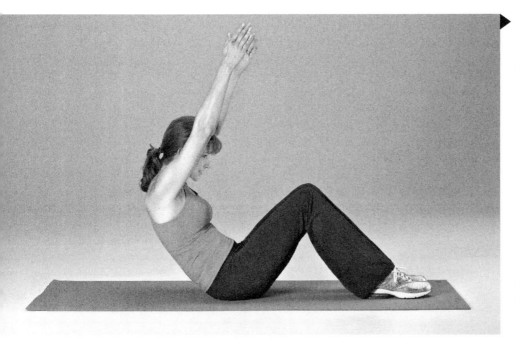

Make it easier:
Do the move with
your knees bent
and your feet flat
on the floor.

Make it harder: Use
a light dumbbell (2
to 5 pounds), hold-
ing it with one hand
on each end, as you
do the exercise.

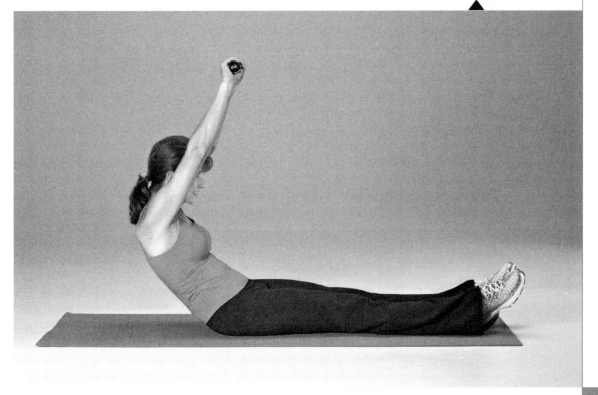

Twist
(targets abs and back)

MAIN MOVE
Sit on the floor with your knees bent and your feet flat on the floor. Hold a dumbbell (2 to 10 pounds) with both hands, with your arms out in front of you at chest height. Keeping your back straight, tighten your abs and lean back slightly. Rotate your upper body to the right, lowering the dumbbell as close to the floor as possible. Return to the center and repeat.

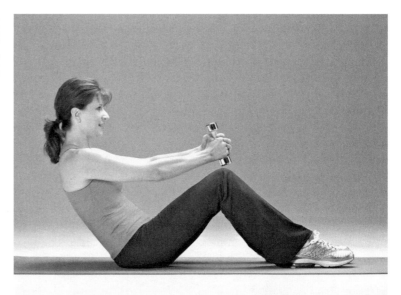

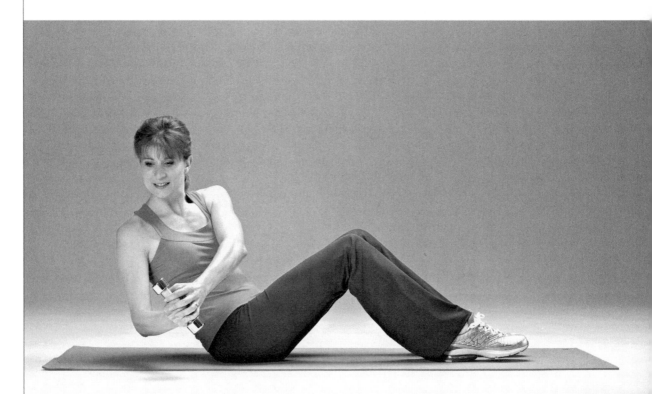

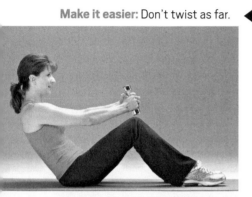

Make it easier: Don't twist as far.

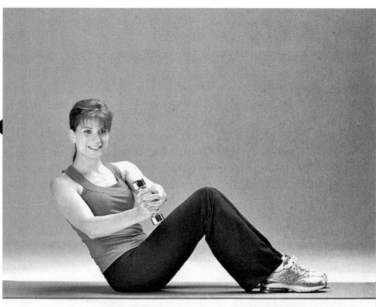

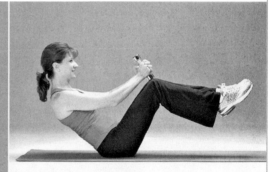

Make it harder: Raise your feet off the floor and balance on your tailbone as you twist.

UPPER-BODY STRENGTH WORKOUT

SINCE THIS WORKOUT REQUIRES DUMBBELLS (which I don't recommend using during your walks), you'll need to do it separately from your walks. The other option for challenging your upper body is to continue to do Toning Walk II (page 119), but use a band with more resistance.

By combining a resistance band with dumbbells for this workout, you'll get stronger and firmer faster. To do this: You can tie the band to the dumbbell, create a loop if you're using tubes with handles, or simply hold both in your hand. Choose what's most comfortable for you.

To make the following moves harder or easier, simply adjust the amount of weight you're lifting and/or adjust your hand position on the bands (choke up for more resistance or make the band more slack for less resistance). Do 1 or 2 sets of 10 to 12 reps of each move.

Chest Press
(targets chest, shoulders, and triceps)

MAIN MOVE
Lie on your back with knees bent, feet flat, and a resistance band looped around your upper back and under your arms. Hold one end of the band and a dumbbell in each hand, with your hands by your chest and your elbows pointing out. Straighten your arms, pressing your hands toward the ceiling. Hold for a second before lowering to the starting position.

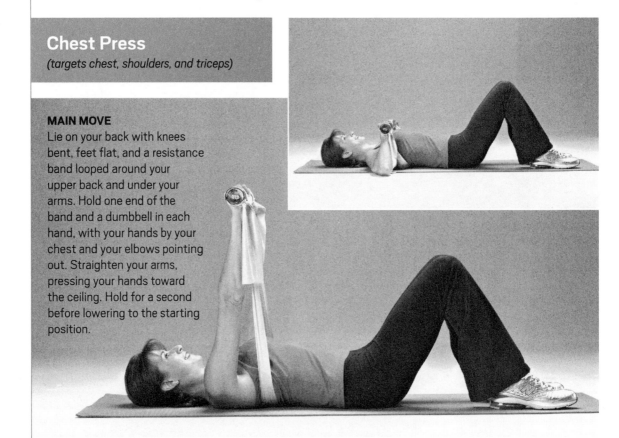

Bent-Over Row
(targets upper back and biceps)

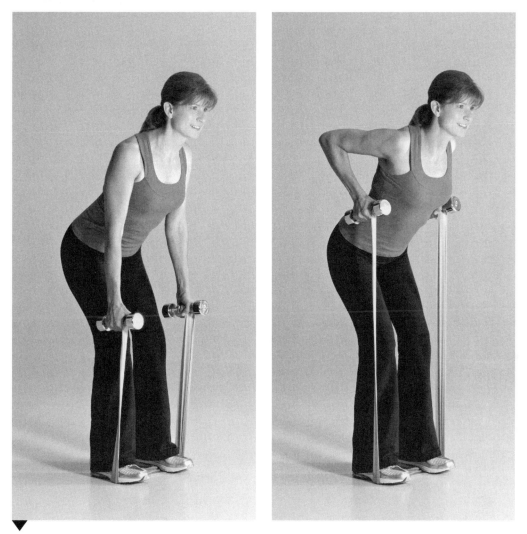

MAIN MOVE

Stand with your feet hip-width apart and a resistance band under both feet. Hold one end of the band and a dumbbell in each hand. Bend forward from your hips about 45 to 90 degrees, knees bent slightly, and let your arms hang beneath your shoulders with your palms facing in toward your body. Keep your abs contracted and your back straight. Squeeze your shoulder blades together, bend your arms, and pull your hands toward your rib cage, with your elbows pointing toward the ceiling. Hold for a second before lowering to the starting position.

Arm Curl
(targets biceps)

MAIN MOVE

Stand with your feet hip-width apart and a resistance band under both feet. Hold one end of the band and a dumbbell in each hand, with your arms down at your sides and your palms facing forward. Bend your elbows, keeping them close to your body. Curl your hands up toward your shoulders, keeping your wrists in line with your forearms. Hold for a second before lowering to the starting position.

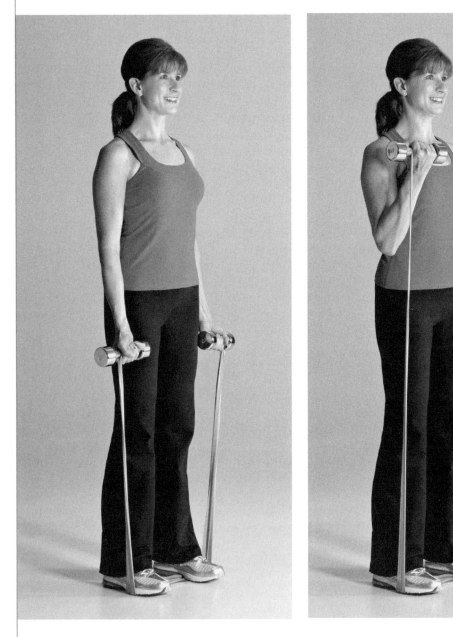

MAIN MOVE

Stand with your feet hip-width apart and a resistance band under both feet. Hold one end and a dumbbell in each hand, with your palms facing in toward your body. Bend forward from your hips about 45 to 90 degrees, knees bent slightly, and bend your elbows 90 degrees, keeping your upper arms by your sides. Straighten your arms so that your hands are near your hips. Hold for a second before lowering to the starting position.

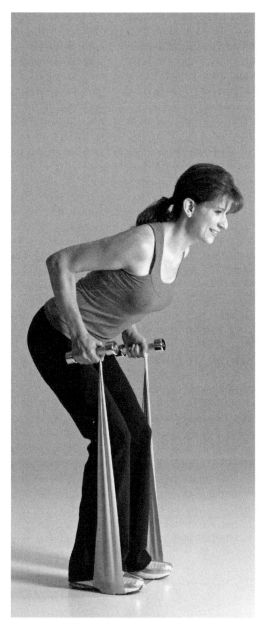

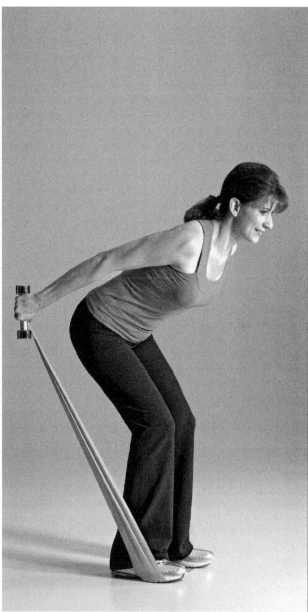

Lateral Raise
(targets shoulders)

MAIN MOVE

Stand with your feet hip-width apart and a resistance band under your right foot. Hold one end of the band and a dumbbell in your right hand, with your arm down at your side and your palm facing in toward your body. Rest your left hand on your hip. Keeping your abs tight, raise your right arm out to the side until it is at shoulder height. Hold for a second before lowering to the starting position.

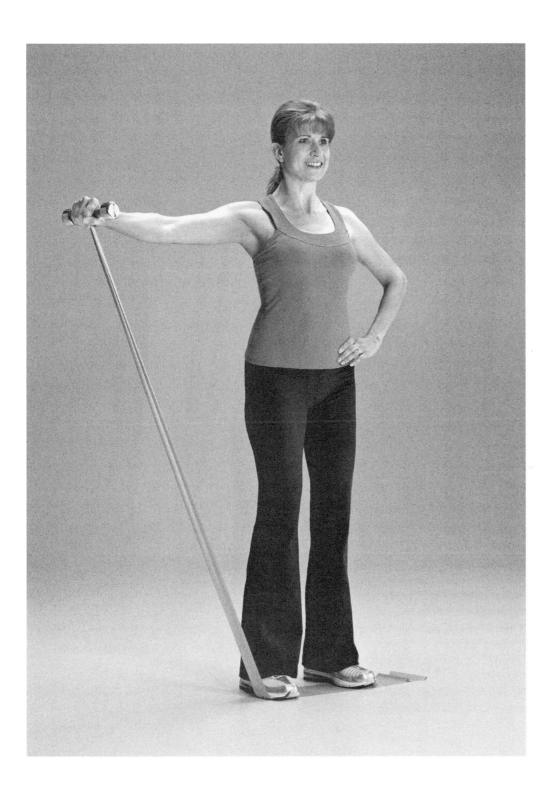

TOTAL-BODY STRENGTH WORKOUT II

THE MULTIMUSCLE MOVES IN THIS ROUTINE are identical to the original Total-Body Strength Workout, but this time you'll use weights. Combining dumbbells with a resistance band provides three times more sculpting power, according to research from Ithaca College.[4] You can tie the band to the dumbbell, create a loop if you're using tubes with handles, or simply hold both in your hand. Do 1 or 2 sets of 12 to 15 reps of each move on both sides when appropriate.

Balancing Deadlift with Arm Raise
(targets glutes, legs, abs, and shoulders)

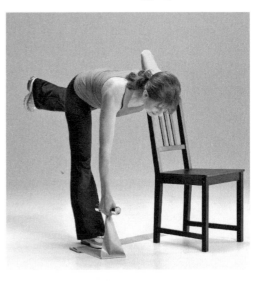

MAIN MOVE
Stand with one end of a band under your right foot; hold the other end and a dumbbell in your right hand. Lightly hold onto a chair for balance with your left hand. Slowly hinge forward from your hips, lowering your upper body toward the floor as your left leg rises behind you, as far as comfortable or until your body and leg are parallel to the floor. Squeeze your glutes as you stand back up, raising your left knee in front of you and simultaneously raising your right arm out to the side. Then slowly lower.

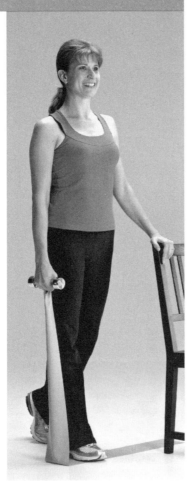

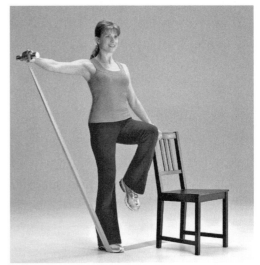

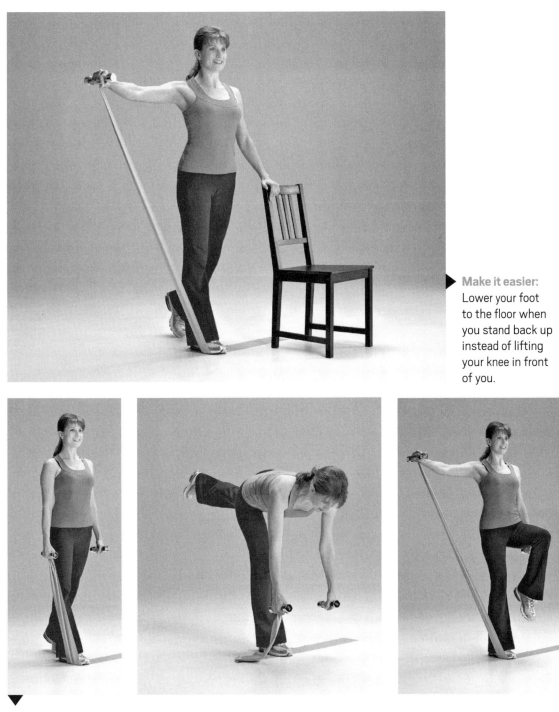

Make it easier: Lower your foot to the floor when you stand back up instead of lifting your knee in front of you.

Make it harder: Do the move without holding onto a chair and hold a dumbbell in your left hand.

Bridge with Press
(targets chest, arms, abs, glutes, and legs)

MAIN MOVE

Lie on your back with your knees bent and your feet flat. Loop a resistance band around your upper back and under your arms. Grasp each end and a dumbbell with your hands near your chest, with your elbows pointing out. Contract your abs and glutes and lift your butt off the floor so that your body forms a straight line from shoulders to knees. At the same time, straighten your arms, pressing your hands toward the ceiling. Hold for a second before lowering your arms, then your body.

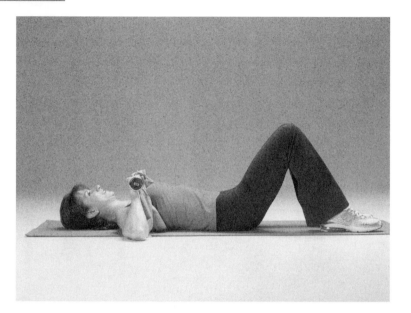

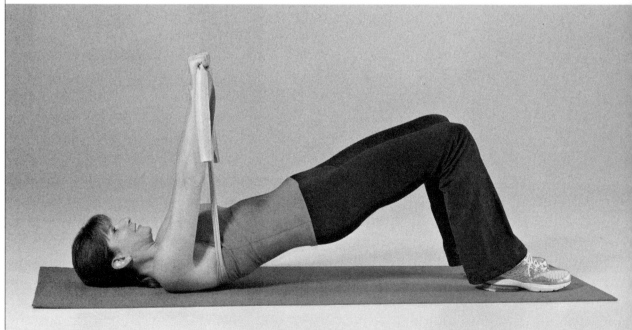

Make it easier: Do the moves separately. Keeping your butt on the floor, press your arms straight up and then lower for the recommended number of reps. Next, keep your arms still as you lift your butt off the floor for the recommended number of reps.

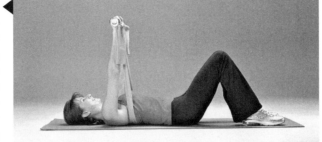

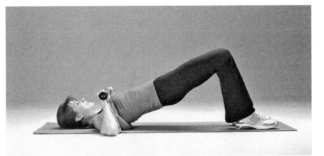

Make it harder: Raise your left foot off the floor, extending your leg, and perform the exercise. Switch legs halfway through the reps.

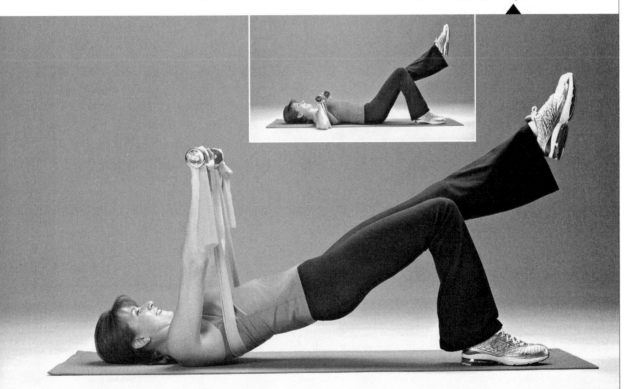

Crunch and Extend
(targets abs and arms)

MAIN MOVE

Anchor the center of a resistance band near the floor (see page 129 for more information) and lie so that it's behind your head. Grasp each end along with a dumbbell in each hand and bend your arms so that your elbows point up and your hands are on either side of your head. Contract your abs and curl your head and shoulders off the floor, keeping your arms stationary. Hold the crunch position and extend your arms. Hold, then slowly bend your arms and lower your head.

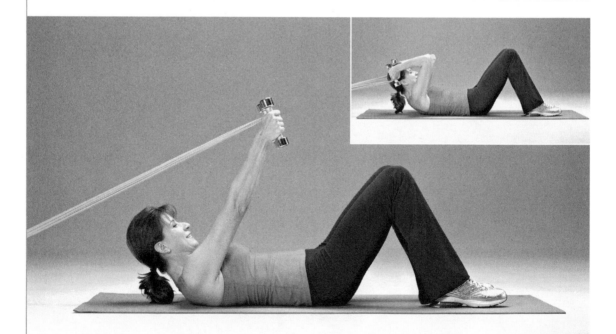

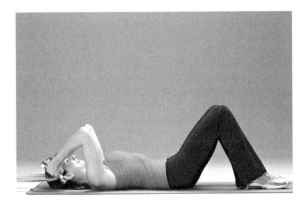

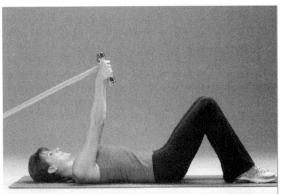

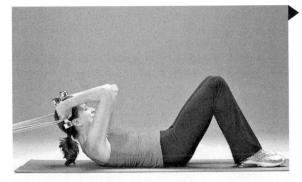

▼

Make it easier:
Do the moves separately. Keeping your head on the floor, extend and bend your arms only. Perform all the reps. Next, keeping your arms bent the entire time, contract your abs, curl your head and shoulders off the floor, and then lower.

Make it harder: Extend your legs up toward the ceiling, keeping them raised throughout all of the reps.

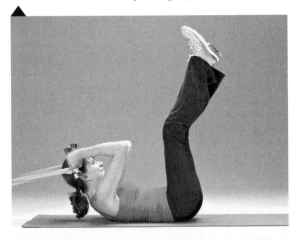

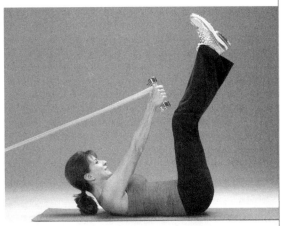

Rotating Lunge
(targets legs, glutes, and obliques)

MAIN MOVE

Anchor the center of a resistance band at about waist level (see page 129 for more information). Stand facing the band with your feet together. Hold the ends and a dumbbell with both hands, with your arms out in front, your elbows bent, and your hands just below chest height. Step your left foot behind you 2 to 3 feet, with your toes pointing forward. Bend your knees and lower until your right knee is bent 90 degrees, keeping your knee over your ankle. At the same time, rotate your torso to the right. Hold, then press into your right foot to stand back up and rotate back to center. Perform all of the reps on one side, then switch legs and repeat.

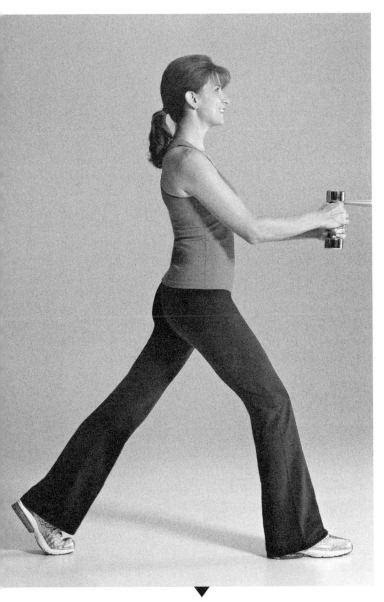

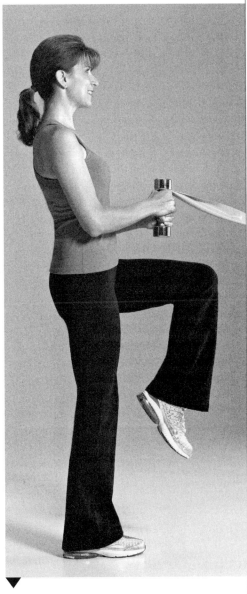

Make it easier: Do the move with your feet stationary, one in front of the other, 2 to 3 feet apart.

Make it harder: As you stand back up, raise your left knee in front of you before stepping back into the next lunge.

Row with Leg Swing

(targets upper back, hips, glutes, and biceps)

MAIN MOVE

Anchor the center of a resistance band at about waist level. Stand facing the band with your feet together. Hold an end and a dumbbell in each hand, with your arms extended in front of you. Bend your elbows and pull your arms back, squeezing your shoulder blades together and keeping your arms close to your body, until your hands are near your hips with your elbows pointing behind you. At the same time, raise your right knee in front of you to hip height. Then extend your arms in front of you and swing your right leg behind you, flexing your foot and squeezing your glutes as you do. Continue without lowering your right foot to the floor.

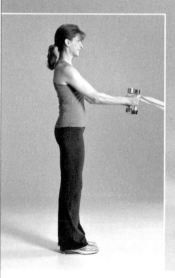

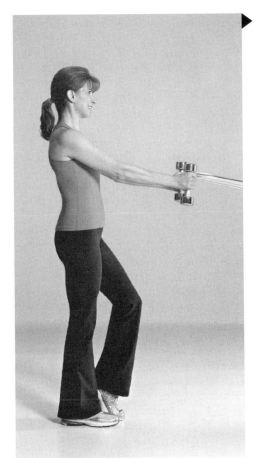

Make it easier:
Skip the backward leg swing and instead lower your foot to the floor after each knee lift. Or, keep doing the backward leg swing, but touch your foot down to the floor in between the knee lift and the leg swing to stabilize you.

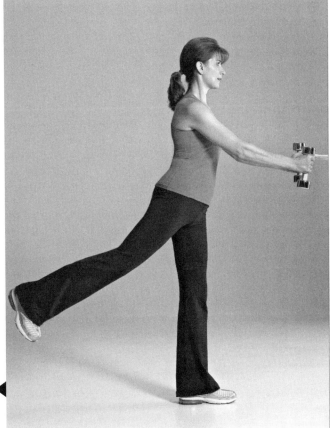

Make it harder: When your leg is extended behind you, pulse it three times, raising and lowering it an inch or so, before bringing it forward into the knee lift.

Elevated Squat with Curl
(targets legs, butt, and arms)

MAIN MOVE

Stand with a resistance band under the balls of your feet, with your feet about shoulder-width apart, your toes pointing forward, and your arms at your sides. Holding an end of the band and a dumbbell in each hand, bend your hips and knees, sitting back as if you were lowering into a chair. Hold; then as you stand up, bend your elbows and raise your hands toward your shoulders, lifting your heels off the floor so that you're balancing on your toes. Lower your heels and repeat, lowering into a squat and extending your arms.

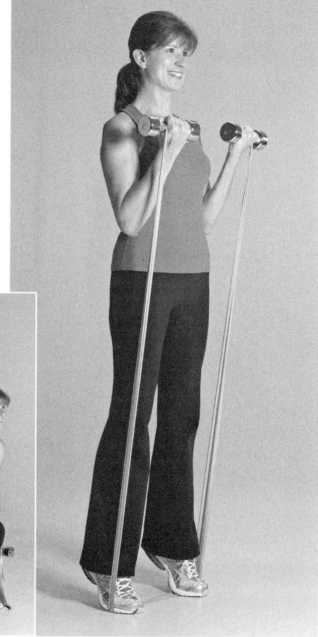

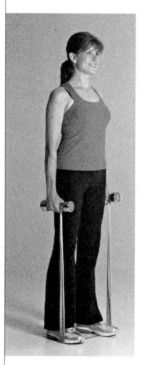

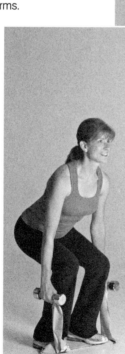

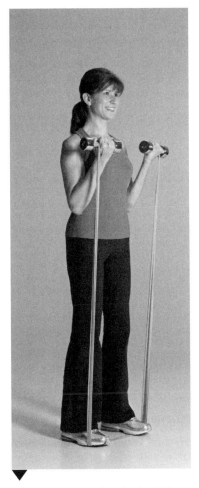 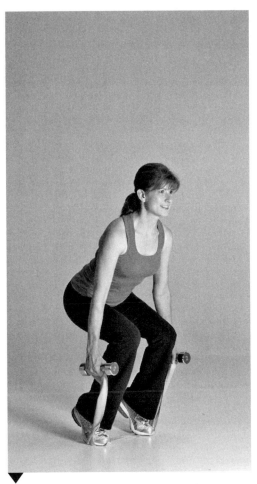

Make it easier: Skip the heel lift, keeping your feet flat on the floor the entire time.

Make it harder: Do the heel lift in the squat position instead. Stand up while balancing on your toes, then lower heels before doing the curl.

Now you are all set for continued success.
Using these various routines, aim to change your workouts every 6 to 8 weeks to avoid boredom, challenge your body in new ways, and avoid a plateau. The results will enable you to enjoy a healthier life.
Good luck!

WOW Winner
Yvonne Shorb
GROUP: Exercise Only

AGE: 61 **HEIGHT:** 5'5½"
POUNDS LOST: 14
INCHES LOST: 6½ overall, including 2½ from her waist
MAJOR ACCOMPLISHMENT: Biggest loser in the Exercise-Only group. Clocked 4.6 MPH during the 1-mile walk test. Lowered blood pressure from a dangerous 138/84 to a healthier 124/76. Cut triglyerides by 55 points.

Superfit Grandma

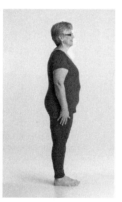

BEFORE

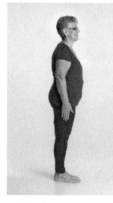

AFTER

YVONNE SHORB, a self-proclaimed yo-yo dieter, was in rewind mode (once again) when she heard about the WOW program. "I was 20 pounds back up from an almost 50-pound weight loss," Yvonne recalled. Even though she felt fairly well-versed in the art of dieting, Yvonne had never been able to keep the pounds off permanently. "I didn't know what to do, so I was thrilled to be a part of this program."

Yvonne had always done just a brisk walk, so the idea of intervals or resistance bands was foreign to her. But she always felt secure on WOW. "I saw how each week of the program builds you up for the following week's schedule," she explained. "I felt educated and informed, so if something new was being introduced, I was ready to go faster or longer."

Yvonne was amazed to find herself enjoying even the longest walk on the program. "I had never, ever walked for 90 minutes in my entire life, not for exercise," said Yvonne. "I was blown away because I actually loved every second." Not only did the grandma of two have a blast on her trek, she felt great the entire time. "I used to have so many aches and pains, especially in my knees and joints. But now I'm 100 percent pain free. I can run after my grandkids so much better, and I feel as young as most 50-year-olds I know—and even some in their 40s!"

Along with getting stronger, Yvonne was sleeping like a baby and enjoying a healthy spike in her energy level by Week 3. And she felt sturdier by Week 4. "It was easier to balance while putting on pants," she said.

Yvonne wasn't just feeling better; she was also seeing less of herself—and liking it. Right before she started WOW, Yvonne had tried on some of her summer clothes and couldn't even begin to get them closed. "By Week 5, I had my whole wardrobe back," she reported. Her doctor was pleased with the results, too. "At the beginning of the program, my resting heart rate (an indicator of fitness level) was 80, and I was having palpitations. Now it's 64 (nearly a 25 percent difference!), and my heart never races." Yvonne's blood pressure, cholesterol, and triglyceride numbers all improved, too.

"You know, I'm 61 years old, and I feel like I've finally found something I can do forever."

P.S. *Three months after the official end of the program, Yvonne recorded an additional 7¼-pound weight loss and shaved another 5¾ inches off her figure, for a grand total of 21¼ pounds and 12¼ inches lost in 5 months. Six weeks later Yvonne walked the Philadelphia half marathon, completing the 13.1-mile course in 2 hours 59 minutes and placing 23rd in her age group. Way to go!*

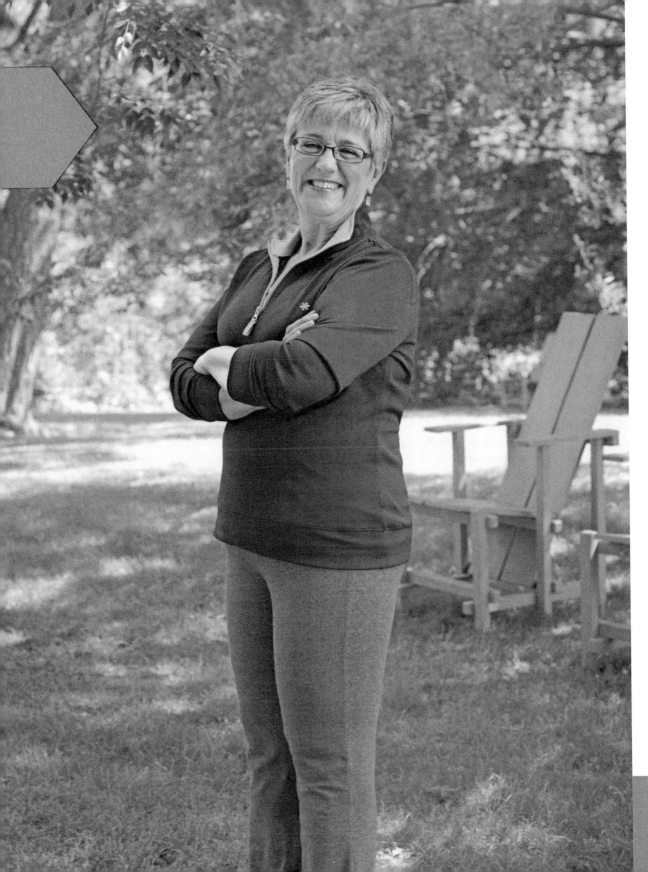

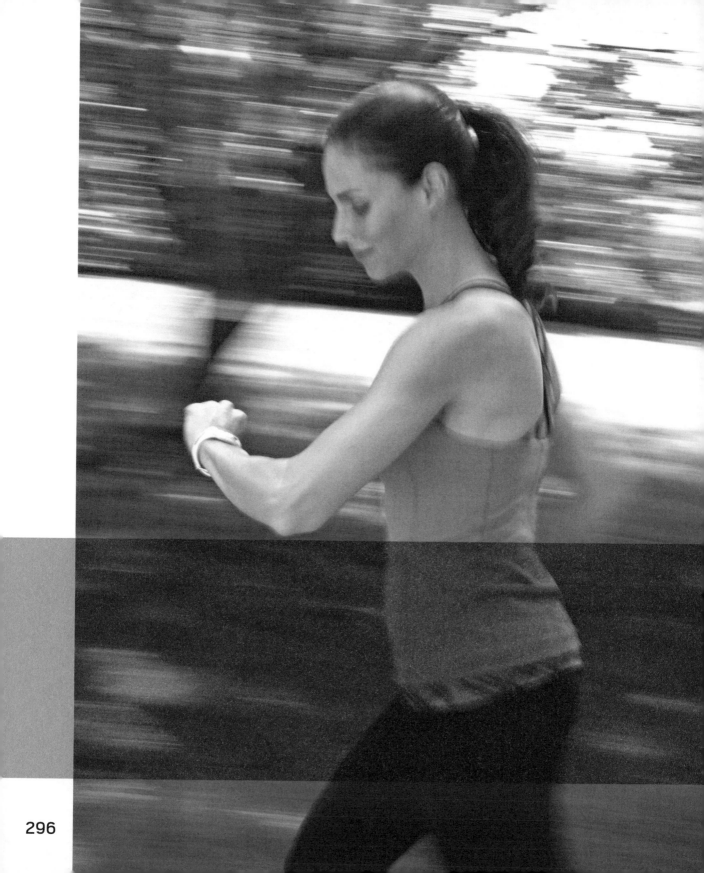

WALK OFF
Weight
JOURNAL

How to Use This Journal

When it comes to starting a new diet and exercise program, no tool has more power to impact long-term habits than keeping a journal.

The WOW journal is easy to use! We've included a week's worth of journal pages to get you started; you can photocopy the blank pages and make your own binder. (If you prefer, you can order the *Walk Off Weight Journal*. See Resources on page 320 for ordering information.)

Each day, record your exercise in the Workout Log and note how it went. Remember to write down which routines you do each day, the time you start your workout, and how long you exercise, including warm-up and cool-down. Finally, at the end of the day, tally up how much you exercised. This is also a good time to plan for when you'll fit in your next day's workouts. Don't forget to rate your energy and self-confidence levels for the day, too. Reviewing your answers periodically can help you overcome obstacles and remind you of just how far you've come.

On the Food Log, write down the foods you eat and your portion sizes. This record will also help you make sure you are getting proper nutrition—enough fiber, calcium, fats, and protein to keep your engine running, and especially enough water and green tea. If you're following our menu plan, rest easy knowing we've selected the right meals to help you meet your daily targets. Use the Daily Nutrition Goals row to check off the number of servings of each food group you consume throughout the day: grains/starches, fruits, vegetables, dairy, healthy fats, and lean proteins. These details will ensure that you are getting the daily recommended doses of essential vitamins and minerals.

At the end of each week, use the Weekly Measurements Log to track your progress. All you need are a bathroom scale and a measuring tape. Try to weigh and measure yourself around the same time on the same scale each week. For the most accurate results, ask someone else to help with the measuring tape. There are also two places to rate your average energy and self-confidence, each day and for the week.

On the page opposite each Weekly Measurements Log, you'll find a blank sheet of lined paper so you can add any other thoughts or observations about your week, including benefits or improvements you're noticing (such as sleeping better, not getting winded when climbing stairs) or whether you've had some difficulties following the plan.

Remember, the Walk Off Weight plan is a fitness guide, not a set-in-stone schedule. You can adjust the routines to make them easier or more challenging and move workouts around during the week to fit everything into your busy lifestyle.

Starting Stats

Record these measurements before you begin the program so you have a baseline from which to assess your progress. Seeing changes in these measurements can help you to stay motivated. If the numbers aren't improving as much as you'd like, this information can help you to modify the program to maximize your results.

TODAY'S DATE/TIME	
NAME:	
AGE:	HEIGHT:
WEIGHT:	
BODY MASS INDEX (BMI):	

You can calculate your BMI using the following formula: Multiply your weight in pounds by 703. Divide that number by your height in inches. Divide that number by your height in inches again.

Example: A woman who weighs 145 pounds and is 67 inches tall (5'7") has a BMI of 22.7. A BMI of 25 or higher is considered overweight; a BMI of 30 or higher is obese. You want to aim for a healthy BMI between 18.5 and 24.9. Alternately, use our online BMI calculator in just a few quick clicks! Go to www.prevention.com, then search for "BMI calculator."

INCHES

Accurately measuring your own limbs and torso can be a challenge, so we recommend that you find a partner to help. Be sure to stand up straight, relax your arms, and follow these guidelines: Measure your chest at the fullest point of your bust. Take your waist measurement at the narrowest part of your torso, or about 2 inches above your navel. Measure your hips at the fullest part. Make sure the tape measure is parallel to the ground. Measure at the fullest part of each thigh and upper arm when arms and legs are relaxed, shoulder-width apart.

CHEST		LEFT THIGH		RIGHT THIGH	
WAIST		LEFT BICEPS		RIGHT BICEPS	
HIPS					

BLOODWORK

(Optional. Please consult your physician to have these measurements taken.)

RESTING HR		TOTAL CHOLESTEROL	
BP (SYSTOLIC)		HDL CHOLESTEROL	
BP (DIASTOLIC)		LDL CHOLESTEROL	
TRIGLYCERIDES		GLUCOSE	
OTHER			

1-MILE WALK

Map out a 1-mile route. Do your warm-up and cool-down separate from the 1-mile route so in total you'll be walking a little over a mile. During the 1-mile route, go at a pace that you feel you can maintain for the entire distance. You should be breathing heavy (about a 6 to 8 intensity level) but not panting. Note your time below.

TOTAL TIME	MIN

Here are some sample daily journal pages to help you get the right idea:

JOURNAL TIP: Don't forget to pencil in your rest day! You might decide to schedule it for when your calendar is so jam-packed that trying to exercise would feel like just one more thing you need to do. Or use it as a reward at the end of the week for doing all the recommended workouts.

WEEK **2** DAY **5** ▶ DATE _April 5, 2011_

WORKOUT LOG

WORKOUTS	TIME	DURATION
Basic Interval 1	6:30 a.m.	30 min
Lower-Body Strength Workout	8:00 p.m.	30 min
	DAILY TOTAL EXERCISE TIME	1 hour

WORKOUT NOTES

How did you feel before? _I was pretty tired when I got up this morning, but once I started walking, I felt energized!_

How did you feel after? _That was better than a cup of coffee!_

Any obstacles? _I had to review the exercises for the lower-body workout several times until I got it, so it took me longer than expected_

Major accomplishment? _I did all the "make it harder" versions of the exercises in the lower-body strength workout!_

Other notes: _Eating according to the guidelines today was tricky, but I'm surprised how much better I feel. I can't wait to see what I feel like this time next week!_

PERSONAL NOTES

ENERGY LEVEL (circle one)
1 being "I'm so tired I can't get out of bed" and **10 being** "I could dance all night!"

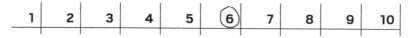

| 1 | 2 | 3 | 4 | 5 | (6) | 7 | 8 | 9 | 10 |

SELF-ESTEEM/SELF-CONFIDENCE (circle one)
1 being "I can't do anything right" and **10 being** "I'm ready to change the world!"

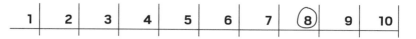

| 1 | 2 | 3 | 4 | 5 | 6 | 7 | (8) | 9 | 10 |

GET THE RIGHT NUTRITION by following the guidelines below. Use the checkboxes in the Daily Nutrition Goals row to help you. **GRAINS/STARCHES:** 5 or 6 servings; **FRUITS:** 3 servings; **VEGETABLES:** 4 or 5 servings; **DAIRY:** 3 servings; **HEALTHY FATS:** 3 or 4 servings; **LEAN PROTEINS:** 3 servings; **WATER:** at least 5 cups; **GREEN TEA:** at least 3 cups; **CALORIES:** 1,600–1,800.

FOOD LOG

	FOOD/DRINKS	TIME	CALORIES
Breakfast	2 whole-grain waffles, 1 tbsp powdered sugar, ¾ cup strawberries, 1 cup green tea 1 glass water before breakfast	9:00 a.m.	345
Lunch	1 egg made into egg salad with 2 tsp light mayo on 2 slices whole-grain toast, 1 large orange, ½ cucumber, sliced; 1 cup skim milk	1:00 p.m.	450
Snack	6 oz nonfat vanilla yogurt, ½ cup blueberries, 1 cup green tea + 2 glasses of water in the afternoon	3:30 p.m.	197
Dinner	4 oz salmon, sautéed in 2 tsp olive oil, 1 cup steamed carrots, ½ cup brown rice, 1 cup skim milk	7:45 p.m.	550
Optional Snack	3 cups light microwave popcorn drizzled with 1 tbsp peanut butter, + 2 glasses of water in the evening	9:00 p.m.	172
	DAILY CALORIE TOTAL		1,714

DAILY NUTRITION GOALS:	Grains/Starches	Fruits	Vegetables	Dairy	Healthy Fats	Lean Proteins
	☒☒☒☒☒☒	☒☒☒	☒☒☒☐☐	☒☒☒	☒☒☒☐	☒☒☒
	Water	Green Tea	Optional (amount per day)			
	☒☒☒☒☒	☒☒☐	Fiber _30_ g Calcium _1,186_ mg Vitamin D _298_ IU			

BONUS TRACKER (*Record your blood sugar, track your medications, gauge your hunger, or make other notes here.*)

I got 7 hours of sleep last night.

I was only going to have 1 snack today, but the popcorn after dinner helped me go to bed without feeling hungry

Here are some sample weekly journal pages to help you get the right idea:

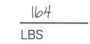 **WEEK 2**   DATE/TIME _04/7/11   8:30 a.m._

WEEKLY MEASUREMENTS LOG

WEIGHT   <u>164</u>
LBS

INCHES   <u>34"</u>   <u>21 3/4"</u>   <u>21 1/4"</u>
            CHEST   LEFT THIGH   RIGHT THIGH

            <u>36"</u>   <u>9"</u>   <u>9 1/4"</u>
            WAIST   LEFT BICEPS   RIGHT BICEPS

            <u>38 1/2"</u>
            HIPS (at fullest part)

PERSONAL NOTES

ENERGY LEVEL (circle one)
1 being "I'm so tired I can't get out of bed" and **10 being** "I could dance all night!"

| 1 | 2 | 3 | 4 | 5 | 6 | 7 | (8) | 9 | 10 |

SELF-ESTEEM/SELF-CONFIDENCE (circle one)
1 being "I can't do anything right" and **10 being** "I'm ready to change the world!"

| 1 | 2 | 3 | 4 | 5 | 6 | (7) | 8 | 9 | 10 |

Additional observations, challenges, notes:

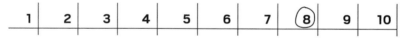
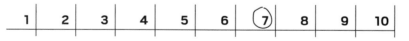
This week, I really pushed myself on the lower body and core exercises. I feel it in my legs for sure! But I noticed I also felt it all week on the sides of my abs. Even sitting at my office desk feels like a workout.

Additional observations, challenges, notes (cont'd):

I'm loving the Peachy Pork Olé from the 2-week menu and ate it twice this week! Cauliflower is surprisingly good... I probably wouldn't have touched it before trying this recipe, but now I'm definitely going to eat it more often.

It's hard to believe how much energy I've had this week, too! I focused better at work, had no problem waking up in the morning, and just feel better than usual. I hope it lasts!

DATE _____

WORKOUTS	TIME	DURATION
	DAILY TOTAL EXERCISE TIME	

WORKOUT NOTES

How did you feel before? _____

_____

How did you feel after? _____

_____

Any obstacles? _____

_____

Major accomplishment? _____

_____

Other notes: _____

_____

PERSONAL NOTES

ENERGY LEVEL (circle one)
1 being "I'm so tired I can't get out of bed" and **10 being** "I could dance all night!"

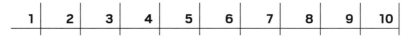

SELF-ESTEEM/SELF-CONFIDENCE (circle one)
1 being "I can't do anything right" and **10 being** "I'm ready to change the world!"

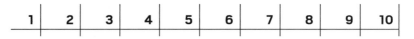

FOOD LOG

	FOOD/DRINKS	TIME	CALORIES
Breakfast			
Lunch			
Snack			
Dinner			
Optional Snack			
	DAILY CALORIE TOTAL		

DAILY NUTRITION GOALS:	Grains/Starches	Fruits	Vegetables	Dairy	Healthy Fats	Lean Proteins
	☐☐☐☐☐☐	☐☐☐	☐☐☐☐☐	☐☐☐	☐☐☐☐	☐☐☐
	Water	Green Tea	*Optional* (amount per day)			
	☐☐☐☐☐	☐☐☐	Fiber _____g **Calcium** _____mg **Vitamin D** _____IU			

BONUS TRACKER *(Record your blood sugar, track your medications, gauge your hunger, or make other notes here.)*

_____

_____

_____

DATE _____

WORKOUT LOG

WORKOUTS	TIME	DURATION
	DAILY TOTAL EXERCISE TIME	

WORKOUT NOTES

How did you feel before? _____

_____

How did you feel after? _____

_____

Any obstacles? _____

_____

Major accomplishment? _____

_____

Other notes: _____

_____

PERSONAL NOTES

ENERGY LEVEL (circle one)
1 being "I'm so tired I can't get out of bed" and **10 being** "I could dance all night!"

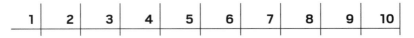

| 1 | 2 | 3 | 4 | 5 | 6 | 7 | 8 | 9 | 10 |

SELF-ESTEEM/SELF-CONFIDENCE (circle one)
1 being "I can't do anything right" and **10 being** "I'm ready to change the world!"

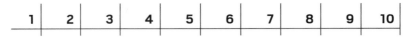

| 1 | 2 | 3 | 4 | 5 | 6 | 7 | 8 | 9 | 10 |

FOOD LOG

	FOOD/DRINKS	TIME	CALORIES
Breakfast			
Lunch			
Snack			
Dinner			
Optional Snack			
	DAILY CALORIE TOTAL		

DAILY NUTRITION GOALS:	Grains/Starches □□□□□□	Fruits □□□	Vegetables □□□□□	Dairy □□□	Healthy Fats □□□□	Lean Proteins □□□
	Water □□□□□	Green Tea □□□	*Optional* (amount per day) Fiber _____ g **Calcium** _____ mg **Vitamin D** _____ IU			

BONUS TRACKER *(Record your blood sugar, track your medications, gauge your hunger, or make other notes here.)*

_____

_____

_____

DATE _____

WORKOUT LOG

WORKOUTS	TIME	DURATION
	DAILY TOTAL EXERCISE TIME	

WORKOUT NOTES

How did you feel before? _____

_____

How did you feel after? _____

_____

Any obstacles? _____

_____

Major accomplishment? _____

_____

Other notes: _____

_____

PERSONAL NOTES

ENERGY LEVEL (circle one)
1 being "I'm so tired I can't get out of bed" and **10 being** "I could dance all night!"

1	2	3	4	5	6	7	8	9	10

SELF-ESTEEM/SELF-CONFIDENCE (circle one)
1 being "I can't do anything right" and **10 being** "I'm ready to change the world!"

1	2	3	4	5	6	7	8	9	10

FOOD LOG

	FOOD/DRINKS	TIME	CALORIES
Breakfast			
Lunch			
Snack			
Dinner			
Optional Snack			
		DAILY CALORIE TOTAL	

DAILY NUTRITION GOALS:	Grains/Starches ☐☐☐☐☐☐	Fruits ☐☐☐	Vegetables ☐☐☐☐☐	Dairy ☐☐☐	Healthy Fats ☐☐☐☐	Lean Proteins ☐☐☐
	Water ☐☐☐☐☐	Green Tea ☐☐☐	*Optional* (amount per day) Fiber _____ g Calcium _____ mg Vitamin D _____ IU			

BONUS TRACKER (*Record your blood sugar, track your medications, gauge your hunger, or make other notes here.*)

_____

_____

_____

WORKOUT LOG

WORKOUTS	TIME	DURATION
	DAILY TOTAL EXERCISE TIME	

WORKOUT NOTES

How did you feel before? _____

_____

How did you feel after? _____

_____

Any obstacles? _____

_____

Major accomplishment? _____

_____

Other notes: _____

_____

PERSONAL NOTES

ENERGY LEVEL (circle one)
1 being "I'm so tired I can't get out of bed" and **10 being** "I could dance all night!"

1	2	3	4	5	6	7	8	9	10

SELF-ESTEEM/SELF-CONFIDENCE (circle one)
1 being "I can't do anything right" and **10 being** "I'm ready to change the world!"

1	2	3	4	5	6	7	8	9	10

FOOD LOG

	FOOD/DRINKS	TIME	CALORIES
Breakfast			
Lunch			
Snack			
Dinner			
Optional Snack			
	DAILY CALORIE TOTAL		

DAILY NUTRITION GOALS:	Grains/Starches	Fruits	Vegetables	Dairy	Healthy Fats	Lean Proteins
	☐☐☐☐☐☐	☐☐☐	☐☐☐☐☐	☐☐☐	☐☐☐☐	☐☐☐
	Water	Green Tea	*Optional* (amount per day)			
	☐☐☐☐☐	☐☐☐	Fiber _____ g **Calcium** _____ mg **Vitamin D** _____ IU			

BONUS TRACKER (*Record your blood sugar, track your medications, gauge your hunger, or make other notes here.*)

_____

_____

_____

DATE _____

WORKOUT LOG

WORKOUTS	TIME	DURATION
	DAILY TOTAL EXERCISE TIME	

WORKOUT NOTES

How did you feel before? _____

_____

How did you feel after? _____

_____

Any obstacles? _____

_____

Major accomplishment? _____

_____

Other notes: _____

_____

PERSONAL NOTES

ENERGY LEVEL (circle one)
1 being "I'm so tired I can't get out of bed" and **10 being** "I could dance all night!"

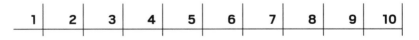

SELF-ESTEEM/SELF-CONFIDENCE (circle one)
1 being "I can't do anything right" and **10 being** "I'm ready to change the world!"

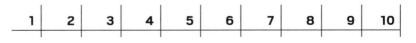

FOOD LOG

	FOOD/DRINKS	TIME	CALORIES
Breakfast			
Lunch			
Snack			
Dinner			
Optional Snack			
	DAILY CALORIE TOTAL		

DAILY NUTRITION GOALS:	Grains/Starches	Fruits	Vegetables	Dairy	Healthy Fats	Lean Proteins
	☐☐☐☐☐☐	☐☐☐	☐☐☐☐☐	☐☐☐	☐☐☐☐	☐☐☐
	Water	**Green Tea**	*Optional* (amount per day)			
	☐☐☐☐☐	☐☐☐	Fiber_____g **Calcium**_____mg **Vitamin D**_____IU			

BONUS TRACKER *(Record your blood sugar, track your medications, gauge your hunger, or make other notes here.)*

_____

_____

_____

WEEK ____ DAY ____ ▶ WORKOUT LOG

WORKOUTS	TIME	DURATION
	DAILY TOTAL EXERCISE TIME	

WORKOUT NOTES

How did you feel before? _____

_____

How did you feel after? _____

_____

Any obstacles? _____

_____

Major accomplishment? _____

_____

Other notes: _____

_____

PERSONAL NOTES

ENERGY LEVEL (circle one)
1 being "I'm so tired I can't get out of bed" and **10 being** "I could dance all night!"

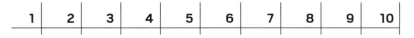

SELF-ESTEEM/SELF-CONFIDENCE (circle one)
1 being "I can't do anything right" and **10 being** "I'm ready to change the world!"

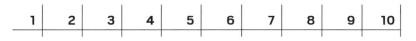

FOOD LOG

	FOOD/DRINKS	TIME	CALORIES
Breakfast			
Lunch			
Snack			
Dinner			
Optional Snack			
		DAILY CALORIE TOTAL	

DAILY NUTRITION GOALS:	Grains/Starches ☐☐☐☐☐☐	Fruits ☐☐☐	Vegetables ☐☐☐☐☐	Dairy ☐☐☐	Healthy Fats ☐☐☐☐	Lean Proteins ☐☐☐
	Water ☐☐☐☐☐	Green Tea ☐☐☐	Optional (amount per day) Fiber _____g Calcium _____mg Vitamin D _____IU			

BONUS TRACKER *(Record your blood sugar, track your medications, gauge your hunger, or make other notes here.)*

_____

_____

_____

DATE _____

WORKOUT LOG

WORKOUTS	TIME	DURATION
	DAILY TOTAL EXERCISE TIME	

WORKOUT NOTES

How did you feel before? _____

_____

How did you feel after? _____

_____

Any obstacles? _____

_____

Major accomplishment? _____

_____

Other notes: _____

_____

PERSONAL NOTES

ENERGY LEVEL (circle one)
1 being "I'm so tired I can't get out of bed" and **10 being** "I could dance all night!"

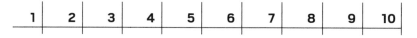

| 1 | 2 | 3 | 4 | 5 | 6 | 7 | 8 | 9 | 10 |

SELF-ESTEEM/SELF-CONFIDENCE (circle one)
1 being "I can't do anything right" and **10 being** "I'm ready to change the world!"

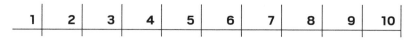

| 1 | 2 | 3 | 4 | 5 | 6 | 7 | 8 | 9 | 10 |

316

FOOD LOG

	FOOD/DRINKS	TIME	CALORIES
Breakfast			
Lunch			
Snack			
Dinner			
Optional Snack			
	DAILY CALORIE TOTAL		

DAILY NUTRITION GOALS:	Grains/Starches	Fruits	Vegetables	Dairy	Healthy Fats	Lean Proteins
	☐☐☐☐☐☐	☐☐☐	☐☐☐☐☐	☐☐☐	☐☐☐☐	☐☐☐
	Water	Green Tea	*Optional* (amount per day)			
	☐☐☐☐☐	☐☐☐	Fiber _____ g Calcium _____ mg Vitamin D _____ IU			

BONUS TRACKER *(Record your blood sugar, track your medications, gauge your hunger, or make other notes here.)*

_____

_____

_____

WEIGHT _____
LBS

INCHES _____   _____   _____
CHEST   LEFT THIGH   RIGHT THIGH

_____   _____   _____
WAIST   LEFT BICEPS   RIGHT BICEPS

_____
HIPS (at fullest part)

PERSONAL NOTES

ENERGY LEVEL (circle one)
1 being "I'm so tired I can't get out of bed" and **10 being** "I could dance all night!"

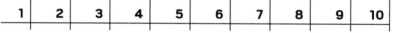

| 1 | 2 | 3 | 4 | 5 | 6 | 7 | 8 | 9 | 10 |

SELF-ESTEEM/SELF-CONFIDENCE (circle one)
1 being "I can't do anything right" and **10 being** "I'm ready to change the world!"

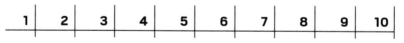

| 1 | 2 | 3 | 4 | 5 | 6 | 7 | 8 | 9 | 10 |

Additional observations, challenges, notes:

_____

_____

_____

_____

_____

Additional observations, challenges, notes (con't):

_____

_____

_____

_____

_____

_____

_____

_____

_____

_____

_____

_____

_____

_____

_____

_____

_____

_____

_____

_____

_____

_____

Resources

Throughout this book, I recommend products and equipment that can help maximize your WOW experience—and your results. Many of these items are widely available at sporting goods stores and from other retailers, as well as online. I've listed a number of sources here, but by all means, feel free to shop around to find the best quality and price.

Get Gear

BUNION AID (for bunion pain relief)
www.alphaorthotics.com

CALORIE BURN TRACKING DEVICES
These gadgets come with different features, so be sure to shop around. Here are three quality brands: **Bodybugg** www.bodybugg.com, **Fitbit** www.fitbit.com, and **Gruve** www.gruve.com.

DAZER II (to repel dogs)
For more information, go to www.dazer.com. For online retailers, search "dog dazer."

DISTANCE TRACKING DEVICES
You can find these GPS-powered trackers at sporting goods and electronic stores, as well as online. A high-quality brand that I use is **Garmin**. (For product information, visit www.garmin.com.)

EARBAGS
www.earbags.com

HEART RATE MONITORS
You can find a variety of brands at www.amazon.com or by searching "heart rate monitors" online. A quality brand that I recommend is **Polar** (www.shoppolar.com).

HYDRATION PACKS
Available at sporting goods stores and online. A high-quality brand that I recommend is **CamelBak** (visit www.camelbak.com for product information).

MP3 PLAYERS
Available at electronics stores such as Best Buy and Radio Shack or in the electronics department at retailers such as Target.

PEDOMETERS
You can find a variety of brands at www.amazon.com or by searching "pedometers" online. Quality brands that I recommend are **Yamax** (www.yamaxx.com), **Accusplit** (www.accusplit.com), **Omron** (www.omronhealthcare.com), and **Oregon Scientific** (www.oregonscientific.com).

REFLECTIVE APPAREL
IllumiNITE www.illuminite.com

Night-Gear www.night-gear.com

RESISTANCE BANDS AND TUBES
Balls 'n' Bands www.ballsnbands.com

Spri www.spriproducts.com

YogaDirect www.yogadirect.com

Or search "exercise bands" or "resistance tubes" online for a variety of retailers.
    Some resistance band and tube packages include a door anchor/attachment. If you need to purchase one separately, check the online retailers above or search "resistance band door anchor."

SHOES
Since you need to try on your shoes, look for specialty walking or running shoes in your area. Some national chains to try are **Finish Line**, **Foot Solutions**, and **The Walking Company**.

SOCKS

Amazing Socks www.amazingsocks.com

FootSmart www.footsmart.com

Road Runner Sports
www.roadrunnersports.com

Also visit the Web sites for these specific brands: **Adidas Aloe** www.finishline.com (search "aloe socks") and **Cocona** (made from coconut shells) www.coconafabrics.com

New Balance Marathon Trainer Left/Right www.newbalance.com

Thorlo www.thorlo.com

SPORTS BRAS

You'll find a variety of brands in sporting goods and department stores as well as online. High-quality brands that I recommend are **Champion** (www.championusa.com), **Enell** (www.enell.com), and **Moving Comfort** (www.movingcomfort.com).

SPORTS WATCHES

Our **WOW test panelists** used the **Timex Ironman 50-Lap Mid** (www.timex.com). You can find a variety of brands at sporting goods stores or by searching online.

STABILITY BALL

These large inflatable balls are sold at many department stores and sporting goods stores. Or search "stability ball" for online retailers.

TRACTION FOOTWEAR

You can find traction footwear, including **Stabilicers**, **Yaktrax**, and other brands, at www.noslipstore.com.

WALKING DVDS

For a variety of indoor walking workouts that don't require a treadmill, including *Prevention*'s **Walk Yourself Fit**, visit www.collagevideo.com. I also recommend **Leslie Sansone's** walking DVDs.

WEIGHTS

Dumbbells are readily available in department and sporting goods stores. Buying in person will save on shipping charges. If you want varying weights, consider adjustable dumbbells. I recommend the **Reebok Speed Pack**. It's available at Target for about $70 or search online for other retailers.

WALK OFF WEIGHT JOURNAL, PODCASTS, AND WORKOUT DVD

Order at www.prevention.com/shop. I designed these to complement the WOW program. The DVD offers more toning workouts.

Find a Professional

American Academy of Orthopaedic Surgeons www.aaos.org
An orthopedist is a medical doctor who specializes in musculoskeletal disorders.

American Academy of Physical Medicine and Rehabilitation www.aapmr.org
Click on "Find a PM&R Physician" to locate a physiatrist, a medical doctor who specializes in nonsurgical treatments for pain and injury.

American Physical Therapy Association www.apta.org
Physical therapists specialize in rehabilitation using exercise and other nonsurgical modalities.

American Podiatric Medical Association www.apma.org
A podiatrist specializes in the diagnosis and treatment of foot and ankle problems.

For More Information

Mark Fenton, *The Complete Guide to Walking, New and Revised: For Health, Weight Loss, and Fitness* (Connecticut: The Lyons Press, 2008)

Casey Meyers, *Walking: A Complete Guide to the Complete Exercise* (New York: Ballantine Books, 2007)

Lee Scott, **Simple Secrets for a Great Walking Workout DVD**, www.wowpowerwalking.com

Endnotes

INTRODUCTION

1 E. G. Trapp, et al., "The effects of high-intensity intermittent exercise training on fat loss and fasting insulin levels of young women," *International Journal of Obesity* 32 (2008): 684–91.

2 K. Sykes, et al., "Accumulating aerobic exercise for effective weight control," *Journal of the Royal Society for the Promotion of Health* 124 (2004): 24–28.

3 C. R. Richardson, et al., "A meta-analysis of pedometer-based walking interventions and weight loss," *Annals of Family Medicine* 6 (January/February 2008): 69–77.

4 M. A. Tully, et al., "Brisk walking, fitness, and cardiovascular risk: a randomized controlled trial in primary care," *Preventive Medicine* 41 (August 2005): 622–28.

5 A. E. Ready, et al., "Walking program reduces elevated cholesterol in women postmenopause," *Canadian Journal of Cardiology* 11 (November 1995): 905–12.

6 S. K. Park, et al., "The effect of combined aerobic and resistance training on abdominal fat in obese middle-aged women," *Journal of Physiological Anthropology and Applied Human Science* 22, no. 3 (May 2003): 129–35.

CHAPTER 1

1 Mediamark Research, Inc. National syndicated survey of media and consumer choices, Fall 2008.

2 Sporting Goods Manufacturing Association. insight08 Sports Participation in America.

3 R. Clinghan, et al., "Do you get value for money when you buy an expensive pair of running shoes?" *British Journal of Sports Medicine* 42 (March 2008): 189–93.

4 T. M. Asikainen, et al., "Exercise for health for early postmenopausal women," *Sports Medicine* 39, no. 11 (2004): 753–78.

5 Abby C. King, et al., "Long-term effects of varying intensities and formats of physical activity on participation rates, fitness, and lipoproteins in men and women aged 50 to 65 years," *Circulation* 91 (1995): 2596–604.

6 P. Ekkekakis, et al., "Walking in (affective) circles: Can short walks enhance affect?" *Journal of Behavioral Medicine* 23, no. 3 (2000): 245–75.

7 J. E. Manson, et al., "A prospective study of walking as compared with vigorous exercise in the prevention of coronary heart disease in women," *New England Journal of Medicine* 241, no. 9 (1999): 650–58.

8 F. B. Hu, et al., "Physical activity and risk of stroke in women," *Journal of the American Medical Association* 283, no. 22 (2000): 2961–67.

9 ———, "Walking compared with vigorous physical activity and risk of type 2 diabetes in women: a prospective study," *Journal of the American Medical Association* 282, no. 15 (1999): 1433–39.

10 B. Rockwell, et al., "A prospective study of recreational physical activity and breast cancer risk," *Archives of Internal Medicine* 159, no. 19 (1999): 2290–96.

11 V. A. Catenacci, et al., "Physical activity patterns in the National Weight Control Registry," *Obesity* 16 (2008): 153–61.

12 F. Amati, et al., "Separate and combined effects of exercise training and weight loss on exercise efficiency and substrate oxidation," *Journal of Applied Physiology* 105 (2008): 825–31.

13 R. Ross, et al., "Exercise-induced reduction in obesity and insulin resistance in women: a randomized controlled trial," *Obesity Research* 12 (2004): 789–98.

14 A. H. Taylor and A. J. Oliver, "Acute effects of brisk walking on urges to eat chocolate, affect, and responses to a stressor and chocolate cue," *Appetite* 52 (February 2009): 155–60.

15 M. M. Riordan, et al., "The effects of caloric-restriction and exercise-induced weight loss on left ventricular diastolic function," *American Journal of Physiology —Heart and Circulatory Physiology* 294, no. 3 (2008): H1174–82.

16 C. A. Slentz, et al., "Effects of the amount of exercise on body weight, body composition, and measures of central obesity: STRRIDE—a randomized controlled study," *Archives of Internal Medicine* 164, no. 1 (2004): 31–39.

17 M. Hamer and A. Steptoe, "Walking, vigorous physical activity, and markers of hemostasis and inflammation in healthy men and women," *Scandinavian Journal of Medicine and Science in Sports* 18 (2008): 736–41.

18 Cathie J. Bloem and Annette M. Chang, "Short-term exercise improves Ð-cell function and insulin resistance in older people with impaired glucose tolerance," *Journal of Clinical Endocrinology and Metabolism* 93 (2008): 387–92.

19 H. Himmelreich, et al., "Gluteal muscle recruitment during level, incline, and stair ambulation in healthy subjects and chronic low back pain patients," *Journal of Back and Musculoskeletal Rehabilitation* 21, no. 3 (2008): 193–99.

20 D. C. Nieman, "Current perspective on exercise immunology," *Current Sports Medicine Reports* 5 (2003): 239–42.

21 L. F. Callahan, et al., "A randomized controlled trial of the People with Arthritis Can Exercise program: symptoms, function, physical activity, and psychosocial outcomes," *Arthritis and Rheumatism* 59, no. 1 (2008): 92–101.

22 Diane Feskanich, Walter Willett, and Graham Colditz, "Walking and leisure-time activity and risk of hip fracture in postmenopausal women," *Journal of the American Medical Association* 288 (2002): 2300–2306.

23 Jeremy S. Sibold and Kathy Berg, "Mood enhancement persists for up to 12 hours following aerobic exercise" (annual meeting, American College of Sports Medicine, Seattle, WA, May 2009).

24 A. A. Eyler, et al., "The epidemiology of walking for physical activity in the United States," *Medicine and Science in Sports and Exercise* 35, no. 9 (2003): 1529–36.

25 J. B. Bartholomew, D. Morrison, and J. T. Ciccolo, "Effects of acute exercise on mood and well-being in patients with major depressive disorder," *Medicine and Science in Sports and Exercise* 37, no. 12 (2005): 2032–37.

26 Laiz Helena de Castro Toledo Guimaraesa, et al., "Physically active elderly women sleep more and better than sedentary women," *Sleep Medicine* 9, no. 5 (2007): 488–93.

27 L. Duane, et al., "Association of physical activity and human sleep disorders," *Archives of Internal Medicine* 158 (1998): 1894–98.

28 Steriani Elavsky and Edward McAuley, "Exercise and self-esteem in menopausal women: a randomized controlled trial involving walking and yoga," *American Journal of Health Promotion* 22, no. 2 (2007): 83–92.

29 Philip D. Chilibeck, et al., "Physical activity level and menopausal symptoms," *Medicine and Science in Sports and Exercise* 40, no. 5 (2008): s482–83.

30 G. Ravaglia, et al., "Physical activity and dementia risk in the elderly: findings from a prospective Italian study," *Neurology* 6, no. 70 (2008): 1786–94.

31 Matthew B. Pontifex, et al., "The effect of acute aerobic and resistance exercise on working memory," *Medicine and Science in Sports and Exercise* 41, no. 4 (2009): 927–34.

32 Parinda Khatri, et al., "Effects of exercise training on cognitive functioning among depressed older men and women," *Journal of Aging and Physical Activity* 9, no. 1 (2001): 43–57.

33 Kathleen Hutchinson and Helaine Alessio, "Miami researchers find link between cardiovascular fitness and hearing sensitivity," Miami University Graduate School. www.miami.muohio.edu/graduate/research/speech_physed.cfm (accessed September 9, 2009).

34 P. T. Williams, "Prospective epidemiological cohort study of reduced risk of incident cataract with vigorous physical activity and cardiorespiratory fitness during 7-year follow-up," *Investigative Ophthalmology and Visual Science* 50, no.1 (2009): 95–100.

35 P. T. Williams, "Prospective study of incident age-related macular degeneration in relation to vigorous physical activity during a 7-year follow-up," *Investigative Ophthalmology and Visual Science* 50, no. 1 (2009): 101–6.

36 M. S. Al-Zahrani, E. A. Borawski, and N. F. Bissada, "Increased physical activity reduces prevalence of periodontitis," *Journal of Dentistry* 33, no. 9 (2005): 703–10.

37 Oscar H. Franco, "Effects of physical activity on life expectancy cardiovascular disease," *Archives of Internal Medicine* 165 (2005): 2355–60.

38 Elavsky and McAuley (2007).

CHAPTER 2

1 J. Laforgia, et al., "Comparison of energy expenditure elevations after submaximal and supramaximal running," *Journal of Applied Physiology* 82, no. 2 (1997): 661–66.

2 M. McGinnis, "The fastest way to sculpt," *Prevention* (November 2007): 164–73.

3 K. E. Chad, et al., "The effect of exercise duration on the exercise and post-exercise oxygen consumption," *Canadian Journal of Sport Sciences* 13, no. 4 (1988): 2.

4 M. Segar, et al., "Type of physical activity goal influences participation in healthy midlife women," *Women's Health Issues* 18, no. 4 (July/Aug. 2008): 281–91.

5 J. S. Greiwe and W. M. Kohrt, "Energy expenditure during walking and jogging," *Journal of Sports Medicine and Physical Fitness* 40 (December 2000): 297–302.

6 L. V. Billat, "Interval training for performance: a scientific and empirical practice," *Sports Medicine* 31 (2001): 13–31.

7 E. F. Coyle, "Very intense exercise-training is extremely potent and time efficient: a reminder," *Journal of Applied Physiology* 98 (2005): 1983–84.

8 C. P. Earnest, "Exercise interval training: an improved stimulus for improving the physiology of pre-diabetes," *Medical Hypotheses* 71 (2008): 752–61.

9 Ibid.

10 D. A. Hood, "Invited Review: Contractile activity-induced mitochondrial biogenesis in skeletal muscle," *Journal of Applied Physiology* 90, no. 3 (March 2001): 1137–57.

11 Earnest (2008).

12 Trapp (2008).

13 Caroline R. Richardson, et al., "A meta-analysis of pedometer-based walking interventions and weight loss," *Annals of Family Medicine* 6 (2008): 69–77.

14 D. M. Bravata, et al., "Using pedometers to increase physical activity and improve health," *Journal of the American Medical Association* 298, no. 19 (November 21, 2007): 2296–2304.

15 S. J. Marshall, "Translating physical activity recommendations into a pedometer-based step goal," *American Journal of Preventive Medicine* 36 (2009): 410–15.

16 Laforgia (1997).

17 A. Tremblay, et al., "Impact of exercise intensity on body fatness and skeletal muscle metabolism," *Metabolism* 43 (July 1994): 814–18.

18 E. L. Melanson, "Exercise improves fat metabolism in muscle but does not increase 24-h fat oxidation," *Exercise and Sports Sciences Reviews* 37 (2009): 93–101.

19 J. L. Talanian, "Two weeks of high-intensity aerobic interval training increases the capacity for fat oxidation during exercise in women," *Journal of Applied Physiology* 102 (2007): 1439–47.

20 Melanson, "Exercise improves fat metabolism."

21 King (1995).

22 K. A. Burgomaster, "Six sessions of sprint interval training increases muscle oxidative potential and cycle endurance capacity in humans," *Journal of Applied Physiology* 98 (2005): 1985–90.

23 J. C. Colada and N. T. Triplett, "Effects of short-term resistance program using elastic bands versus weight machines for sedentary middle-aged women," *Journal of Strength and Conditioning Research* 22, no. 5 (September 2008): 1441–48.

24 R. Ogai, et al., "Effects of petrissage massage on fatigue and exercise performance following intensive cycle pedaling." *British Journal of Sports Medicine*, 42, no. 10 (Oct. 2008): 534–38.

25 L. C. Dalleck, et al., "Dose-response relationship between moderate-intensity exercise duration and coronary heart disease risk factors in postmenopausal women," *Journal of Women's Health* 18 (2009): 105–13.

26 S. N. Blair, et al., "Changes in physical fitness and all-cause mortality," *Journal of the American Medical Association*, 273 (1995): 1093–98.

27 Chad (1988).

28 B. A. Irving, et al., "Effect of exercise training intensity on abdominal visceral fat and body composition," *Medicine and Science in Sports and Exercise* 40 (2008): 1863–72.

29 J. F. Phelan, et al., "Post-exercise energy expenditure and substrate oxidation in young women resulting from exercise bouts of different intensity," *Journal of the American College of Nutrition* 16, no. 2 (April 1999): 140–46.

30 K. Cullinen, "Weight training increases fat-free mass and strength in untrained young women," *Journal of the American Dietetic Association* 98 (1998): 414–18.

31 A. M. Tester, et al., "Effect of machine and stability strength training on the walking speed of postmenopausal women" (annual meeting, American College of Sports Medicine, Seattle, WA, May 2009).

CHAPTER 3

1 Clinghan (2008).

2 D. T. McMaster, et al., "Forms of variable resistance training," *Strength and Conditioning Journal* 31 (February 2009): 50–63.

3 Colado and Triplett (September 2008).

4 J. L. White, J. C. Scurr, and N. A. Smith, "The effect of breast support on kinetics during overground running performance," *Ergonomics* 52, no. 4 (2009): 492–98.

5 Neider, M. B., et al., "Pedestrians, vehicles, and cell phones," *Accident Analysis and Prevention* (2009), doi:10.1016/j.aap.2009.10.004.

6 C. V. Zegeer, et al., "A guide for reducing collisions involving pedestrians," National Cooperative Highway Research Program Report 500 (2004).

7 M. Buchowski, et al., "Seasonal changes in amount and patterns of physical activity in women," *Journal of Physical Activity and Health* 6, no. 2 (March 2009): 252–61.

8 J. M. Jakicic, et al., "Effects of intermittent exercise and use of home exercise equipment on adherence, weight loss, and fitness in overweight women," *Journal of the American Medical Association* 282, no. 16 (October 27, 1999): 1554–60.

CHAPTER 4

1 W. Westcott et al., "Stretching for strength," *Fitness Management* 16, no. 6 (1999): 44–6.

2 D. Cipriani , B. Abel, and D. Pirrwitz, "A comparison of two stretching protocols on hip range of motion: implications for total daily stretch duration," *Strength and Conditioning Journal* 17, no. 2 (2003): 274–78.

CHAPTER 5

1 W. L. Haskell, et al., "Physical activity and public health: updated recommendations for adults from the American College of Sports Medicine and the American Heart Association," *Medicine and Science in Sports and Exercise* 39 (2007): 1423–34.

2 Tester (2009).

3 S. Kimitake and M. Mokha, "Does core strength training influence running kinetics, lower-extremity stability, and 5000-M performance in runners?" *Journal of Strength and Conditioning Research* 23 (January 2009): 133–40.

4 D. M. Williams, et al., "Comparing psychosocial predictors of physical activity adoption and maintenance," *Annals of Behavioral Medicine* 36 (2008): 186–94.

5   N. A. King, et al., "Individual variability following 12 weeks of supervised exercise: identification and characterization of compensation for exercise-induced weight loss," *International Journal of Obesity* (2007): 1–8.

6   K. E. Foster-Schubert, et al., "Human plasma ghrelin levels increase during a one-year exercise program," *Journal of Clinical Endocrinology and Metabolism* 90 (2005): 820–25.

7   R. A. Carels, et al., "The relationship between self-monitoring, outcome expectancies, difficulties with eating and exercise, and physical activity and weight loss treatment outcomes," *Annals of Behavioral Medicine* 30 (2005): 182–90.

8   E. P. Meijer, et al., "Effect of exercise training on total daily physical activity in elderly humans," *European Journal of Applied Physiology* 80 (1999): 16–21.

9   J. A. Levine, et al., "Interindividual variation in posture allocation: possible role in human obesity," *Science* 307 (January 28, 2005): 584–86.

10 M. T. Hamilton, et al., "Role of low energy expenditure and sitting in obesity, metabolic syndrome, type 2 diabetes, and cardiovascular disease," *Diabetes* 56 (November 2007): 2655–67.

CHAPTER 6

1   R. R. Wing and R. W. Jeffrey, "Prescribed 'breaks' as a means to disrupt weight control efforts," *Obesity Research* 11 (February 2003): 287–91.

2   K. Spiegel, et al., "Sleep curtailment in healthy young men is associated with decreased leptin levels, elevated ghrelin levels, and increased hunger and appetite," *Annals of Internal Medicine* 141 (2004): 846–50.

CHAPTER 7

1   L. A. Tucker and K. S. Thomas, "Increasing total fiber intake reduces risk of weight and fat gains in women," *Journal of Nutrition* 139, no. 3 (2009): 576–81.

2   K. H. Poddar, et al., "Low-fat dairy intake and body weight and composition changes in college students," *Journal of the American Dietetic Association* 109 (2009): 1433–38.

3   J. M. Poothullil, "Recognition of oral sensory satisfaction and regulation of the volume of intake in humans," *Nutritional Neuroscience* 8, no. 4 (2005): 245–50.

4   D. Parra, et al., "A diet rich in long chain omega-3 fatty acids modulates satiety in overweight and obese volunteers during weight loss," *Appetite* 51, no. 3 (2008): 676–80.

5   L. C. Tapsell, et al., "Increasing PUFA intake with walnuts in a low fat diet supports long term weight loss in diabetes," *Federation of American Societies for Experimental Biology Journal* 22, no. 2 (2008): 1b 708.

6   M. A. Veldhorst, et al., "Effects of high and normal soy protein breakfasts on satiety and subsequent energy intake, including amino acid and 'satiety' hormone responses," *European Journal of Nutrition* 48, (2009): 92–100.

7   J. D. Stookey, et al., "Drinking water is associated with weight loss in overweight dieting women independent of diet and activity," *Obesity* 16 (2008): 2481–88.

8   K. C. Maki, et al., "Green tea catechin consumption enhances exercise-induced abdominal fat loss in overweight and obese adults," *Journal of Nutrition* 139 (2009): 264–70.

9   R. J. Green, et al., "Common tea formulations modulate in vitro digestive recovery of green tea catechins," *Molecular Nutrition and Food Research* 59, no. 9 (2007): 1152–62.

10 B. Stephens, et al., "Effects of inactivity and energy status on appetite regulation in men and women," American College of Sports Medicine Annual Meeting, Seattle, WA, May 2009.

11 P. J. Geiselman, et al., "Effects of chewing gum on specific macronutrient and total caloric intake in an afternoon snack," *Federation of American Societies for Experimental Biology Journal* 23 (2009): 101–3.

12 J. F. Hollis, et al., "Weight loss during the intensive intervention phase of the weight-loss maintenance trial," *American Journal of Preventive Medicine* 35, no. 2 (2008): 118–26.

13 A. K. Kant, et al., "Association of breakfast energy density with diet quality and body mass index in American adults: National Health and Nutrition Examination Surveys, 1999–2004," *American Journal of Clinical Nutrition* 88 (2008): 1396–1404.

14 E. J. Stevenson, et al., "Fat oxidation during exercise and satiety during recovery are increased following a low-glycemic index breakfast in sedentary women," *Journal of Nutrition* 139 (2009): 890–97.

CHAPTER 8

1   B. F. Benedict, et al. "Plantar fascia-specific stretching exercise improves outcomes in patients with chronic plantar fasciitis," *Journal of Bone and Joint Surgery* 88A, no. 8 (August, 2006): 1775–81.

2   Klaus A. Milachowski, "Comparing radiological examinations between hallux valgus night brace and a new dynamic orthosis for correction of the hallux valgus," *Fuß & Sprunggelenk* [*German Journal of Foot and Ankle Surgery*] (February 2008): 14–18.

3   K. Glavind, "Use of a vaginal sponge during aerobic exercises in patients with stress urinary incontinence," *International Urogynecology Journal of Pelvic Floor Dysfunction* 8, no. 6 (1997): 351–53.

4   J. Carlson, et al., "Exercising at work as self-reported work performances," *International Journal of Workplace Health Management* 1, no. 3 (2008): 176–97.

5   Samuele M. Marcora, Walter Staiano, and Victoria Manning, "Mental fatigue impairs physical performance in humans," *Journal of Applied Physiology* 106 (2009): 857–64.

6   J. B. Unger and C. A. Johnson, "Social relationships and physical activity in health club members," *American Journal of Health Promotion* 9, no. 5 (1995): 340–43.

7   T. E. Duncan and E. McAuley, "Social support and efficacy cognitions in exercise adherence: a latent growth curve analysis," *Journal of Behavioral Medicine* 16, no. 2 (1993): 199–218.

8   C. I. Karageorghis, et al., "Psychophysical and ergogenic effects of synchronous music during treadmill walking," *Journal of Sport and Exercise Psychology* 31, no. 1 (2009): 18–36. .

9   Christopher Capuano, et al. October 18, 2005. Study presented at the annual meeting of the North American Association for the Study of Obesity, The Obesity Society, Vancouver, British Columbia.

10 Wing (2003).

11 E. Foley, R. Matheis, and C. Schaefer, "Effect of forced laughter on mood," *Psychological Reports* 90, no. 1 (2002): 184.

12 Oliver J. Webb and Frank F. Eves, "Effects of environmental changes in a stair climbing intervention: generalization to stair descent," *American Journal of Health Promotion* 22, no. 1 (2007): 38–44.

13 J. Lee, et al., "Cold drink ingestion improves exercise endurance capacity in the heat," *Medicine and Science in Sports and Exercise* 40, no. 9 (August 2008):1637–44.

CHAPTER 9

1   L. J. DiStefano, et al., "Gluteal muscle activation during common therapeutic exercise," *Journal of Orthopaedic and Sports Physical Therapy* 39 (July 2009): 532–40.

2   R. Escamilla, et al., "An electromyographic analysis of plank and Swiss ball exercises: training and rehabilitation implications," *Medicine and Science in Sports and Exercise* 39, no. 5 (May 2007): S259.

3   M. S. Olson, et al., "Prediction of superficial versus deep abdominal muscle activity during selected Pilates exercises," *Medicine and Science in Sports and Exercise* 40, no. 5 (May 2008): S426.

4   E. Anderson, et al., "The effects of combining elastic and free weight resistance on strength and power in athletes," *Journal of Strength and Conditioning Research* 22, no. 2 (March 2008): 567–74.

Index

Boldface page references indicate photographs. <u>Underscored</u> references indicate boxed text.

Shoes
  breaking in, 36
  cost of, 32, 34
  design of, 32–33
  extra pair, 241
  foot health, effect on, 232
  heels, 232
  lacing, 38
  last (bottom) of, 33
  mesh, 44
  reflective, 45
  replacement of, 37
  running shoes, use for walking, 37
  selecting
    fit, checking, 34
    foot tracings, use of, 33, 34
    testing shoes, 33, 36
    wet walking test, use of, 35
    when to shop, 34
    where to shop, 35
  shin pain and, 228
  strap-on cleats for, 45
  toning shoes, 37
  waterproof, 44, 45
  where to buy, 37
Shoulders
  exercises for
    balancing deadlift with arm
      raise, 130, 130–31, 282–83,
      282–83
    chest press, 276, 276
    elevated plank, 266–67, 266–67
    front pull, 95, 95
    lateral raise, 280, 280–81
    overhead press, 94, 94
    plank, 98–99, 98–99
    tabletop balance, 100–101,
      100–101
  injury from walking with
    dumbbells, 23
Shrimp
  Honey Baked Shrimp, 200
Side abdominals (obliques),
  exercises for
  bicycle, 106–7, 106–7
  rotating lunge, 134–35, 134–35,
    288–89, 288–89
  side plank, 102–3, 102–3
Side leg lift, 260–61, 260–61

Side lunge, 258–59, 258–59
Side plank, 102–3, 102–3
Side stitch, 234
Sit back (stretch), 56, 56
Skillpower, 240
Sleep
  health benefits of, 151
  improvement with exercise, 7,
    151
  required amount of, 151
  tips for improving, 151
Sleep apnea, 151
Slipups, surviving, 143
SmartWool socks, 36
Smile, benefits of, 240–41
Smoothie recipes
  Banana Smoothie, 214
  Touch-of-Honey Smoothie, 194
Snacks. See also Menus
  calorie goal for, 177
  recipes
    Bananaberry Bread, 185
    Cream Cheese–Filled Carrot
      Cake Gems, 199
  timing of, 172, 173
  Week 1 groceries, 180
  Week 2 groceries, 182
Sneakers. See Shoes
Snowshoeing, 46
Socks, 32, 34, 36, 38, 232
Sodas, 164–65
Sodium intake, 173, 177
Speed, calculating by number of
  steps per minute, 68
Speed Walks
  description of, in WOW program,
    15, 26
  workouts
    Phase 2: Week 5, 145
    Phase 2: Week 6, 149
    Phase 2: Week 7, 153
    Phase 2: Week 8, 157
SPF clothing, 44
Sports bra, 41, 41, 234
Sports drink, 80
Sprint intervals. See Intervals
Squat
  elevated squat with curl, 140–41,
    140–41

moving, 88, 88–89
one-leg, 84–85, 84–85
with resistance band, 89
stationary, 89
STABIL-icers, 45
Stability exercises
  ball balance, 268–69, 268–69
  elevated plank, 266–67, 266–67
  twisting crunch on a ball,
    270–71, 270–71
Standing tall, 18
Stationary lunge, 87, 87
Steps
  intensity of, 20
  speed calculation by number of
    steps per minute, 68
  tracking count with pedometers,
    42–43
Stomach cramps, 235
Strength training
  Core Strength Workout, 97–107,
    98–107
  Core Strength Workout II,
    266–75, 266–75
  dumbbell weight, choosing
    correct, 249
  Lower-Body Strength Workout,
    81–89, 82–89
  Lower-Body Strength Workout II,
    258–65, 258–65
  muscle building with, 26–27
  resistance band use, 40, 41
  Total-Body Strength Workout,
    129–41, 130–41
  Total-Body Strength Workout II,
    281–93, 281–93
  Upper-Body Strength Workout,
    276–81, 276–81
  WOW program, use in, 15,
    26–27
Stretching
  for Achilles tendonitis, 231
  after cool-down, 55–56
  before workout, 55
  benefits of
    muscle tone, 54
    pain/tightness relief, 55
    strength, 54
  bent-leg balance, 57, 57

INDEX

339